Essential Simulation in Clinical Education

Essential Simulation in Clinical Education

Edited by

Kirsty Forrest
Professor
Director of Medical Education
Australian School of Advanced Medicine
Macquarie University
Sydney, Australia

Judy McKimm
Dean and Professor of Medical Education
Swansea University
Swansea, UK

Simon Edgar
Consultant Anaesthetist
Education Coordinator, Scottish Clinical Simulation Centre
Director of Medical Education at NHS Lothian
Edinburgh, UK

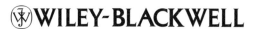
WILEY-BLACKWELL

A John Wiley & Sons, Ltd., Publication

Library of Congress Cataloging-in-Publication Data

Essential simulation in clinical education / edited by Kirsty Forrest, Judy McKimm, Simon Edgar.
   p. ; cm.
   Includes bibliographical references and index.
   ISBN 978-0-470-67116-0 (softback : alk. paper) – ISBN 978-1-118-65934-2 (eMobi) -- ISBN 978-1-118-65935-9 (ePDF) – ISBN 978-1-118-65936-6 (ePub)
   I. Forrest, Kirsty. II. McKimm, Judy. III. Edgar, Simon.
   [DNLM: 1. Education, Medical–methods. 2. Computer Simulation. 3. Patient Simulation. W 18]
   R735.A1
   610.71–dc23
                              2013003063

A catalogue record for this book is available from the British Library.

Wiley also publishes its books in a variety of electronic formats. Some content that appears in print may not be available in electronic books.

Cover image: Northwestern Simulation
Cover design by Visual Philosophy

Set in 10/12 pt Adobe Garamond Pro by Toppan Best-set Premedia Limited
Printed and bound in Malaysia by Vivar Printing Sdn Bhd

1 2013

Contents

Contributors

Mark Adler MD
Associate Professor of Pediatrics and Medical
Education
Center for Education in Medicine
Northwestern University Feinberg School of
Medicine
Ann & Robert H. Lurie Children's Hospital of
Chicago
Division of Emergency Medicine
Chicago, USA

Rajesh Aggarwal MA PhD FRCS
NIHR Clinician Scientist in Surgery
Imperial College London
London, UK

Joanne Barrott RN RM BSc (Hons) MMedSci
Regional Clinical Skills Manager
Leeds Metropolitan University
Leeds, UK

Bryn Baxendale MB ChB FRCA FAcadMedEd
Consultant Anaesthetist and Director
Trent Simulation and Clinical Skills Centre
Nottingham University Hospitals NHS Trust;
Honorary Professor of Clinical Simulation
School of Psychology
University of Nottingham
Nottingham, UK

Fernando Bello PhD
Senior Lecturer in Surgical Graphics and
Computing
Imperial College London
London, UK

Andrew Buttery MSc
Specialist Trainer
Trent Simulation & Clinical Skills Centre
Nottingham University Hospitals NHS Trust
Nottingham, UK

Aidan Byrne MBBCh MSC MD
Professor
Medical School
Cardiff University
Cardiff, UK

**Frank Coffey MB DCH MMedSci Dip Sports
Med MRCPI FRCSEd FCEM**
Consultant in Emergency Medicine
Nottingham University Hospitals NHS Trust;
Associate Professor
University of Nottingham
Nottingham, UK
Academic-Residence
Royal College of Surgeons in Ireland
Dublin, Ireland

**Ara Darzi KBE FMedSci HonFREng MD
FRCSI FRCS FACS FRCPSG**
Professor of Surgery
Imperial College London
London, UK

Peter Dieckmann PhD DiplPsych
Director of Research
Danish Institute for Medical Simulation (DIMS)
Capital Region of Denmark
Herlev Hospital
Herlev, Denmark

Simon Edgar MBChB FRCA MSC Med Ed
Consultant Anaesthetist
Director of Medical Education at NHS Lothian
Edinburgh, UK;
Educational Co-ordinator
Scottish Clinical Simulation Centre
Larbert, UK

Walter J. Eppich MD MEd
Assistant Professor of Pediatrics and Medical
Education
Center for Education in Medicine
Northwestern University Feinberg School of
Medicine
Ann & Robert H. Lurie Children's Hospital of
Chicago
Division of Emergency Medicine
Chicago, USA

**Kirsty Forrest MBChB BSc Hons FRCA
MMEd FAcadMed**
Professor
Director of Medical Education
Australian School of Advanced Medicine
Macquarie University
Sydney, Australia

Thomas Gale BM BS FRCA MEd
Associate Professor;
Director of Clinical Skills
Peninsula Schools of Medicine and Dentistry
Plymouth, UK

**Ronnie Glavin MB ChB MPhil FRCA FRCP
(Glas)**
Consultant Anaesthetist
Victoria Infirmary
Glasgow, UK

Stanley J. Hamstra PhD
Research Director, University of Ottawa Skills and
Simulation Centre
Assistant Dean, Academy for Innovation in
Medical Education
Associate Professor, Departments of
Anesthesiology, Medicine, Surgery
University of Ottawa
Ottawa, Canada

Iliana Harrysson BSc
Honorary Research Fellow
Imperial College London
London, UK

Jean Ker BSc MD FRCGP FRCPE FHEA
Professor of Medical Educations
Director Clincal Skills Centre
University of Dundee
Dundee, UK

**Roger L Kneebone PhD FRCS FRCSEd
FRCGP**
Professor of Surgical Education
Imperial College London
London, UK

Jimmy Kyaw Tun MBChB MA
Clinical Research Fellow
Imperial College London
London, UK

Nikki Maran MB ChB FRCA
Consultant Anaethetist
Associate Medical Director Patient Safety
NHS Lothian
Educational Co-ordinator
Scottish Clinical Simulation Centre
Larbert, UK

Alistair May MBChB FRCA FCARCSI
Educational Co-ordinator
Scottish Clinical Simulation Centre;
Consultant in Anaesthesia
NHS Greater Glasgow and Clyde
Glasgow, UK

Michelle McKenzie Smith MSc
Senior Clinical Educator/Deputy Manager
Montagu Clinical Simulation Centre
Montagu Hospital
Mexborough, UK

**Judy McKimm MBA, MA (Ed), BA (Hons),
CertEd, DipH&SW, SFHEA, FAcadMed**
Dean of Medical Education
Swansea University
Swansea, UK

Amit Mishra MBBS, BSc (Hons)
Honorary Research Fellow
Imperial College London
London, UK

Viren N. Naik MD Med FRCPC
Vice Chair Education;
Associate Professor
University of Ottawa
Ottawa, Canada

Jane P. Micklin MA PGCE RODP
Clincal Skills Project Worker
Leeds Metropolitan University
Leeds, UK

Lanty O'Connor BA
Manager of Simulation Technologies
Northwestern University Feinberg School of
Medicine
Chicago, USA

Doris Østergaard MD PhD
Associate Professor of Anaesthesiology
Danish Institute for Medical Simulation
Herlev University Hospital
Herlev, Denmark

Charlotte Ringsted MD, MHPE, PhD
Professor of Medical Pedagogy
Director of Centre for Clinical Education
University of Copenhagen and Capital Region
Copenhagen, Denmark

Martin Roberts MSc
Research Fellow
Institute of Clinical Education
Peninsula Schools of Medicine and Dentistry
Plymouth, UK

Jacob Rosenberg MD DSc FRCS FACS
Professor
Herlev Hospital
University of Copenhagen
Copenhagen, Denmark

**Ann B. Sunderland RGN BSc (Hons) NPDip
PGCHE MMedSci**
Academic Lead for Simulated Practice and
Clinical Skills;
Simulation Development Officer for Yorkshire
and Humber
Leeds Metropolitan University
Leeds, UK

Jessica Janice Tang PhD
Research Psychologist
Imperial College London
London, UK

**Jennifer M. Weller MD MClinEd MBBS
FANZCA FRCA**
Associate Professor
Head of Centre for Medical and Health Sciences
Education;
Specialist Anaesthetist
University of Auckland
Auckland, New Zealand

Foreword

When a new scientific or technical advance begins everyone laughs at it, downplays its significance and applicability to progress or real-world application. Manuscript submissions to journals are rejected because reviewers and editors just don't 'get it'. As the field matures these things abate, until everyone agrees that of course it makes sense and we knew it all along. Ultimately, of course, one of the best signs that a field is maturing – or has downright matured – is that textbooks on the topic appear. This book: *Essential Simulation in Clinical Education*, edited by Kirsty Forrest, Judy McKimm and Simon Edgar, is an interesting member of a new wave of textbooks on simulation in healthcare that is just coming on the market.

I am proud that two of the editors are from my own clinical field of anesthesiology – or given the British editors of this book, perhaps I should say 'anaesthetics'. Many people ask why anesthesia professionals have had such a large role to play in simulation in healthcare, both in the early days (for me at least going back to the mid-1980s) and in the current period almost 30 years later? There are indeed several reasons, and I suspect the editors of this book would agree with them. First, anesthesia (excluding management of acute and chronic pain outside the operating theatre) is almost never therapeutic in itself; it is a means to facilitate needed surgery. Second, anesthesia is a very abnormal state for the human body – evolution didn't mean for people to be temporarily rendered unconscious, insensitive to pain, and paralyzed only to be restored to normalcy a few minutes or hours later. And, to date, nearly every form of making this happen is dangerous, and in fact can readily harm or even kill patients. This made anesthesia professionals very, very interested in patient safety, in minimizing risk, and in finding ways of training that best prepared the practitioners of this arcane art (as well as their coworkers in surgery) to handle all the kinds of adverse event that nature, or their own inevitable mistakes, might throw at them. Thus, surgery and anesthesia along with a host of other clinical domains, qualify as endeavors that I classify as being of 'high intrinsic hazard'. Others in this class include aviation and spaceflight (evolution certainly didn't prepare human beings to travel in the air or outer space, and at least for the former, what goes up must come down), production of electricity via nuclear reactions, or military combat with increasingly long-range and lethal weaponry. All these other endeavors of high-intrinsic hazard adopted simulation as a core component of the initial and recurrent training of their personnel and teams. Thus, it should come as no surprise that anesthesia professionals facing similar problems were, and are, in the vanguard of leadership in clinical simulation, not only for our own fields of operative anesthesia and intensive care, but now extending to a whole host of clinical domains, for nearly all disciplines of healthcare personnel, at all levels of training and experience.

This book is interesting in part because it leans heavily on editors and authors from the UK, with a small set of authors from areas that were former British colonies, provinces, or dominions (the USA, although Chicago was not under British control, Canada, and New Zealand). Several authors are from Denmark – which Britain never ruled; instead the Great Danish Army conquered major parts of England in 865 CE, so it is perhaps only fitting that these authors also join this work. The authors include many very-well-known names in the world's pantheon of simulation experts. The UK has been a hotbed of simulation for many years, and the integration of simulation into some components of their healthcare system has outstripped that in many other parts of the world. Moreover, their take on simulation – while appropriately represented in the peer-reviewed literature – has not been thoroughly disseminated to the rest of the world (and certainly not to my side of "the pond"). The book is also interesting in covering the full panoply of simulation – as the editors put it in their introduction: overview, history, evidence, teaching learning and assessment, people, skills, the places, doing it (meaning actually conducting simulation, not the more colloquial connotation of the term), complete with some fascinating real-life examples, and some viewpoints on the future of clinical simulation. Hence it is with pleasure that I mark the publication of this book and hope that it will thoroughly teach and fascinate (and perhaps even once in a while astonish or exasperate?) its readers.

February, 2013
David M. Gaba, MD
Associate Dean for Immersive and Simulation-based Learning
Professor of Anesthesiology, Pain, and Perioperative Medicine
Stanford University School of Medicine
Co-Director, Simulation Center at VA Palo Alto Health Care System
Founding and current Editor-in-Chief, *Simulation in Healthcare*
Los Altos, California, USA
(a part of the country which was once under the rule of Spain, but never of Great Britain)

Glossary and abbreviations

ACLS	Advanced Cardiac Life Support.
ANTS	Anaesthetists' Non-Technical Skills.
ASPiH	Association of Simulated Practice in Healthcare.
Behavioural marker systems	A list or matrix of observable, non-technical behaviours linked to specific social or cognitive criteria that contribute to superior or substandard performance within a work environment.
BEME	Best Evidence Medical Education.
Blueprinting	The process of identifying the particular outcomes or parts of a curriculum that are assessed by specific components of an assessment.
BodySim	Uses clinician-assessors rather than independent judges. After scoring each candidate, assessors grade them as pass, fail or borderline and the pass score is the average score obtained by those in the borderline group.
Borderline groups method	Assessment method in which appropriately qualified and experienced individuals are first asked to describe the competence of individuals deemed to be on the borderline between competence and incompetence. Next specific individuals predicted to lie in this zone are identified and their test scores analysed.
CASE	Comprehensive Anesthesia Simulation Environment.
Cavalier attitudes	Casual, dismissive manner: 'It's only a plastic dummy!'.
Checklist	A list of observable actions and/or outcomes that contribute to competent clinical performance in an assessed scenario.
Contrasting groups method	Judges are asked to examine the overall performance of a sample of candidates and award each one a pass or fail, regardless of the actual scores awarded. The score distribution within the pass group is then compared with that for the fail group and used to establish a cutpoint where the distributions overlap.
CPD	Continuing Professional Development.
CRM	Crew Resource Management.
DS	Distributed Simulation.
EBAT	Event-based approach to training.
Fixed percentage method	Relative method whereby the proportion of examinees who will pass is predetermined for each cohort.
GAS	Gainesville Anesthesia Simulator.
GasMan	A software-based tool allowing for the clinical simulation of volatile anesthesia uptake and distribution within the body.
Global rating scale	An list of increasing levels of clinical performance in an assessed scenario to which numerical scores may be attributed.
GTAs	Gynaecology Teaching Associates.
Haptics	Tactile feedback technology which takes advantage of the sense of touch by applying forces, vibrations, or motions to the user to develop and enhance motor skills (e.g. in surgical techniques).

HEA	Higher Education Academy.
Hofstee method	A cutpoint is created by combining the Angoff and fixed percentage methods. The panel of expert judges is asked to set minimum and maximum pass scores and minimum and maximum acceptable failure rates. A graphical method is then used to identify a cutpoint that falls between these extremes.
Hybrid simulation	Process of attaching part-task trainers to simulated patients so that assessment of clinical skills can include added complexity to measure aspects of the doctor–patient interaction.
Hypervigilance	An enhanced state of sensitivity combined with an exaggerated intensity of behaviours whose purpose is to detect threats.
ICEPS	Imperial College Evaluation of Procedure-specific Skill.
Internal metrics	Physical measurements, recorded by instruments in the simulation environment, that can be related to aspects of clinical performance.
ISBAR (Identify self, Situation, Background, Assessment, Recommendations)	A tool to improve information sharing in patient handover between team members, or when referring a patient to another health profession for their input.
KISMET (Kinematick Simulation, Monitoring and off-line Programming Environment for Telerobotics)	A software tool for planning, simulation, programming and monitoring of remote handling equipment, industrial robots and various types of mechanisms.
Maastricht Assessment of Simulated Patients (MaSP)	Tool designed to assess and develop the quality of the SPs feedback to the student at the end of a simulation session.
MATTUS	Minimal Access Therapy Training Unit.
Mini-CEX	Mini-Clinical Evaluation Exercise.
Mini-Clinical Evaluation Exercise (Mini-CEX)	A structured workplace based assessment of an observed clinical encounter designed to help focus trainer feedback on skills essential to the provision of good clinical care by the learner.
Minimally Invasive Surgical Trainer (MIST)	A part task trainer utilising haptic feedback and either real or virtual (MIST-VR) targets allowing for the development of minimally invasive or laparoscopic skills.
MISTELS	McGill Inanimate System for Training and Evaluation of Laparoscopic Skills.
MOC	Maintenance of Certification.
Modified Angoff process	A panel of expert judges determine a score that would be achieved by a borderline ('just passing') candidate. The average of these scores is then the final pass mark.
Moulage	Make-up and other products are applied to the simulator to augment the realism of a scenario in a relevant way by creating physical manifestations of disease (a rash) or injury (abrasions, lacerations, burns, or other trauma). The moulage only needs to be sufficiently realistic to trigger a target response.
NOTSS	Non-Technical Skills for Surgeons.
OSATS	Objective Structured Assessment of Technical Skills.
OSCE	Objective Structured Clinical Examination.

PACER (Probe, Alert, Challenge, Emergency, Response)	PACER and the Two Challenge Rule Tools to assist team members to speak up or challenge decisions by the team leader.
Postgraduate Ward Simulation Exercise (PgWSE)	Provides direct evidence of performance using simulation based education. It lasts for twenty minutes and during the exercise the doctor receives timed interruptions whilst dealing with a new admission, an emergency situation and a specific communication issue.
RAPIDS	Rescuing a Patient in Deteriorating Situations.
RCRS	Rochester Communication Rating Scale.
Resusci Anne	A training mannequin first introduced in 1960 by Norwegian toy maker Åsmund Laerdal designed to accurately simulate the human respiratory system and external body landmarks in order to facilitate training and used for teaching cardiopulmonary resuscitation (CPR) to both emergency workers and members of the general public.
SAGES	American Gastrointestinal Endoscopic Surgeons.
SBAR	Situation, Background, Assessment, Recommendation.
SBCE	Simulation-based Clinical Education.
SBTT	Simulation-based Team Training.
Selective abstraction	A key concept that highlights the notion that elements of a given scenario need to be recreated with greater or lesser degrees of authenticity to heighten perceived realism depending on how central a certain element is to the case.
Sequential Simulation (SqS)	A method of condensing an extended clinical pathway into a shorter time frame. Achieved by selecting representative components and linking then across different sectors of the healthcare system and different time frames.
Sim One	The first realistic anesthesia simulator produced in the late 1960's at the University of Southern California. It was used mainly for the training of endotracheal intubation and the induction of anesthesia. The mannequin had outputs for peripheral pulses and heart sounds, but no outputs for electronic monitors.
Simulated patient (SP)	An individual who is trained to act as a real patient in order to simulate a set of symptoms or problems providing reliable and reproducible clinical material for training and assessment of skills in communication and physical examination.
SNAPPI (Stand back and get attention, Notify team of the situation, Assessment of situation, Plan and Priorities, Invite ideas)	A tool to structure a team call out, where the team is brought together to ensure shared situational assessment, shared goals and inviting team input into the problem.
SPLINTS	Scrub Practitioners' List of Intra-operative Non-Technical Skills.
Spotlight Model	Proposes that a shift of visual attention corresponds to a shift in processing resources among several analysed locations, like moving a spotlight.
Standardized patient	An individual who typically has real clinical signs and symptoms and who has been trained to provide a standardized history and/or feedback to learners.

Storyboard	A template populated with the integral components relating to the design, running and debrief of a simulation scenario.
Team-oriented medical simulation	Simulation-based developmental activity where the learning outcomes of the scenario are focused on group interaction, team dynamics and overall performance rather than at an individual level.
Utstein	Utstein is an abbey in Norway, which has hosted several meetings, where a group of international experts come up with recommendations or guidelines for a given topic. Utstein is now synonymous with reporting guidelines for resuscitation.
Vocal cues	Addition of a patient's voice in manikin-based simulation can be particularly helpful to help participants engage with the simulation. Learners can gather relevant information for clinical decision-making and management as well as assess the patient's mental status.
WBA	Workplace-based Assessment.
Zoom Lens Model	Utilizes the properties of the Spotlight Model, but also includes the property of changing size in visual attention. This property was inspired by the zoom lens function on a camera in which there is a trade off between the size of the visual attention region and processing efficiency.

Features contained within your textbook

Every chapter begins with an overview of the topic.

Key point, Summary and Case study boxes highlight important features to remember.

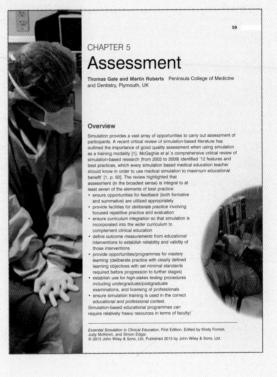

CHAPTER 5
Assessment

Thomas Gale and Martin Roberts Peninsula College of Medicine and Dentistry, Plymouth, UK

Overview

Simulation provides a vast array of opportunities to carry out assessment of participants. A recent critical review of simulation-based literature has outlined the importance of good quality assessment when using simulation as a training modality [1]. McGaghie et al.'s comprehensive critical review of simulation-based research (from 2003 to 2009) identified '12 features and best practices, which every simulation based medical education teacher should know in order to use medical simulation to maximum educational benefit' [1, p. 50]. The review highlighted that assessment (in the broadest sense) is integral to at least seven of the elements of best practice:
* ensure opportunities for feedback (both formative and summative) are utilized appropriately
* provide facilities for *deliberate practice* involving focused repetitive practice and evaluation
* ensure *curriculum integration* so that simulation is incorporated into the wider curriculum to complement clinical education
* define *outcome measurements* from educational interventions to establish reliability and validity of those interventions
* provide opportunities/programmes for *mastery learning* (deliberate practice with clearly defined learning objectives with set minimal standards required before progression to further stages)
* establish use for *high-stakes testing* procedures including undergraduate/postgraduate examinations, and licensing of professionals
* ensure simulation training is used in the correct *educational and professional context*.
Simulation-based educational programmes can require relatively heavy resources in terms of faculty/

Essential Simulation in Clinical Education, First Edition. Edited by Kirsty Forrest, Judy McKimm, and Simon Edgar.
© 2013 John Wiley & Sons, Ltd. Published 2013 by John Wiley & Sons, Ltd.

✓ Key points

* Simulation has a long history with its development closely tied to technological advances in computer and materials science.
* Simulation is now recognized as adding value to training and education and enabling practice of a range of skills and competencies in a safe environment.
* Many countries and regions have established simulation centres, although these are inequitably distributed around the world.
* Simulation-based education enables the delivery of a continuum of learning throughout a doctor's career.
* More research is needed to determine the impact of simulation training on improving health outcomes.

SUMMARY

We hope that the ideas, thoughts and concepts in this book will stimulate readers to think about how they can improve learning with simulation. Those who are involved in the development and delivery of simulation healthcare education need to have a better understanding and the most recent evidence of its use. If simulation education is used by those that are not aware of its challenges or previous work, the outcomes could be costly and lead to the technique being abandoned. Keeping pace with the implications of published research, new technologies and influences from other disciplines is important.

Discussion in the literature can tend towards the sceptic, such as editorial headlines of 'High fidelity and fun: but fallow

Case study 7.1 Laparoscopic cholecystectomy

Laparoscopic cholecystectomy (LC) remains the gold standard treatment of symptomatic gallstone disease and will represent one of the most common procedures a junior surgical trainee will perform. Hence technical skills training in this procedure is of great importance.

A hypothetical training ladder, which would impart these skills, would involve the following steps.
1. Theoretical and anatomical teaching of principles underlying procedure and technical skills required.
2. Basic training using a box trainer/endotrainer using the FLS course

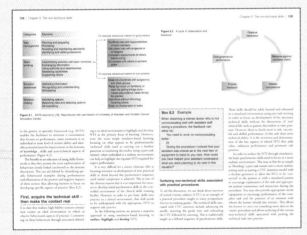

Your textbook is full of illustrations, tables and useful hints.

① Hints and tips

Simulators *per se* are just tools; they may enhance training if their use is aligned with learning objectives. Educators should pay careful attention to integration of simulation methods within the overall curriculum, provision of feedback and opportunities for deliberate practice of skills, and other evidence-based features of simulation to improve educational practice and, ultimately, patient care.

We hope you enjoy using your new textbook. Good luck with your studies!

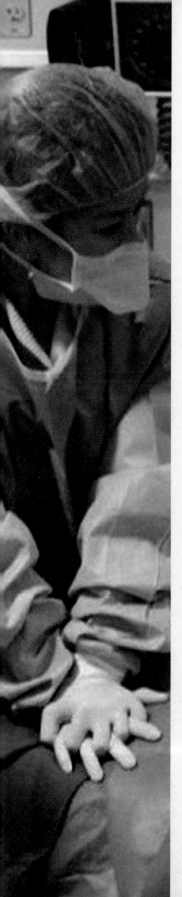

CHAPTER 1
Essential simulation in clinical education

Judy McKimm[1] and Kirsty Forrest[2]   [1]Swansea University, Swansea, UK; [2]Australian School of Advanced Medicine, Macquarie University, Sydney, Australia

'The use of patient simulation in all its forms is widespread in clinical education with the key aims of improving learners' competence and confidence, improving patient safety and reducing errors. An understanding of the benefits, range of activities that can be used and limitations of simulation will help clinical teachers improve the student and trainee learning experience.' [1]

Overview

The use of simulation for the training of healthcare professionals is becoming more and more popular. The drivers of improved patient safety and communication have led to a significant investment in the expansion of facilities and equipment across Western healthcare organizations. For example, Royal Colleges in the UK are including mandatory training using simulation within their curricula and politicians have also jumped on to the bandwagon extolling the virtues of simulation training. The use of simulation in training is becoming synonymous with effective learning and safer care for patients and is fast becoming a panacea for all the perceived ills of teaching and training. However, simulation is not a substitute for health professionals learning with and from real patients in real clinical contexts. As Gaba reminds us:

'simulation is a technique, not a technology' [2, p. 2]

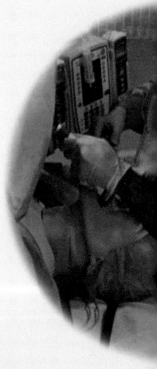

Overview (ctd)

Other authors [3,4,5] note that we must take care in case the seductive powers of simulation lead to dependency, become self-referential and produce a 'new reality'. Simulation must not become an end in itself, disconnected from professional practice.

Ongoing and outstanding discussions include the following questions: What do participants learn from simulation? How are they expected to learn? How will the knowledge and skills be transferred to clinical practice? Will general or specific aspects of performance be transferred? Do our current methods and techniques make this transfer possible? When in a clinician's training should simulation be used? How should simulation be introduced into the curriculum? When should the team be trained as opposed to the individual? Can simulation impact on patient safety? Can and should we look for a return on investment when talking about simulation education?

This book will provide the reader with evidence around these questions and much more. The contents of the chapters build from the broader themes of history, best practice and pedagogy through to the practical aspects of how to teach and train with simulation and ends with examples and possible future developments. However each chapter can stand alone for those who wish to explore a single topic. Each is written by authors who are highly experienced in the development of simulation-based education. Our thoughts on and synopses of the various chapters follow.

History

Simulation in medical training has a long history, which started with the use of very basic models to enable learners to practice skills and techniques (e.g. in obstetrics). In spite of this early start, medical simulators did not gain widespread use in the following centuries, principally for reasons of cost and a reluctance to adopt new teaching methods. With advances in materials and computer sciences, a wide range of modalities have developed including virtual reality and high-fidelity manikins, often located in dedicated simulation centres. Chapter 2 describes these developments in detail, reminding us that the combination of increased awareness of patient safety, improved technology and increased pressures on educators have promoted simulation as an option to traditional clinical skills teaching. The chapter also defines and describes a classification for stimulation. Although a wide range of simulation activities exist, these are still often linked with specific medical specialities rather than 'centrally' managed or resourced. How simulation can best be supported in low-income countries, where the need is great but resources are not always available, is an issue still to be addressed. The impact of simulation on patient safety and health care improvements is still relatively under-researched although an evidence base is growing.

Evidence

There is widespread agreement, supported by robust research, systematic reviews and meta-analyses, on what makes for effective simulation. This theme is further explored in Chapter 3, which considers the evidence base underpinning the widespread use of simulation-based training in undergraduate and postgraduate contexts, general and specialty-based curricula, and clinical and non-clinical settings. Simulation supports the acquisition of procedural, technical skills through repetitive, deliberate practice with feedback, and also supports the acquisition of non-technical skills, such as communication, leadership and team working. The evidence base for the former is more extensive and robust than for the latter, which has been identified as an area for further research. The value of embedding or integrating simulation within curricula or training programmes is highlighted, as is the benefit of a programmatic, interval-based approach to simulation. In addition, workplace-based simulation for established multiprofessional teams (when supported by the institution's leaders) is seen as effective way of embedding sustainable changes in practice.

Teaching, learning and assessment

Simulation is no different from many other forms of education and training: instructors or facilitators need to be skilled and knowledgeable about educational theory and how this relates to their teaching practice. As with any educational intervention, activities need to be designed to enable learners to achieve defined learning outcomes and meeting their own learning needs. However, simulation offers particular challenges to both facilitators and participants: it requires some suspension of disbelief; it may feel threatening, challenging and unsafe (particularly for experienced health professionals); and it requires skills in giving feedback, both 'in the moment' and through more structured debriefings. Chapter 4 considers some of the most relevant learning theories and educational strategies that help to provide effective training and overcome some of the inherent barriers to learning through simulation.

Providing high-quality educational experiences is vital if learners are to engage in simulation with all its challenges; however, assessment drives much of learning, and simulation has a huge role to play in ensuring that health professionals are fit, safe and competent to practise. In Chapter 5, the authors consider the important elements which contribute towards effective assessment of both technical and non-technical skills at all stages of education and training. As with any assessments, those using simulation should possess the attributes of reliability, validity, feasibility, cost-effectiveness, acceptability and educational impact. Assessments need to be integrated within the curriculum and within an overall assessment scheme which utilizes a range of methods. Simulation can provide opportunities for both formative (developmental) and summative (contributing to grade or score) assessments, although appropriate levels of fidelity and realism need to be selected based on the specific context.

Well-designed simulation provides excellent opportunities for learners to receive timely and specific feedback from educators and real, virtual and simulated patients and so helps develop and hone clinical and communication skills. Simulation also enables those involved in assessment to consistently and reliably assess clinical performance by using increasingly sophisticated technology such as haptic trainers which incorporate internal metrics and can measure fine motor skills and give in the moment feedback, or combinations of simulations (such as simulated patients and part task trainers) which can assess complex clinical activities or team working.

A large number of checklists and global rating scales have been developed, tested and validated in various settings which give rise to both opportunities and challenges for educators. Chapter 5 describes some of the most widely used instruments. The ability to measure performance more consistently and reliably provides assurances for patients and the public that healthcare professionals are safe to practice. However, the more reliable simulated assessments become, the possibilities of using such assessments in selection, relicensing and performance management increase. For such assessments, and also for high-stakes 'routine' assessments, educators must be satisfied that the assessment instruments selected are appropriate and validated, that the personnel and equipment involved and scenarios chosen are appropriate and that all those involved in delivering the assessment (including standard setting, development of checklists, marking and giving feedback) are suitably trained.

The people

Although the range and potential of simulation equipment and computer-based technologies seems almost infinite, without the continued involvement of trained, enthusiastic and skilled people, simulation education will not flourish and grow. Chapter 6 considers the recruitment, education, training and professional development of two of the main groups involved in simulation-based education: the educators or faculty, and simulated (or standardized) patients (SPs). As with any type of education, simulation facilitators (trainers, instructors or educators) need to be trained to teach, assess, give

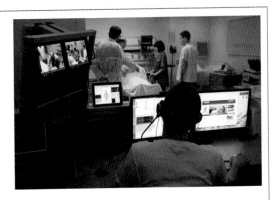

Figure 1.1 Teaching using simulation requires an ability to use technical equipment and be able to work with simulated, real and virtual patients. Photo by Laura Seul, copyright Northwestern Simulation.

feedback and evaluate the effect of the education alongside other teachers on healthcare programmes. As a learning modality, simulation has some unique features in which teachers require development so that they can provide high quality educational experiences, such as using technical equipment and computers and working with simulated, real and virtual patients (Figure 1.1).

The challenging nature of some simulation encounters also requires educators to be explicit about and adhere to high professional standards and values so as to maintain a safe atmosphere which encourages learning. Educators also need to be able to adopt a range of styles, such as an instructing style for novices learning a technical skill or a coaching or facilitative style for an expert group, and be proficient in techniques such as giving feedback and the debrief. Educators must also be credible, whether they are clinically qualified or not; this may mean acquiring new skills or knowledge or team teaching with clinical colleagues. In common with many areas of practice, professional standards of educators are now being widely adopted alongside increasing regulation and quality assurance. Educators therefore need to be aware of these changes and prepared to take a lifelong learning approach to their own development.

SPs have been widely used in both the teaching and assessment of health professionals and provide a valuable adjunct to involving both real and virtual

patients. SP interaction with learners can vary from fairly minimal interaction with limited responses to a highly standardized and scripted encounter, in which the SP might have a lot of flexibility in how they respond to the learner. The role of SPs in providing timely and accurate feedback from the 'patient's perspective' is one of the key advantages of involving SPs. Many SPs are also trained as educators who can work unsupervised in both teaching and assessment situations. As with any involvement in education, it is important that SPs are selected, trained and supported in their role, particularly when they are involved in high-stakes assessments or in evaluating qualified doctors' performance. SPs have also been used as covert patients to evaluate health services and the practice of individual doctors. Although planning and managing an SP service is time-consuming and can be costly in the initial stages, experienced SPs can replace clinicians in both teaching and assessments, which can lead to more standardized experiences for learners and cost savings over time. Recent international developments include consideration of SP accreditation, standards and certification as part of a drive to ensure high-quality education and training.

The skills: technical, non-technical and team working

Simulation takes place in a range of settings, but is probably most widely used and has had the most measurable impact in surgical settings, led by anaesthetists and surgeons. Taking an historical approach, Chapter 7 looks at surgical technical skills, highlighting some of the key drivers behind the introduction of simulation training and its impact on patient safety and error reduction. This chapter describes some of the key developments in developing and enhancing surgical skills. The need for further training and development via simulation training has been driven by the need to ensure higher standards of patient safety and error reduction; patient expectations of healthcare; the introduction of new operating procedures (such as laparoscopy); and technological advances (e.g. endoscopes, miniaturization of equipment and imaging technology). Technological advances have also enabled simulation to utilize different materials

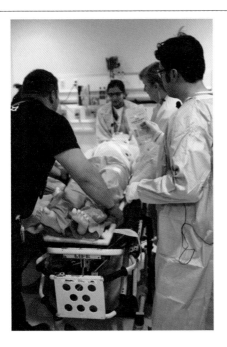

Figure 1.2 Simulations enable doctors to improve their operating techniques. Photo by Laura Seul, copyright Northwestern Simulation.

and harness computing power in the form of virtual reality simulators and other devices that facilitate and measure haptic (tactile) feedback in real time in order to ensure surgical technical skills are of a required standard. Such simulations enable doctors to improve operating techniques, particularly in the learning curve stage, when patients are deemed most at risk (Figure 1.2).

As the dividing line between surgeons, radiologists and other physicians becomes increasingly blurred with the more widespread use of minimally invasive procedures and interventional radiology, virtual reality simulators are being used to train a variety of health professionals. This brings its own challenges and opportunities. For example, as we are better able to measure fine response times and technique, simulation-based proficiency tests that incorporate 'real-time' pressures and stressors (as used in aviation and military settings) may well be used to discriminate between applicants for specific posts. If the use of simulation training and assessment expands, then new simulation centres may

need to be established that can efficiently utilize resources, equipment and expertise to train and assess large numbers of doctors and other health professionals. This would require a 'whole-system' approach to simulation.

Chapter 8 considers and explores the training and development of non-technical (social and cognitive) skills and the way in which human factors impact on patient safety. In many high-risk industries, human factors have been shown to cause the majority of errors and often these are not due to lack of knowledge or inability to perform a technical skill, but due to lack of so-called 'softer' skills like team working, communication, leadership and decision-making. This chapter describes the development and implementation of Crew Resource Management (CRM) and behavioural marker systems to observe, assess and give feedback to individuals and teams. Examples are given of scenarios and details of each of the steps required in designing training in alignment with defined behavioural markers.

The healthcare team has been called the 'cornerstone' of health services, yet teamwork failures are widely viewed as a major contributor to adverse health outcomes and errors. Chapter 9 explores some of the reasons why this is the case and discusses how simulation-based team training (SBTT) delivered by trained instructors can help address some of the common issues concerning poor or ineffective communication and differing perceptions about the goals of healthcare, team roles and leadership. A number of models and strategies are discussed in the chapter, along with their application and relevance for training uni- and multiprofessional teams. These strategies focus on improving team performance through enhancing team cognition, developing shared mental models and problem-solving approaches, and facilitating team members to challenge the attitudes and perceptions of other professional groups. Structured observation charts that focus on assessing behaviours help instructors and team members to give more helpful feedback. Because most teams are multidisciplinary, SBTT should also aim to involve different professional groups, ideally in authentic work situations, both in the actual workplace and in simulation centres.

The places

In many contexts, a dedicated simulation centre (whether established on a local or regional scale) is seen as an efficient and effective way of centralizing resources and expertise, particularly those around high-fidelity simulators or when large numbers of people are to be trained. For those involved in, or considering, establishing a simulation centre, Chapter 10 provides a highly detailed, step-by-step guide to all the factors that need to be considered. The authors draw from their own experience of running a large-scale simulation centre, providing many 'hints and tips' and ideas applicable to many contexts. Factors that need attention include securing initial and ongoing funding; determining training needs and the numbers of users of the centre; recruiting, training and retaining faculty; identifying the right equipment and ensuring that this is maintained well; providing high-quality training that is pedagogically sound that meets learners' (and funders') needs; and quality assuring all activities. Collaboration with key stakeholders is vitally important, especially to ensure sustainability of the centre and its activities, as is engagement with national and international simulation and clinical skills networks, whose members have wide expertise. At the operational level, administrative and technical staff are central to the effective and efficient delivery of training and maintenance of equipment and, as other writers have stressed, it is essential that simulation activities are embedded within curricula or training programmes so that learners gain the most benefit.

As health service and education budgets become increasingly constrained, many simulation groups are starting to explore more cost-effective solutions to delivering high-quality simulations away from dedicated simulation centres. Distributed simulation (DS) is one solution to these problems. Chapter 11 describes the work of the Imperial College London team in researching into the most effective ways of setting up effective 'portable' simulation activities in a range of settings and specialties. Working with a multidisciplinary team, the research group has drawn on the psychological theories of selective attention and applied these in the development of a range of DS models which can be applied in a variety of settings. This 'selective abstraction' is

what makes DS so useful when resources are limited as only the most important features are used which help to generate a realistic scenario in any given context. Portability is achieved through the use of simple, user-friendly equipment for observing, recording, playback and debriefing, similar to that used in static simulation centres and practical, lightweight and easily transportable components which can be erected quickly by a minimal team. This gives the flexibility to recreate a range of clinical settings according to individual requirements.

DS could herald the way forward for future developments as it can provide a cost-effective, accessible and versatile approach to teaching and learning tailored to the needs of individual groups at the right level of fidelity. Although the preliminary exploration and validation work of the DS was conducted in a surgical setting with clinicians at different levels of experience and different surgical procedures, DS is now starting to be utilized in different hospital and community-based settings such as emergency medicine and, utilizing concepts such as sequential simulation, considering how to simulate care pathway modelling in different domains of medicine and support services. This has potential for widespread application in low income countries or contexts in which static, expensive simulation centres are unlikely to be established.

Doing it

Although the context and nature of the simulation activity might vary, including the types of participants, the locality and the purpose of the training, it is essential that simulation education provides a safe environment in which participants can actually learn. Because simulation is often perceived as challenging and sometimes threatening, simulation educators need to pay close attention not only to the achievement of learning outcomes, but to the process of group dynamics and individuals' psychological safety. In Chapter 12, the authors take a structured approach to designing effective simulation education, considering each of the components of the simulation setting, and suggest ways in which educators can help support learners gain the most from the encounter. As we have mentioned, simulation educators need to utilize best practice from other areas of education, including small group facilitation skills, giving constructive feedback and defining clear learning outcomes. However, the simulation encounter also benefits from attention to specific elements such as scenario design and the structured debrief. Ensuring that participants are appropriately introduced to the scenario, the simulation context and the other people involved in the simulation is very important. Also important is setting ground rules and either using a structured approach to simulation design and delivery, such as the event-based approach to training (EBAT), or making sure that educators have the skills and expertise to deliver training on-the-fly. The chapter also discusses the use of confederates, moulage and audiovisual equipment and provides an in-depth guide to the use of the debrief as part of the provision of effective and useful simulation.

Real-life examples

Chapter 13 introduces a fascinating insight into the practice of simulation 'on the ground' through a series of nine short, structured case examples of simulation teaching, learning and assessment activities in a range of different clinical settings with learners from various health professions at different stages of education and training. Examples are from Australia, the Netherlands, the USA, Africa and the UK, and from both primary and secondary care. Each worked example describes the background and context; what was done; the results and outcomes; take home messages; and hints and tips.

The case studies cover a range of topics and uses of simulation:

• using the simulator Harvey™ to teach cardiology
• assessing leadership skills in medical undergraduates
• interprofessional learning of airway management
• a multicountry and multicultural study using simulation in emergency care
• clinical skills assessment of postgraduate paediatric trainees
• a national assessment programme for 'doctors in difficulty'
• the use of incognito standardized patients in general practice
• team-based simulation for rural and remote practice
• trauma team training in a university hospital.

All the case studies demonstrate the importance of evaluating interventions so that practice can be improved. Evaluation needs to be not just of the simulation activity itself, but also aimed at improving health outcomes. The case studies also indicate the clear links between simulation, policy and practice and that simulation-based education needs to be located as near as possible to the workplace (at the very least to workplace needs and involving clinicians) and that interprofessional and multiprofessional working enhances the experience for all. The case studies also demonstrate the value of, and indeed the need for, collaboration: among professions, disciplines, organizations, teams and countries. Lessons learned and hints and tips provide valuable ideas for those developing and establishing simulation-based activities.

The future

The final chapter comprises three sections. In each section the authors give their personal perspective on what they see as some of the key developments in simulation and how these will impact on future development and implementation.

The first section focuses on the use of simulation technologies, specifically in surgical training and education, to improve patient safety and reduce errors in the operating theatre and associated settings. Taking the concepts of a patient's and surgeon's journey, the section considers how simulation can help provide more seamless care as well as support the professional development of surgeons throughout their working lives. The use of virtual patients, three-dimensional high-definition holographic technology to simulate real patients' anatomy and physiology and team-based training will enable the surgical team to plan and deliver personalized optimum pre-operative, surgical and postoperative interventions, to practise complex skills and manoeuvres, and to rehearse strategies should complications arise (Figure 1.3). As technologies develop, the use of laparoscopic, miniaturized and robotic surgery will increase; thus surgeons will need regular updating, training and refreshment of skills and techniques. Selection (for general surgery or for sub-specialties) might also involve simulation once technologies can provide reliable, consistent and accurate estimation of performance. Simulated

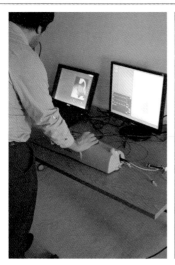
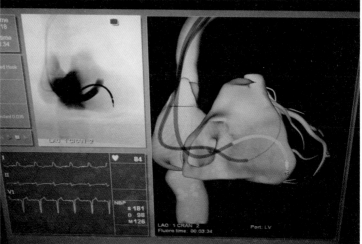

Figure 1.3 Coronary angiography simulator (a) and screen shot (b). Courtesy of Jivendra Gosai, Hull Institute of Learning and Simulation.

environments or worlds such as SecondLife™ will enable non-technical skills and activities (such as handover or discharge planning) to be practised safely using avatars (Figure 1.4). Over time, as part of the drive to reduce error and improve performance, 'black box' recorders might be placed in all theatres to measure and record real time performance.

The second section takes a different look at simulation-based education and its role and place within a changing education and training context. Taking two main paradigm shifts in medical education, the shift from time-based to competency-based education and the move towards lifelong learning, the authors explore how simulation can help to support and drive these shifts. The move towards competency-based education is more goal oriented and requires deliberate practice and ongoing measurement and assessment of skills, both technical and non-technical, or competencies at all stages of training. To demonstrate mastery at defined levels, accurate, reliable assessments are needed. Simulation is well placed to help provide opportunities for deliberate practice, integration and mastery and assess defined competencies through formative and summative assessments without the need for practice on real patients all the time. This can help accelerate learning and skills,

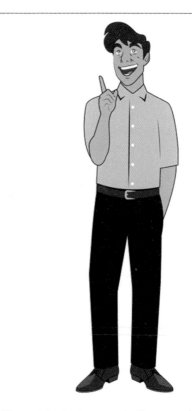

Figure 1.4 Avatar example. Courtesy of Henry Fuller. http://secondlife6750.wordpress.com.

and thus move away from a time-based model of education towards one that acknowledges and is responsive to the needs and attributes of individual learners throughout life. To evaluate the high-level impact of simulation interventions, more scholarly research is required and educators need to be supported and equipped with the expertise and time needed to develop research, evaluation and writing skills. Medical education research units that are populated with qualified and experienced educators can support education scholarship by collaborating with and mentoring clinician educators. The importance of gathering the right evidence to evaluate interventions is highlighted, and the Kirkpatrick evaluation hierarchy is cited as helping guide the rationale for education interventions and the quality and impact of teaching innovations.

The final section considers the future of training in simulation through consideration of three inter-linked elements: curriculum integration, resources and faculty development. As many writers have emphasized, simulation needs to be integrated within a curriculum or programme to enable learners to achieve defined learning outcomes. It is suggested that simulation should be thought of not just as a method of learning or assessing 'content', but as significantly influencing the content of the curriculum. Through engagement with simulation activities, educators from many disciplines (e.g. psychology, anthropology, computer and materials sciences, as well as biomedical scientists and clinicians) have together co-created curricula and learning interventions that would not have been considered possible decades ago. A vision for the future of simulation training is of groups of healthcare workers coming together to rehearse and practice and prepare for the introduction of new clinical challenges or new protocols or ways of safely implementing new practices. Faculty development will also continue to be informed by simulation through involvement of multiple stakeholders including those from performing arts, psychology and business.

In common with all areas of education, increasing constraints on resources mean that educators and managers have to provide robust evidence of value for money and efficiency. As well as essential resources such as time, space, administrative and practical support, simulation activities require specialised (and often expensive) equipment and technology. Many developments have only been made possible because of close collaboration between simulation users, commissioners, manufacturers and even regulators. In the future this will require more robust mechanisms to ensure that the resources required for investment are likely to bring about a significant return and that transparent and meaningful quality assurance mechanisms are established. It is also important to ensure that resources are focused towards areas of need, such as low-income countries, where well-designed simulation can have great impact. The final challenge highlighted is that of continuing to develop and understand the theoretical basis that underpins simulation-based education and devise models and explanatory frameworks that can be used in scholarly practice and research. Taking a programmatic approach to this work through international collaboration provides the best way forward to ensure simulation-based education trains and prepares health professionals to deliver safe, high-quality healthcare and meet tomorrow's global challenges.

SUMMARY

We hope that the ideas, thoughts and concepts in this book will stimulate readers to think about how they can improve learning with simulation. Those who are involved in the development and delivery of simulation healthcare education need to have a better understanding and the most recent evidence of its use. If simulation education is used by those that are not aware of its challenges or previous work, the outcomes could be costly and lead to the technique being abandoned. Keeping pace with the implications of published research, new technologies and influences from other disciplines is important.

Discussion in the literature can tend towards the sceptic, such as editorial headlines of 'High fidelity and fun: but fallow ground for learning?' [6]. The article the editorial refers to concludes that some participants do not perform as well as others if under too much stress during simulated scenarios [7]. Other published research discusses how surprising or unanticipated events (which are inherently stressful) in an immersive virtual reality game can foster deeper learning [8]. Both these results, though conflicting at first, emphasize that learners are individuals; however, current research tends to look at how groups respond to simulation education. Which brings us back to the question: what is simulation education for? The range of modalities, uses and applications means that simulation based education cannot be purely labelled as good and bad for any one healthcare professional or team.

Evidence suggests that simulated scenarios have to be distinct, novel and incremental in their learning objectives for those who have repeated exposure to simulation training. This has been described as 'episodic' training and been postulated as the way forward for sustainable improved clinical performance [9]. The use of social media in clinical simulation education and training programmes, for example the use of smart phones to provide short, sharp 'teaching points' either with blogs, podcasts or interactive questions before and after training is increasing. When it comes to new technologies, the pace of development is probably not matched by those who develop and deliver simulation education. We are often constrained by our own education, experience and imagination when it comes to truly utilizing the full range and benefits of simulation education. With rapid advances in technology and expanding research programmes in simulation in clinical education, one might speculate that the best is yet to come.

REFERENCES

1. Forrest K, McKimm J (2010) Using simulation in clinical education. *British Journal of Hospital Medicine*, **71:** 345–349.

2. Gaba DM (2004) The future vision of simulation in healthcare. *Quality and Safety in Health Care* **13:** i2–i10.

3. Bligh D, Bleakley A (2006) Distributing menus to hungry learners: can learning by simulation become simulation of learning? *Medical Teacher* **28:** 606–613.

4. Kneebone RL, Kidd J, Nestel D, Barnet A, Lo B, King R, Yang GZ, Brown R (2005) Blurring the boundaries: scenario-based simulation in a clinical setting. *Medical Education* **39:** 580–587.

5. Kneebone RL, Scott W, Darzi A, Horrocks, M (2004) Simulation and clinical practice: strengthening the relationship. *Medical Education* **38:** 1095–1102.

6. Basu Roy R, McMahon, GT (2012) High fidelity and fun: but fallow ground for learning? *Medical Education* **46:** 1022–1023.

7. Fraser K, Ma I, Teteris E, Baxter H, Wright B, McLaughlin K (2012) Emotion, cognitive load and learning outcomes during simulation training. *Medical Education* **46:** 1055–1062.

8. van der Spek ED, van Oostendorp H, Meyer J-J Ch (2012) Introducing surprising events can stimulate deep learning in a serious game. *British Journal of Educational Technology* **44:** 156–169.

9. Reader T (2011) Learning through high-fidelity simulation in anaesthesia: The role of episodic memory. *British Journal of Anaesthesia* **107:** 483–487.

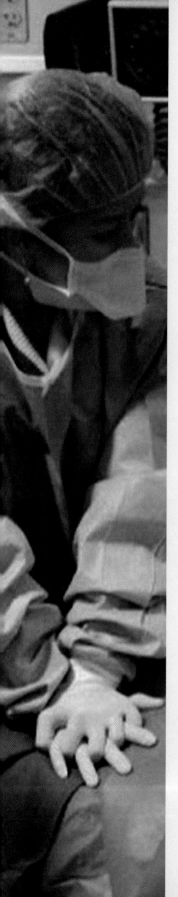

CHAPTER 2

Medical simulation: the journey so far

Aidan Byrne   Cardiff University, Cardiff, UK

Overview

The story of simulation is dominated by the efforts of pioneers who have struggled to improve training by using the resources available to them. These individuals have, however, largely worked in isolation and often failed to identify prior, related work that would have provided them with valuable guidance [1]. It is therefore difficult to write a definitive history of simulation, as any one innovation can rightly be ascribed to multiple groups and publication of results has often followed many years after the development of the technique. As Rosen suggests:

Many great ideas are ignored or dismissed only to be rediscovered at a future date with better understanding and acceptance [2, p. 157].

The published work on medical simulation highlights that the main aim of those developing simulators has been to improve the performance of students or trainees and thereby to improve the quality of healthcare delivery and patient safety. The view of what performance is, how learning occurs and how performance should be measured does, however, take many different forms.

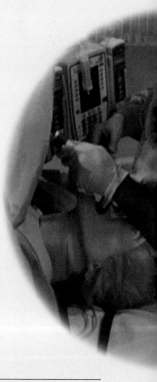

   Throughout the early history of simulation, advocates and pioneers were often derided, by those wedded to the apprenticeship model of learning and the practice of medicine as an art, for 'playing with dolls' and taking the students away from 'real' patients and by implication, 'real' learning.

   This chapter takes a selective dip in and out of the history of medical simulation, focusing on some of the key innovators and the technological developments that allowed innovation to take place. Apologies are offered to those innovators whose efforts have been unintentionally omitted.

Essential Simulation in Clinical Education, First Edition. Edited by Kirsty Forrest, Judy McKimm, and Simon Edgar.
© 2013 John Wiley & Sons, Ltd. Published 2013 by John Wiley & Sons, Ltd.

Definition

Simulation has been defined as:

The technique of imitating the behaviour of some situation or process (whether economic, military, mechanical, etc.) by means of a suitably analogous situation or apparatus, especially for the purpose of study or personnel training [3].

Taxonomy

Attempts to produce a useable taxonomy of medical simulators have focused on the physical appearance of the simulator, in terms of scope, realism or fidelity. However, the way a simulator is used depends greatly on the educational context and one physical simulator can be used in a variety of contexts. For example, an intravenous access training arm is usually cited as an example of a simple, 'part task trainer'; however, such arms are often now incorporated into much more sophisticated manikins or used alongside human actors to provide so called 'hybrid' simulation. The definitions listed in

Table 2.1 will be used in this chapter and defines each simulator according to specific educational contexts and processes.

Early simulators

It is difficult to determine the origin of medical simulators as they probably pre-date modern medicine and even recorded history. Anyone embarking on a new venture in simulation is strongly advised to make a detailed study of the literature as many have found that the planned 'innovation' has been already been described before. There is evidence that models were used to describe the process of childbirth from the ninth century, with manikins, 'phantoms', used to teach midwives the process of childbirth in the 1600s [4]. Perhaps most notably, Madame du Coudray, the midwife to the court of King Louis XV developed 'the Machine', a life-sized and anatomically correct model made of cloth, leather and sponge with which she travelled the countryside teaching techniques to aid childbirth [4]. Such basic models have been refined and developed, gradually incorporating more realistic features

Table 2.1	A simple classification of simulators		
	Appearance	**Interaction with the learner**	**Educational context**
Part task trainer	Realistic, but of a single body part	Feels realistic but limited or no response	Repetitive practice of isolated skill
Full body simulator	Realistic body, often with associated physiological modelling	Allows examination (for example, pulses) and realistic interactions	Realistic practice of whole scenarios
Screen simulator	2D image of patient, equipment or staff	Realistic response to input via keyboard or mouse	Cognitive exploration of a variety of situations
Virtual reality	3D image of patient, equipment or staff	Realistic response to input via a variety of methods	Realistic practice, often of a defined task
Real people as simulators	Real people	Verbal and non-verbal communication	Practice of a variety of clinical skills
Hybrid simulation	Any combination of the above	Verbal and non-verbal communication and interaction	Realistic practice
Simulated environments	An entire clinical environment	Full interaction with patient and team	Realistic practice and team training

and functions as knowledge and, in particular, new materials have allowed. Progress is crucially dependant on material science in determining what is possible to achieve and at what cost. Prior to modern developments, in what many would now regard as an unacceptable practice, the recently dead have not only provided specimens for anatomical dissection (teaching 'models') but also for the active practice of skills such as intubation. Increased public awareness and wider availability of materials and technology has led to reappraisal of such methods and a greater focus on artificial materials and models [5].

Part task trainers

In the late 1950s, it was recognized that external cardiac massage could maintain circulation [6] and that normal oxygen and carbon dioxide levels could be achieved by expired air ventilation [7]. This transformed the practice of a doctor, from careful enquiry and consideration into that of an immediate care provider who might be required to act within seconds. This led to new and very different training requirements which could not be provided through the traditional medical school practices of seminars, lectures or bedside teaching.

Alongside these developments in acute medicine, the development of mouldable soft plastics in America was noticed by Åsmund S. Lærdal, who up to that time had been a manufacturer of greetings cards and plastic toys. He brought samples of the plastic from America and began investigating the possibilities of using the plastic to develop more lifelike toy dolls. A meeting with the anaesthetist Dr Bjørn Lind provided the stimulus to start developing a manikin after attending a demonstration of the effectiveness of mouth-to-mouth resuscitation by Dr Peter Safar [1]. Lærdal's aim was to develop a realistic training aid for teaching mouth-to-mouth resuscitation. In an attempt to stimulate learning, the manikin, Resusci Anne, was made as lifelike as possible using the face of a beautiful girl found floating in the River Seine, presumably after a failed romance. As the girl had not been identified, a death mask was taken, which was widely reproduced and is now famous. The manikin incorporated a mechanism that required the neck to be hyperextended and the chin thrust forward in order

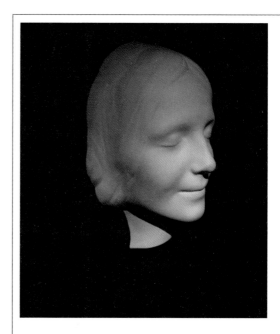

Figure 2.1 Face of Resusci Anne.

to open the airway, in addition to a spring in the chest to allow for the practice of external cardiac massage (Figure 2.1).

In 1968 Dr Michael Gordon demonstrated Harvey [8], a cardiovascular, part task trainer designed to assist in the teaching of cardiovascular examination and diagnostic skills. Harvey consisted of a manikin (minus legs) recumbent on a large cabinet containing the electronic and electromechanical workings. It was able to simulate jugular and radial pulses, precordial impulses and heart sounds in the four auscultatory areas and to vary those sounds with respiration in 50 different cardiac conditions [9].

An important factor in the design of Harvey was that the project started with very clear educational objectives and from the beginning was developed alongside a range of educational materials for use with the simulator. The driver was to produce 'more and better trained physicians in less time, at less cost' and to provide an objective measure of competency [9]. Partly as a result of this focus on educational efficiency, a study of 208 fourth-year medical students showed that training on Harvey led to increased knowledge (using a multiple choice question test) and better performance of skills as tested on Harvey and real patients. Patients did not perceive any difference between students trained on the simulator or through more traditional 'apprenticeship', which demonstrates the potential impact of simulation on transfer into the clinical setting [10].

The original design was limited by the available technology. The pulses and movement of the chest wall were produced by electromechanical devices and the sound produced by a modified stethoscope, activated to receive a series of taped recordings of appropriate sounds. The manikin also allowed students to examine the eyes with an ophthalmoscope after dilating the pupils with drops. Although the system was largely designed as an electromechanical device, later designs have incorporated more sophisticated digital electronic technology. 'Harvey' is still used as a pivotal technology in the focused cardiorespiratory learning for undergraduate students of medicine in hundreds of schools worldwide.

Real people as simulators

In 1964, Barrows and Abrahamson [11] recognized that the ability to interact with real patients was of prime importance when assessing the abilities of medical students, but that traditional clinical clerkships (hospital attachment) posed problems of reliability, standardization and reproducibility. They introduced the idea of a 'programmed patient' or normal person trained to assume and present the history and, on examination, neurological findings of an actual patient in the manner of an actual patient. The need for the person to be repeatedly examined led them to seek a 'young female professional art model with acting ability' who was then given an 'indoctrination program' [11, p. 803] which aimed to make her fully aware of the entire neurological examination procedure and the basic terminology used, along with the findings of specific cases.

The patient was used to assess the abilities of groups of seven students on a neurological clerkship, who were each asked to complete a written case summary as if the patient were real and given 30 minutes to interact with the patient, followed by

4 hours to complete the summary using any source of reference they wished.

The idea was not just ignored by other medical educators, however, but actively resisted by those who found the idea of using 'actors' demeaning to medical education and derided in the press [12] for using 'scantily clad models' to engage their students.

Medical educators persisted in the face of opposition and in 1976, Stillman *et al.* [13] described the use of 'trained mothers' as a method of teaching interviewing skills. In a follow-up study using a group of medical students, those trained using the technique scored higher in an evaluation of their interview skills with a real patient and this difference was still evident a year later. Although the majority of published studies in this area relate to the training of medical students, the technique is now established as a method for further developing the skills of qualified doctors [14].

Kretzschmar [15] noted that during teaching of gynaecological examination, anxiety on the part of the student inhibited learning. In addition, he was concerned that patients were being exploited as 'teaching material' and that there was a lack of accurate feedback to students on their performance. He recognized the equal importance of technical and interpersonal skills and the need to teach and assess both at the same time so in 1978 he recruited a group of 'professional patients' or Gynaecology Teaching Associates (GTAs). The GTAs were trained in common clinical conditions, associated 'personality problems' in recognition that patients and disease states are not synonymous and that doctors should be trained to deal with the complexities of normal clinical life and in giving feedback. This helped students repeatedly practice their technique in a supportive and non-threatening environment.

The programme involved two students working with two GTAs in the setting of a normal outpatient clinic over a two and a half hour session, with demonstration and then practice of breast, abdominal and pelvic examination. Results showed that the students rated the experience highly and that they did not regard the learning experience as artificial [15]. The principle challenge to such methods is the ability to recruit and train adequate numbers of patients who can provide the training and maintain their status as a patient, rather than being seen as medical school staff. GTAs help to avoid the ethically challenging problems of truly informed consent when female patients are examined by students while under anaesthesia for related gynaecological procedures [16].

The use of real patients is now widespread in medical education, both as a part of the assessment process, in recognition of the added realism they provide, but also as active partners in the development of medical education and as experts in their own right [17].

Screen-based simulation

In the early 1960s, Barrow and Abrahamson began to experiment with 8-mm film cassettes [11], which allowed students to observe 4-minute clips of patient signs. This technology was then used to record an actor trained to produce a demonstration of a fictitious case, complete with full clinical details, which students could review and learn from.

The advent of affordable video recorders was recognized and adapted by Briscoe *et al.* [18], who in 1987 developed a system which simulated a psychiatric interview using a microcomputer and videotape system. Although crude, it allowed students to select questions for the patient to answer and then to watch the patient answering the question. The aim was to make the responses of vulnerable psychiatric patients available to a wider audience, without risk to the patient and included a very basic element of diagnostic training. The advent of digital media and more sophisticated interfaces has allowed the development of a wide range of on-screen simulation.

A vast array of e-learning resources are now available, some of which contain interactive and exploratory elements which allow students to work through clinical cases in a manner that mirrors clinical practice. For example, the Air Medic 1 system integrates screen-based teaching/simulation around communication and team working, with biofeedback sensors [19]. The aim is to allow students to manage their own emotional responses in stressful situations. A variety of other resources have been developed and shown to be equally effective as other teaching methods and rated highly by stu-

dents [20]. Whether such systems are regarded as 'simulation' is open to debate and some reviews do not include such systems.

As software developed, advances in physiological modelling were increasingly incorporated into simulated models. For example, in 1981 Fukui and Smith [21] described complex modelling of the ventilation and circulatory systems, initially describing the uptake and distribution of anaesthetic gases. This computerized model incorporated 18 different compartments in which an anaesthetic gas could distribute, the cardiac output was calculated beat to beat, and the blood pressure flow in the cardiovascular system was represented by 52 equations. The software was gradually developed into the commercial BodySim [2] programme, which divided the human body into a series of small discrete models, each with a series of interactions with multiple other models. So, for example, the administration of an anaesthetic gas to the lungs resulted in transfer of the gas to the blood and then the heart, which would then reduce the cardiac output and so reduce the uptake of the gas and so on. The result was an interface where the effect of the administration of treatments could be demonstrated in real time. Other similar computer programmes with a primary educational focus, such as GasMan [22], were developed which included a series of educational exercises with the aim of increasing students delivery of anaesthesia safely. These early computer developers had to work within huge constraints. Software was written in BASIC programming language and had to occupy less than 64 K of memory, which at the time was very close to 100% of the computer memory available. On current computers, this is equivalent to using around 0.000064%. As capacity increased, the BodySim programme added a more complex interface which sought to represent the operating room environment so that students could deliver anaesthesia and deal with complications in a screen-based 'virtual' operating theatre. The system also included the ability to produce a detailed summary of events and an automated 'expert' interpretation. A related programme, using the same components, the ACLS (Advanced Cardiac Life Support) simulator, was able to demonstrate effective learning and retention of basic resuscitation skills [23] based on the ACLS protocols of the American Heart Association.

Simulated environments

In 1967, the first computer-controlled full patient simulator, Sim One, was developed at the University of Southern California School of Medicine [8] by Dr Stephen Abrahamson, a director of an Educational Research Centre and Dr Judson Denson, an anaesthetist physician in collaboration with Sierra Engineering and Aerojet General Corporation. The stimulus appears to have been a military corporation's need to diversify in the face of falling military research income leading them to seek other markets for their expertise [1]. For the time, the manikin was amazingly complex with realistic skin, a moving chest wall and synchronized heart rate and pulses. In addition, it was able to blink its eyes, open its mouth and respond automatically to four intravenously administered drugs with the processing power provided by a hybrid digital and analogue computer. In an initial study, comparing the efficiency of the simulator versus conventional 'on the job training' to teach novice anaesthetists the skill of endotracheal intubation, the simulator showed some evidence of reduced training times.

This development marked the first real attempt to bring the technology and psychology that had already been used successfully in the aviation industry to medicine, with the aim of making simulated practice a major part of both training and assessment. The technology appears to have been too far ahead of its time as there was no demand for such training, and the technology was too expensive and complex for routine use. Only one such simulator was built and no longer exists.

In 1987 Gaba and DeAnda [24] designed the Comprehensive Anesthesia Simulation Environment (CASE), which used a complex manikin combined with an entire operating room environment, complete with monitors, equipment and staff. The system required the students to fully engage in the simulation both by interacting with the 'patient', but also managing the theatre team. Although the simulations were judged to be highly realistic, they initially relied on 'scripted' scenarios, with the 'patient' responding to each intervention in a pre-

determined way. The group later added full physiological modelling from the Anesthesia Simulator Recorder [25] and partnered with an aviation simulation company to produce the fully commercial CAE-Link simulator. The most important development of this group was the recognition that, as in aviation, training only the leader is not enough and that teams need to be trained together to produce effective learning. They took the established techniques of Cockpit (later Crew) Resource Management (CRM) that emphasized the role of such qualities as communication, error management and leadership in addition to technical performance [26]. During this period, an independent group based in Florida designed the Gainesville Anesthesia Simulator (GAS), also using a complex manikin, and sought to recreate the entire anaesthetic environment [2], although the group focused more on individual performance. These two systems developed in competition and after some years the GAS system, developed by the company Medical Education Technologies Inc., ultimately became the most commercially successful system. At the same time several groups in Europe produced less complex simulators with much the same intent [27,28,29].

Those engaged in these projects aimed not just to produce a realistic environment, although the goal of realism was an important principle. Rather the main driver was the understanding that human behaviour is not entirely conscious and that humans often behave in ways that defy logic and sometimes belief. The aim was therefore to provide an environment in which learners could be put under realistic stressful conditions and trained to understand and deal with the consequences of that stress.

In 1994 a team at the University of Basel developed the concept of team oriented medical simulation, which integrated the training of multiple teams with high-fidelity simulators [30]. For example, a surgeon might be operating with a laparoscopic trainer and cause rapid bleeding. The surgeon would then attempt to stop the bleeding, while the anaesthetic team were dealing with the haemodynamic consequences, and both teams hopefully communicating with each other. This approach drew heavily on the concepts of CRM as used by other groups. This method involved two main changes from previous methods. First, there were no actors involved in the simulations, but rather each member of the team played their normal role. Second, the focus was on improving the performance of the team rather than on the performance of individuals. This involved stressing the role of situational awareness, decision-making and conflict resolution rather than adherence to protocols.

Virtual reality

In 1989, Rosen and Delp [31], members of a NASA research team, designed an on-screen three-dimensional (3D) representation of the muscles of the leg designed to allow surgeons to attempt virtual tendon transfers and investigate the resulting changes in gait. Each muscle and tendon in the lower limb was modelled in terms of the forces acting at each joint. Although limited in scope, it had a clear focus on the need for the operator to plan and predict the conduct and outcome of surgery. In particular, it allowed surgeons to visualise the effects of tendon transplantation or shortening on the virtual patient's gait.

Four years later, Savata and Lanier developed the first virtual reality operation environment [32], although the graphics, interaction and surgical interventions were extremely basic. In the same year, Merrill developed a much more sophisticated 3D model which included the property of tissue elasticity, which allowed the organs to be deformed and stretched by the actions of the operator [33]. An early attempt to integrate this visual technology into a realistic laparoscopic training was the based on the KISMET (Kinematick Simulation, Monitoring and off-line Programming Environment for Telerobotics) computer modelling system [34]. The system used real laparoscopic instruments modified to incorporate motion sensors so that any movement of an instrument was detected, transferred to the computer and incorporated into the model, which then produced an image for the trainee. The principle used in these systems is the reduction of the body to a series of distinct virtual components described by properties such as mass and deformability. Any actions of the user are then interpreted as resulting in movement or deformity of these components.

Although simple in principle, the realism of such systems is determined by the resolution, accuracy of modelling and the refresh rate. The resolution is the size of the smallest point used to describe the objects, with more points equating to greater realism. The accuracy of modelling is how close the behaviour of the model relates to the real world and the refresh rate is the number of times per second that the model is updated. A model will work better if it is made up of very fine points, uses realistic modelling and updates more frequently, although increasing any of these aspects requires an increase in computing power. A model which does not react to the input of the operator in real time is clearly not going to provide a useful learning experience, so that developers generally use the most sophisticated models at the highest resolution which produce an acceptable refresh rate. The technological advance that made these systems possible was the high-performance graphical workstation that could provide the massive computational power required to produce realistic 3D images in real time. This capability was greatly enhanced by the release of data from the Visible Human Project in 1994, which provided an open source of data for 3D modelling. Combined with the ability to import data directly from patients' computed tomography scans, a series of patient-specific simulations were developed where natural variations in anatomy and pathology could be represented [35].

By 1997, surgical simulators were being developed by multiple groups [36] which included haptic feedback: the ability of the simulator to apply pressure to the hands of the operator so as to mimic the tactile sensation of instrument and tissue manipulation. That means that when an instrument is pushed forward into virtual soft tissue, the operator 'sees' the virtual instrument deforming the tissue and feels gradually increasing resistance and when the instrument hits a virtual solid substance, the operator feels the instrument come to an abrupt halt. Although expensive and complex, the advantages of haptic systems are that an operation can be simulated in great detail, including anatomical variations, bleeding and the use of a variety of techniques. The main problem with such systems is the sensitivity of human touch. The human eye cannot separate images which change more often than around 24 times per second; therefore, a television only has to produce around 25 images per second for the viewers to perceive the result as a smooth, moving image. In contrast, the touch sensors of the fingers are easily capable of detecting movements at a resolution of hundreds of times per second. In addition, an image produced by a computer is transferred to the screen almost instantaneously and can be changed within a few milliseconds, whereas haptic feedback is provided by motors moving physical objects that inevitably suffer from inertia and longer response times. The result is that the computing power to control the feedback system must be much more powerful and expensive than that required to run an equivalent graphic system [37].

Many systems have now been developed which aim to provide training in a number of surgical contexts, particularly where the operator views the surgical field either through some form of telescope or operating instrument, for example an operating microscope in ophthalmology [38], endovascular therapy [39] and laparoscopic surgery [37]. The major advantage of applying these technologies is that the system captures data on all aspects of the operators' performance as a matter of routine. These data are not limited to such parameters as the 'time to complete' but also include such parameters as the amount of tremor, the force exerted by the instrument on the tissues, the number of movements and (for example) the amount of any cavity visualized. Studies with these VR systems, for example from Mahmood and Darzi [40], have demonstrated that in the absence of haptic feedback, psychomotor performance enhancement is limited.

While the systems described earlier provide realistic images as seen through instruments, there have also been attempts to replicate large-scale environments, for example the CAVE (CAVE Audio Visual Environment) [41]. Recent developments in these large-scale environments consist of rear projection, 3D screens and high-definition sound [42] which provide an immersive environment where, for example, the problem of dealing with casualties at the side of the road next to moving cars can be simulated.

In 2007, the interactive web-based software, 'Second Life' was first reported in use for medical educational purposes [43]. In Second Life, individuals can access a virtual online world as computer-generated avatars or virtual self, with the physical characteristics of the individual chosen by the user. Each individual explores the virtual world usually using a keyboard or mouse, interacting with both the virtual environment and other individuals through their own avatars. The primary attraction of such simulated environments is that large numbers of individuals in distant locations can interact as if they were physically present in the virtual world. There are now large numbers of medical resources in Second Life, including neurological examination and heart murmur training as well as more traditional libraries [44]. It is also possible to attend virtual seminars and conferences and in virtual learning centres, individuals can consult with experts or those suffering from disease, attend lectures or interact with a range of virtual learning materials [45]. Although it is too early to judge how successful these ventures will be in the long term, with the advent of 3D screens and headsets, possibilities are offered of almost full immersion into an artificial world; however, there is some evidence that such environments may offer a poor learning experience for some students [46].

A summary of these innovations is portrayed pictorially in Figure 2.2 as a timeline.

Development of simulation education centres

Early simulation facilities were often the product of individuals working alone or in small groups within clinical departments, with most of the equipment developed 'in-house' or adapted from commercial products [27,28,29] based in clinical areas. However, after 1990, 'simulation centres' began to be established. Few centres have been funded entirely through public sources. Personal communication indicates that centres have been funded by a variety of start-up and ongoing sources, including private capital, charitable donation, through undergraduate and postgraduate education funds, the military, drug company support, equipment manufacturer support and revenue from courses.

The variety of stimuli for the building of centres is also reflected in their surroundings, with some

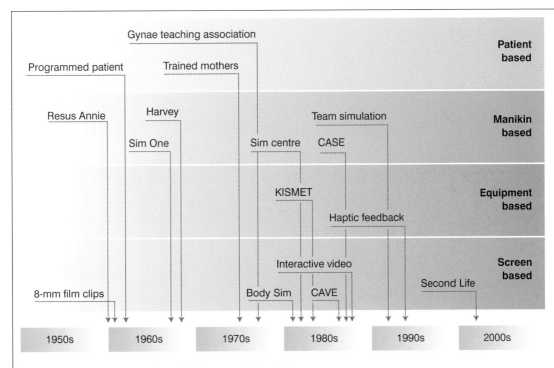

Figure 2.2 Key innovations in simulation over the last 50 years.

centres working in commercial premises without directly linked healthcare organizations and others sited within hospitals/clinics or on University campuses. Chapter 10 describes the key features of simulation centres in more detail.

The growth in the numbers of centres in Europe is shown in Figure 2.3. These data were based on the database maintained by Alan Jones at the Bristol Medical Simulation Centre [47] and show a massive expansion over the last 20 years. The numbers must be interpreted with caution however as the process is voluntary and there are no defined criteria for inclusion as a 'simulation centre', so that those centres included may not include features that some regard as essential aspects of simulation. It is also difficult to determine whether the slowing of increase in numbers is due to a genuine decline in the number of centres opening each year or to a delay in centres registering with the database.

The expansion of simulation has not been confined to Europe, with the number of centres in each region shown in Figure 2.4. Although these numbers must again be interpreted with caution as they are collected by a European organization whose website is in English, it is clear that simulation centres are not evenly distributed around the world and the differences shown are even more striking when population numbers are taken into account. For example, in North America there is a simulation centre for each 0.5 million people. In Africa there is a centre for each 100 million people.

Guidelines and regulation

As described earlier, advances in simulation have been driven largely by the efforts of individuals and not as the result of external regulation or policy change. In addition, the different branches of simulation have rarely worked effectively together, with manikin-based training led by anaesthesia, haptic and virtual reality training led by surgery and the use of patients/actors by community medicine. However, there has been a concerted effort to build links between these communities led by organizations such as the Association of Simulated Practice in Healthcare (ASPiH) in the UK [48], the Society

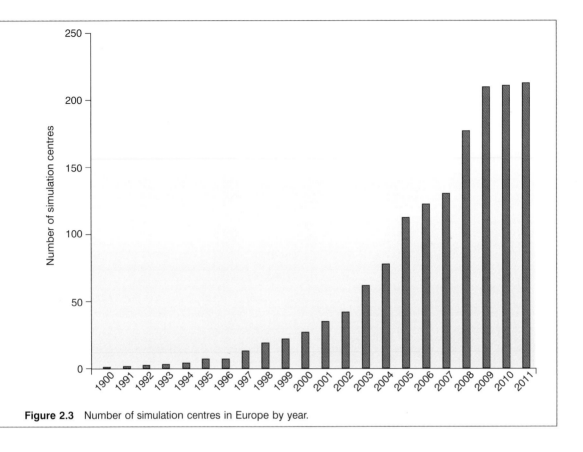

Figure 2.3 Number of simulation centres in Europe by year.

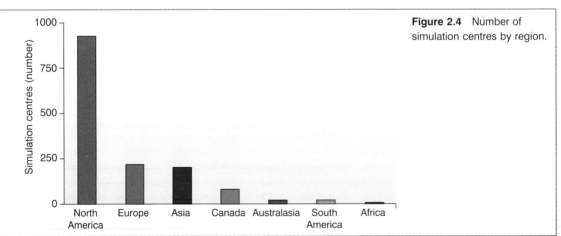

Figure 2.4 Number of simulation centres by region.

for Simulation in Healthcare in the United States [49] and the Society in Europe for Simulation Applied to Medicine.

At the same time, the benefits of simulation to patient safety have been recognized, with regulatory bodies increasingly supporting the concept of simulation in their training programmes and providing accreditation to training centres. For example, by 1990, it had become well recognized in laparoscopic surgery that surgical mortality was linked to operator skill, and that adequate levels of skill could not be acquired by the traditional apprenticeship model in the operating theatre [50], leading to the society of American Gastrointestinal Endoscopic Surgeons (SAGES) guidelines [51], which provide both operators and trainers with standards that include knowledge and defined levels of technical skill. Although laparoscopic cholecystectomy was the operation on which training focused, other centres were established to train surgeons. One example is the Minimal Access Therapy Training Unit (MATTUS) in Scotland, which provided simulation skills and an associated teaching and assessment package that looked to define trainability and assess the level of skill exhibited by trainees [52].

In 1996, the Royal Colleges of Surgeons initiated the Basic Surgical Skills course, which used basic simulation techniques to teach skills including suturing, wound management and endoscopic surgery. The course is mandatory for trainees starting their surgical career and now appears to be an accepted requirement for progression [53]. The American Society of Anesthesiologists [54] now accredit simulation centres and endorse courses which provide credit directly linked to accreditation provided by the American Board of Anesthesiology [55], and in 2012 a Canadian simulation centre in Toronto was the first in the country to receive accreditation from the Royal College of Physicians and Surgeons of Canada. In addition to these national developments, there is now a concerted effort in many regions for simulation centres to be accredited by regional or national bodies in order to improve the quality of education and its links to the curricula of professional bodies.

These events mark the gradual progression in many specialties from initial endorsement of simulation as a teaching method, through the recommendation of simulation in published curricula, with the final step being the acceptance of simulation based assessment as a required part of licensing. While such simulation based assessment is common in industries such as aviation, the long-standing questions of the validity of such assessments in the more complex world of medicine is likely to result in a continued slow uptake in other specialities [56].

These developments mirror a change in governmental guidance, for example in the UK, in 2002 the report *An organisation with a memory* [57], which focused on the problem of human error in healthcare, does not contain the word 'simulation'. However, by 2009, the House of Commons Health Committee Patient Safety Report includes the recommendation that Human Factors training must be fully integrated into undergraduate and postgraduate medical education and includes the word 'simulation' 12 times [58]. In 2011 the Department of Health report *A framework for technology enhanced learning* [59] contains the word simulation 106 times and has as its first recommendation:

As part of a managed learning process and where appropriate, healthcare professionals should learn skills in a simulation environment and using other technologies before undertaking them in supervised clinical practice.

Over the last 25 years, the development of simulation as a technology and educational methodology has been remarkable, with outstanding achievements in many fields allowing students to practice and learn in a variety of environments. In most cases the focus of the designers and developers has been on the subjective experience of the learner. The main challenge now seems to be to define how this technology needs to be used to produce the greatest improvement in patient outcomes and safety. A further challenge is to ensure that change is supported by high-quality research focused not just on improved educational efficacy, but also on improved patient outcomes. Whether technological interventions help achieve these improvements seems most likely if simulation becomes fully embedded in the curriculum and assessment process of all aspects of medical training and practice.

SUMMARY

✓ Key points

- Simulation has a long history with its development closely tied to technological advances in computer and materials science.
- Simulation is now recognized as adding value to training and education and enabling practice of a range of skills and competencies in a safe environment.
- Many countries and regions have established simulation centres, although these are inequitably distributed around the world.
- Simulation-based education enables the delivery of a continuum of learning throughout a doctor's career.
- More research is needed to determine the impact of simulation training on improving health outcomes.

REFERENCES

1. Cooper JB, Taqueti VR (2008) A brief history of the development of mannequin simulators for clinical education and training. *Postgraduate Medical Journal* **84**: 563–570.

2. Rosen K (2008) The history of medical simulation. *Journal of Critical Care* **23**: 157–166.

3. Oxford English Dictionary. Available from www.oed.com (accessed 6 March 2013).

4. Gardner R, Raemer DB (2008) Simulation in obstetrics and gynecology. *Obstetrics and Gynecology Clinics of North America* **35**: 97–127.

5. Ardagh M (1997) May we practise endotracheal intubation on the newly dead? *Journal of Medical Ethics* **23**: 289–294.

6. Kouwenhoven WB, Jude JR, Knickerbocker GG (1960) *Closed-chest cardiac massage. Journal of the American Medical Association* **173**: 1064–1067.

7. Safar P, Brown TC, Holtey WJ, Wilder RJ (1961) Ventilation and circulation with closed-chest cardiac massage in man. *Journal of the American Medical Association* **176**: 574–576.

8. Denson JS, Abrahamson SA (1969) Computer-controlled patient simulator. *Journal of the American Medical Association* **208**: 504–508.

9. Michael SG (1974) Cardiology patient simulator: development of an animated manikin to teach cardiovascular disease. *American Journal of Cardiology* **34**: 350–355.

10. Ewy GA, Felner JM, Juul D, *et al.* (1987) Test of a cardiology patient simulator with students in fourth-year electives. *Academic Medicine* **62**: 738–743.

11. Barrows HS, Abrahamson S (1964) The programmed patient: a technique for appraising student performance in clinical neurology. *Academic Medicine* **39**: 802–805.

12. Wallace P (1997) Following the threads of innovation: this history of standardised patients in medical education. *Caduceus* **13**: 5–28.

13. Stillman L, Sabers DL, Redfield DL (1976) The use of paraprofessionals to teach interviewing skills. *Pediatrics* **57**: 769–774.

14. Reinders ME, Blankenstein AH, van der Horst HE, *et al.* (2010) Does patient feedback improve the consultation skills of general practice trainees? A controlled trial. *Medical Education* **44**: 156–164.

15. Kretzschmar R (1978) Evolution of the gynecology teaching associate: an education specialist. *American Journal of Obstetrics and Gynecology* **131:** 367–373.

16. Chamberlain S, Bocking A, McGrath M, *et al.* (2010) Teaching pelvic examinations under anaesthesia: what do women think? *Journal of Obsetrics and Gynaecology* **32:** 539–540.

17. Jha V, Quinton ND, Bekker HL, Roberts TE (2009) Strategies and interventions for the involvement of real patients in medical education: a systematic review. *Medical Education* **43:** 10–20.

18. Briscoe MH, Byrne A, Hicks B, *et al.* (1987) Interactive video teaching using a home microcomputer. *Medical Education* **21:** 15–17.

19. Kalkman C (2012) Air Medic Sky One (AMS1).Available from http://www.airmedicsky1.org/ (accessed 6 March 2013).

20. O'Leary S, Diepenhorst L, Churley-Strom R, Magrane D (2005) Educational games in an obstetrics and gynecology core curriculum. *American Journal of Obstetrics and Gynecology* **193:** 1848–1851.

21. Fukui Y, Smith NT (1981) Interactions among ventilation, the circulation and the uptake and distribution of halothane – use of a hybrid computer multiple model: I. The basic model. *Anesthesiology* **54:** 107–118.

22. Philip J (1986) Gas Man – An example of goal oriented computer-assisted teaching which results in learning. *International Journal of Clinical Monitoring and Computing* **3:** 165–173.

23. Schwid HA (2001) Components of an effective medical simulation software solution. *Simulation & Gaming* **32:** 240–249.

24. Gaba DM, DeAnda A (1988) A Comprehensive Anesthesia simulation environment: re-creating the operating room for research and training. *Anesthesiology* **69:** 387–394.

25. Schwid HA, O'Donnell D (1990) The anesthesia simulator-recorder: a device to train and evaluate anesthesiologists' responses to critical incidents. *Anesthesiology* **72:** 191–197.

26. Howard S, Gaba DM, Fish KJ *et al.* (1992) Anesthesia crisis resource management training: teaching anesthesiologists to handle critical incidents. *Aviation Space Environmental Medicine* **63:** 763–770.

27. Byrne AJ, Hilton J, Lunn JN (1994) Basic simulations for anaesthetists. A pilot study of the ACCESS system. *Anaesthesia* **49:** 376–381.

28. Chopra V, Engbers FH, Geerts MJ, *et al.* (1994) The Leiden anaesthesia simulator. *British Journal of Anaesthesia* **73:** 287–292.

29. Christensen UJ, Andersen SF, Jacobsen J, *et al.* (1997) The Sophus anaesthesia simulator v. 2.0. *International Journal of Clinical Monitoring and Computing* **14:** 11–16.

30. Sexton J, Marsch S, Helmreich R (1998) Participant evaluation of team oriented medical simulation. In: *Simulators in Anesthesiology* (L. Henson and A. Lee, eds). Plenum: New York: 109–110.

31. Delp SL, Loan JP, Hoy MG, *et al.* (1990) An interactive graphics-based model of the lower extremity to study orthopaedic surgical procedures. *IEEE Transactions on Biomedical Engineering* **37:** 757–767.

32. Savata R (1993) Virtual reality surgical simulator: the first steps. *Surgical Endoscopy* **7:** 203–205.

33. Satava R (2001) Accomplishments and challenges of surgical simulation. *Surgical Endoscopy* **15:** 232–241.

34. Kühnapfel U, Çakmak HK, Maaß H (2000) Endoscopic surgery training using virtual reality and deformable tissue simulation. *Computers & Graphics* **24:** 671–682.

35. Levy J (1996) Virtual reality hysteroscopy. *Journal of the American Association of Gynaecological Laproscopy* **3**: S25–26.

36. Gibson S, Fyock C, Grimson E, *et al.* (1997) S*imulating Surgery Using Volumetric Object Representations, Real-time Volume Rendering and Haptic Feedback*. Cambridge, MA: Mitsubishi Electric Research Laboratories.

37. Playter R, Raibert M (1997) A virtual surgery simulator using advanced haptic feedback. *Minimally Invasive Therapy & Allied Technologies* **6**: 117–121.

38. Sinclair M, Peifer JW, Haleblian R, *et al.* (1995) Computer-simulated eye surgery. A novel teaching method for residents and practitioners. *Opthalmology* **102**: 517–521.

39. Medical Simulation Corporation (2012) Simantha. Available from http://www.medsimulation.com/Simantha.asp (accessed 6 March 2013)

40. Mahmood T, Darzi A (2004) The learning curve for a colonoscopy simulator in the absence of any feedback: no feedback, no learning. *Surgical Endoscopy* **18**: 1224–1230.

41. Cruz-Neira C, Sandin D, DeFanti T (1993) Surround-screen projection-based virtual reality: the design and implementation of the CAVE. In 20th Annual Conference on Computer Graphics and Interactive Techniques. Anheim, CA, USA.

42. Lee CH, Liu A, Del Castillo S, *et al.* (2007) Towards an immersive virtual environment for medical team training. *Studies in Health Technology and Informatics* **125**: 274–279.

43. Boulos MNK, Hetherington L, Wheeler S (2007) Second life: an overview of the potential of 3-D virtual worlds in medical and health education. *Health Information & Libraries Journal* **24**: 233–245.

44. Boulos M, Hetherington L, Wheeler S (2007) Second Life: an overview of the potential of 3-D virtual worlds in medical and health education. *Health Information & Libraries Journal* **24**: 233–245.

45. Department of Biosurgery and Surgical Technology at Imperial College London (2007) Available from http://secondhealth.wordpress.com/ (accessed 6 march 2013).

46. Savin-Baden M, Tombs C, Poulton T, *et al.* (2011) An evaluation of implementing problem-based learning scenarios in an immersive virtual world. *International Journal of Medical Education* **2**: 116–124.

47. Jones A (2012) World Simulation Centre Database. Available from http://www.bmsc.co.uk/sim_database/centres_europe.htm (accessed 6 March 2013).

48. Association for Simulated Practice in Healthcare (2010) Available from: www.aspih.org.uk/ (accessed 6 March 2013).

49. Society for Simulation in Healthcare (2012) Available from https://ssih.org/ (accessed 6 March 2013).

50. Royal college of Surgeons (1990) *Minimal Access Surgery*. London: Royal College of Surgeons of England.

51. Deizel D (2006) *The SAGES Manual: Fundamentals of Laparoscopy, Thoracoscopy and GI Endoscopy*, 2nd edn. Springer.

52. Cushchieri A, Wilson RG, Sunderland G, *et al.* (1997) Training initiative list scheme (TILS) for minimal access therapy: the MATTUS experience. *Journal of the Royal College of Surgeons of Edinburgh* **42**: 295–302.

53. Thomas WEG (1999) Basic Surgical Skills Course: an educational success story. *Annals of the Royal College of Sugeons of England* **S81**: 195–196.

54. The American Society of Anesthsiologists (2012) Available from www.asahq.org/ (accessed 6 March 2013).

55. The American Board of Anesthesiology. Available from www.theaba.org/ (accessed 6 March 2013).

56. Byrne AJ, Greaves JD (2001) Assessment instruments used during anaesthetic simulation: review of published studies. *British Journal of Anaesthesia* **86:** 445–450.

57. Department of Health (2000) *An Organisation with a Memory*. London: The Stationery Office: London.

58. House of commons Health Com mittee (2009) *Patient Safety*. London: The Stationery Office.

59. Department of Health (2011) *A Framework for Enhanced Learning*. London: The Stationery Office.

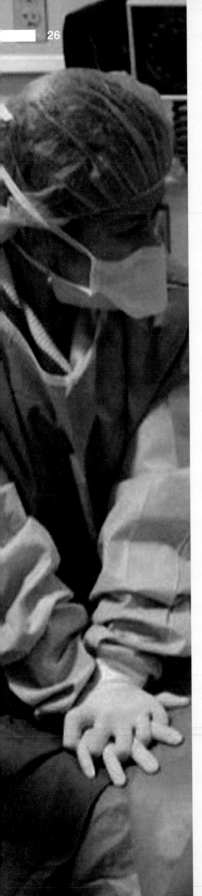

CHAPTER 3

The evidence: what works, why and how?

Doris Østergaard[1] and Jacob Rosenberg[2]   [1]Herlev University Hospital, Herlev, Denmark; [2]University of Copenhagen, Copenhagen, Denmark

Overview

The use of simulation to enhance learning is increasingly used in health profession's education. Simulation-based training can be used to address basic science concepts and clinical medical expertise – both cognitive and practical skills – in an interactive way that reflects the workplace. Training can be arranged for individuals or a multi-professional team of health professionals at any level of education and expertise.

Several reviews have been published with the aim of demonstrating the effect of simulation-based training, but although there is an increasing amount of data indicating the positive effect of simulation-based medical education, research in this field is still in its infancy [1,2,3]. The Best Evidence Medical Education (BEME) review describes the features that leads to effective learning [1] and, based on a range of learning theories (see Chapter 4), simulation seems to be a good learning technique, as it provides the opportunity to plan according to the needs of the learner and incorporate feedback easily. The rationale for using simulation-based training is set out in Box 3.1.

In 2010 and 2011, two influential meetings involving international experts were conducted with the intention to publish a research agenda for simulation-based training. An Utstein-style meeting

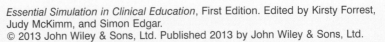

Essential Simulation in Clinical Education, First Edition. Edited by Kirsty Forrest, Judy McKimm, and Simon Edgar.
© 2013 John Wiley & Sons, Ltd. Published 2013 by John Wiley & Sons, Ltd.

Overview (ctd)

was arranged in Copenhagen in 2010. Utstein is an abbey in Norway, which has hosted several meetings, where a group of international experts come up with recommendations or guidelines for a given topic. Utstein is now synonymous with reporting guidelines for resuscitation. The 2010 meeting identified three main areas for research; instructional design, outcome-based assessment and translation to clinical setting [4]. The subthemes and examples of research questions within each theme are listed in Table 3.1. This was followed by a Summit Meeting in 2011 arranged by the International Society for Simulation in Health Care, where 10 topic areas of future research were presented, discussed and published [5]. Overall, bringing together experts with different backgrounds from different countries is beneficial, and meetings like these can serve as guidance for future research.

This chapter follows the headings from the 2005 BEME review and includes lessons learned from the two meetings described earlier. The aim is to give an overview of how the use of simulation-based training can be conducted in order to improve student learning and ultimately patient safety and health outcomes. A review of the existing evidence of what works, why and how is presented and discussed.

Box 3.1   Rationale for using simulation-based training

Pedagogical and patient safety advantages
The simulation setting:
- provides a safe environment where trainees can learn without the risk of harming a patient
- provides an environment that is fully attentive to the learner's needs
- provides an opportunity for repetitive training
- can be adjusted according to learners need
- enables exposure to gradually more complex clinical challenges
- enables exposure to rare emergency situations where time is an important factor
- supports experiential learning

Simulation based medical education provides opportunities for training of the:
- individual
- team of health professions

Simulation based medical education provides an opportunity for
- formative assessment, that includes debriefing and feedback
- stimulating reflection
- learning how to learn
- summative assessment

Table 3.1 Examples of themes and subthemes to be studied. Adapted from Issenberg *et al.* (2011) [4]

Instructional design	Learning acquisition
	Retention of skills
	Cognitive load
	Debriefing
	Learner characteristics
	Impact on learning theory
	Resource requirements and challenges
	Role of instructor
	System requirements
	Simulation program implementation
Outcomes measurements	Reaction level
	Learning level
	Behavioural level
	Organizational level

Essential features for effective learning: what works?

The BEME review on simulation-based training, which analysed 109 articles, addressed the question, 'What are the features and uses of high fidelity medical simulations that lead to most effective learning?' [1]. The authors found that only a few of the studies were performed with enough quality and rigour to yield useful results on the effectiveness of high-fidelity simulations with only 5% of the studies meeting the minimum quality standard. Of note, poor design, inappropriate methods and lack of information made it difficult to compare studies and the quality of the studies varied considerably. The review clearly indicated the need to improve the quality of research on simulation.

The conclusion of the BEME review was that high-fidelity medical simulations are educationally effective and can complement medical education in patient care settings under the right conditions [1]. The three most important conditions are: providing feedback, repetitive practice and curriculum integration and are discussed in detail later. The remaining conditions that can facilitate learning are listed in Table 3.2.

Of note as a prerequisite for effective learning, but not directly addressed in this chapter, is a 'safe'

Table 3.2 Conditions identified to facilitate learning. A total of 109 papers were reviewed (Issenberg *et al.*, 2005) [1]

Conditions	Percentage of the papers identifying the condition
Providing feedback	47
Repetitive practice	39
Curriculum integration	25
Range of difficulty level	14
Multiple learning strategies	10
Capture clinical variation	10
Controlled environment	9
Individualized learning	9
Defined outcomes	6
Simulator validity	3%

learning environment [6]. Adult learners need to feel safe in their professional image and identity. Creating a safe and engaging learning environment is of utmost importance as learners can feel exposed during simulation-based training. Essential factors for success are the preparation of the learners before the simulation, to identify and describe learning objectives and to design learning situations (scenarios) to address these objectives. It is also important to stimulate reflection on individuals' competencies and link these to the clinical setting [7] (see Chapter 4 and 12).

Feedback

The BEME simulation review identified feedback as the single most important condition to facilitate learning using high fidelity medical simulation [1]. Another BEME review (2006) evaluated the evidence on the impact of assessment and feedback on physicians' clinical performance [8] and found that approximately 75% of the studies indicated a positive effect of feedback. Feedback was more likely to be effective when provided by an authoritative source over an extended period of time. Factors, such as doctors' active involvement in the feedback process, the amount of information given, timing and amount of feedback were also important; however, the importance of each of these factors requires further investigation.

Feedback can be provided by the simulator or by the instructor. Advanced surgical simulators provide feedback using a combination of procedural data obtained during the training. Procedure specific checklists are often developed to cover other elements of the procedure. Feedback can be provided either during or after the training session. Using high-fidelity simulations (scenario-based training) feedback is frequently provided after the simulation-based training in a session of equal or longer length than the simulation session. If the scenario has been recorded, clips illustrating good performance and areas for improvement are used to facilitate reflection and learning. The use of video recordings has the potential of strengthening the learners' ability to reflect on action (Figure 3.1). Significant improvements in non-technical skills (NTS) have been demonstrated after oral feedback or video-assisted oral feedback compared with no improvement in a control group [9]. The feedback provided during skills training and scenario-based simulation training comes from different sources, at different times and of varying length – these differ-

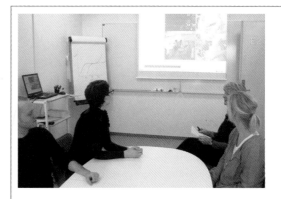

Figure 3.1 Using video recordings during debriefing.

ences may be of importance for the quality of learning and need to be researched.

The session after scenario-based training is often called debriefing (described further in Chapter 12). The term 'feedback' originates from process control and has a connotation that is objective and non-threatening. When a sensor monitoring a process discovers that the output of a process deviates from a target value, a feedback signal is given in order to adjust the system [8]. Providing feedback to a health professional is a much more complex process. In addition to feedback on specific skills, feedback can also be framed to communicate an individuals' performance in relation to a standard of behaviour or professional practice and to guide professional development.

Debriefing is a complex task and a structured approach is therefore recommended. Often a three-phased structure is used consisting of a description, an analysis and an application phase [10]. Here the participants are asked to critically reflect on actions taken in the scenario, explore alternatives and areas for development and discuss the feedback with other team members.

Mezirow [11] describes critical reflection as the process of analysing, questioning and reframing an experience in order to make an assessment of it for the purpose of learning (reflective learning) and/or to improve practice (reflective practice). In contrast to description which may be superficial, deeper reflection includes considerations of how and why

---

Box 3.2   Twelve tips for teaching reflection (Source: Aronson, 2011)

- Define reflection
- Decide on learning goals for the reflective exercise
- Choose an appropriate instructional method for the reflection
- Decide whether you will use a structured approach and create a prompt
- Make a plan for dealing with ethical and emotional concerns
- Create a mechanism to follow up on learner's plan
- Create a conducive learning environment
- Teach learners about reflection before asking them to do it
- Provide feedback and follow up
- Assess the reflection
- Make this exercise plan part of a larger curriculum to encourage reflection
- Reflect on the process of teaching reflection

---

decisions were made [12]. This requires time and willingness to discuss actions and underlying beliefs and values. Although not specifically addressing simulation-based training, the 12 tips for teaching reflection, based on a review of the literature [12], are very useful (Box 3.2).

Adult learners are to some extent capable of evaluating their own skills and analysing performance. A 2008 review of the effectiveness of self-assessment on the identification of learner needs, learner activity and impact on clinical practice indicates that self-assessment can be enhanced with feedback, particularly video and verbal, and by providing explicit assessment criteria [13]. Practical skills seem to be easier to self-assess than knowledge. This is highly relevant for those involved in designing and delivering simulation-based training. Increasing the learner's awareness of the standards to be achieved seems to improve the accuracy of self-assessment, for example adherence to evidence-based guidelines for resuscitation.

In the debriefing session, the facilitator should guide and stimulate the learner's ability to reflect by steering the discussion, conducting the debriefing according to the learner's needs and using a good questioning technique based on gaining insight into the mental model behind the learner's reaction and action [14]. Sometimes this means being able to probe more deeply into a discussion of a specific learning point. The facilitator should, however, be able to shift to the role of instructor if the learner needs guidance, for instance in setting the right diagnosis or initiating the recommended treatment.

Repetitive practice – deliberate practice

In much of medical education, the ultimate goal is expertise or mastery. Acquisition of expertise in medicine as in other areas such as sports and chess is governed by the learner's engagement in deliberate practice of the desired educational outcome [15]. This involves setting clear learning objectives or well-defined tasks, repetitive practice and skills assessment followed by specific feedback from either simulators or instructors in order to improve performance in a controlled setting [16].

Deliberate practice can be difficult in clinical practice due to patient safety issues, a limited number of patients being available when training is needed and production pressure and organisational barriers. Simulation-based training provides an opportunity for learners to train in a safe environment, where errors can be corrected without endangering the patient. Finally, it provides the possibility to individualize training, to train at the time when the competency is required and for as long a time as is needed. This is not always possible in the clinical setting.

Procedural skills

Following the introduction of laparoscopic surgery 30 years ago, reports of an increased incidence of bile duct injury led credentialing societies to develop guidelines for the safe acquisition of laparoscopic skills [17]. The ability of training on a virtual reality simulator to enhance operative skills and reduce technical errors was demonstrated in many publications and summarized in a Cochrane review [18]. Furthermore, repetitive practice has been shown to shorten learning curves for laparoscopic and surgical procedures [19,20] in shorter time periods than exposure to clinical cases.

A review demonstrated that simulation usually leads to improved knowledge and skills [21]. Learners included students and qualified clinicians with training levels ranging ranged from simple procedures to more advanced, such as laparo- and endoscopic procedures. Most of the studies focused on the immediate effect of simulation-based training in the simulated environment. Another 2011 review demonstrated the effectiveness of simulation-based medical education as being superior to traditional clinical education in achieving specific procedural skills [22]. A total of 14 studies were included, representing simple and more advanced procedures. The design of the studies comprised randomized control trials (RCTs), cohort studies, case–control and pre–post baseline studies. Six studies showed improvement in laparoscopic techniques for cholecystectomy, four studies showed improved capability to perform invasive procedures and two studies showed improved performance in cardiac life support [22].

A smaller number of studies have evaluated the transfer of learning to the clinical environment and found a positive effect. Transfer of skills obtained in the simulated environment has been demonstrated from simulator settings to patient care settings. [19,20,23,24]. More studies are needed in order to understand the relationship of timing, duration of training and factors which impact routine and skills decay.

Several variables influencing the impact of simulation-based training have been identified, such as (1) the nature and complexity of the procedural skills, (2) the simulator and the setting, (3) the instructional design and educational theory, (4) context, (5) transferability, (6) accessibility and cost-effectiveness [21]. As with the other reviews mentioned in this chapter, the authors indicated the need for robust research designs to strengthen the evidence. [21].

Although some of the studies mentioned earlier primarily addresses technical procedural skills, some

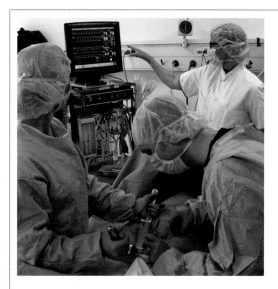

Figure 3.2 Communication between the surgeon and anaesthesiologist.

consider more complex learning, which can be described as the integration of knowledge, skills and attitudes, the coordination of qualitatively different constituent skills and often the transfer of what is learned in training setting to work settings [25]. The question still remains whether simulation-based medical education with deliberate practice can lead to longstanding change and the improvement of professional behaviours and non-technical skills such as decision making, situation awareness, team work, communication and leadership skills (Figure 3.2).

Curriculum integration

In the 2005 BEME review, the integration of simulation-based medical education into the curriculum was seen as vital [1]. It should not be an extraordinary activity, but, to be effective, should be built into the learners' normal training schedule and take place at intervals over time [26].

Many positive examples have been cited about how to implement simulation-based training in both undergraduate and postgraduate education. After 40 years' experience, many educational programmes for nurses in the USA have simulation-based training as an integrated part of the curriculum [27]. A survey conducted by the Association of Medical Colleges in 90 medical schools and 64 hospitals found that >80% of the medical schools have implemented simulation-based training throughout all 4 years, whereas in the teaching hospitals the use of simulation increased from 22% to 69%. More than 85% of the medical schools and teaching hospitals used full-scale manikins and part task trainers. Standardized patients are more frequently used in the university setting than in teaching hospitals [28].

In the Netherlands, the Dutch Society for Simulation in Health Care has provided a platform for sharing experience to facilitate the implementation of proficiency-based training at a national level based on the experience with minimal invasive surgery [29]. One of the important issues is that skills training has to be integrated into the clinical training programme at the right time, and therefore needs to be related to everyday clinical activities. This implies close collaboration between those responsible for the clinical and the simulation programmes. One of the first countries to implement simulation-based training in formal specialist training programmes for anaesthesiologists was Denmark [30]. This example has been taken up by other countries such as the USA, Norway and the Netherlands. Several scientific societies, for example the American Board of Anesthesiologists, have made simulation-based training mandatory in order to achieve certification [31] (Figure 3.3).

Several simulation-based concept courses for different professions have been developed. Some of these are commercially available and represent a standardized educational concept. Multiprofessional obstetric skills programmes have been introduced in hospitals or at regional levels in for example Demark and the United Kingdom [32,33]. They are developed and conducted locally for the real team – the team working together in the clinical setting (Figure 3.4). It should be emphasized that, in general, the real team in their own environment should train together although ensuring some of the team are not called back to clinical work needs to be managed. There are several advantages such as being familiar with the surroundings, and being able to test the organization of roles and tasks.

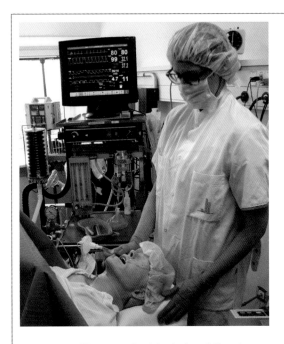

Figure 3.3 The anaesthesiologist in a full-scale simulation.

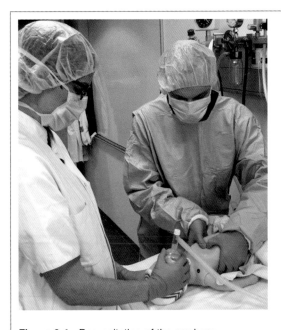

Figure 3.4 Resuscitation of the newborn.

Working with the real team potentially makes transfer from the simulated to the clinical setting easier. Many of these programmes have been developed based on analysis of training needs in areas such as patient safety data or knowledge and skills tests for which the effects of the training can be measured. Institutional commitment and the involvement of leaders is important for sustainability [33]. In order to maximize the benefit of simulation, training needs to be sustained over time.

Internationally, training of established multidisciplinary teams in hospitals is well established, including training for resuscitation, medical emergencies and for trauma teams. At first, training was developed for teams such as emergency or crisis teams, where time is of importance for good patient outcomes. More recently, training of ward teams in identifying the critically ill patient and managing handover has been developed. In general, there is a need for all health professionals to see themselves as part of several teams and simulation can be helpful in providing safe opportunities for different professionals to engage in various teams and their activities (Figure 3.5).

Outcome measurement

In this section, Kirkpatrick's four-level model is used to structure the information [34]. In Kirkpatrick's model:
• Level one, the reaction level, measures the participants' responses to and satisfaction with the inter-vention. Evaluation forms are usually developed to cover this level.
• Level two, the learning level, illustrates the degree of change in the participants' knowledge, skills or attitudes. This is usually measured by formal assessment. Self-assessment has also been used as an indicator of the effectiveness of training, but the reliability of this method has been questioned [13].
• Level three, the behavioural or organizational level, illustrates change of behaviour or impact on operating procedures or both. Work-based assessments can be used as indicators of the effectiveness of transfer to clinical practice and to the organization.
• Level 4, the patient outcome level, describes the benefit for the patients or the consequences of the training programme. A sensitive incident reporting system or patient database may give indications of effect at this level.

Educational activities are typically evaluated by course participants often using written or online forms or audio-response systems. This can be combined with an oral evaluation at the end of a session. The feedback from the instructors is equally important. A detailed evaluation is especially important if new activities are developed for new target groups to find out whether the level of difficulty is right. The evaluation of the effect of simulation-based training can be at the individual or the team level. The studies mentioned later represent different levels of learners, learning objectives (technical, non-technical skills or combinations) and simulators, but lessons learned can be used across institutions and specialties.

Level 1

Overall, there are numerous studies describing the positive effect of simulation-based training at the reaction level independent of the method used (all types of simulation). In undergraduate medical education, simulation has been shown to be a valuable tool with high satisfaction among learners and teachers. The more advanced simulators also make it possible to create relevant training activities for senior staff. Looking at satisfaction with team-training activities, course participants are in general very positive, and simulation-based training seems

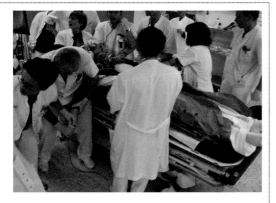

Figure 3.5 Trauma team training.

to change the clinicians' reactions and attitudes in a positive way towards patient safety.

Level 2

At the learning level (level 2), we have to decide which skills are to be measured and how these will be assessed. Validated procedure-specific checklists have been developed to evaluate the effect of skills training programmes. Behavioural marker systems have been developed for anaesthetists and surgeons [35,36] in order to rate an individual or team performance against predetermined skills taxonomy or framework. Systems, such as the Observational Teamwork Assessment for Surgery (OTAS) have been designed for evaluation of team performance in the operating theatre [37] (Figure 3.6). One of the challenges described is how to evaluate the effect of training, and if the team performance varies during the scenario. To ensure reliability, training for evaluators is necessary.

A recent systematic review and meta-analysis concluded that simulation-based training compared with no intervention in health professions' education produced positive effects on knowledge, skills and behaviours [38]. In a 2009 Cochrane review, virtual reality training was shown to supplement or replace clinical laparoscopic surgical training. The review includes 23 trials. Four trials compared virtual reality, video trainer training and no train-

ing, or standard laparoscopic training. Three studies compared different methods of virtual reality training. In trainees without prior surgical experience, virtual reality training decreased the time taken to complete a task, increased accuracy and decreased errors compared with no training; the virtual reality group was more accurate than the video trainer training group. Virtual reality training of participants with limited experience was found to reduce operating time and errors better than standard training. Most of the trials, however, were with a high-risk of bias [18]. The conclusion of the review was that virtual reality training can supplement standard apprenticeship-based laparoscopic surgical training and is at least as effective as video trainer training in supplementing standard laparoscopic training. The review addressed the need for further research of better methodological quality and more patient relevant outcome [18]. Several other reviews support these findings and found clinical improvement following training on laparoscopic simulators, for example residents trained in laparoscopy performed better in the clinical setting than residents trained without exposure to simulation [20].

Although the use of this technology is increasing, only a limited number of high-quality studies demonstrate the positive effect of team training on learning. A positive effect of obstetric team training on knowledge has been demonstrated in two studies [39,40], whereas Robertson *et al.* were unable to demonstrate an effect [41]. Three different teaching methods were used in the study by Birch *et al.* [40], which found that a combination of lectures and simulation seemed to be superior to using either lectures or simulation. Several studies have shown an effect on skills [41,42,43] following obstetric team training. Completion of tasks were done faster [41,43] and fewer mistakes were seen 6 months later in the simulated scenarios [42]. Simulation-based training has also been shown to have an impact on communication skills, for example Siassakos *et al.* [44] found communication to be more directed and tasks more likely to be acknowledged and performed after obstetric team training. Using the administration of an essential drug as a surrogate for team efficiency, efficient teams are more likely to exhibit team behaviours related to better handover and task allocation [45].

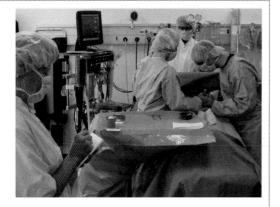

Figure 3.6 Training of the operating theatre team with the instructor in the room.

Levels 3 and 4

In a review looking at the evidence for the utility of simulation in medical education, only a few studies show direct improvement in clinical outcome from the use of simulation-based training [3]. Examples of improved patient care practices linked directly to simulation-based training include studies of better management of obstetric deliveries, endoscopic surgery and bronchoscopy. Several studies using historical control groups have shown that simulation-based training can reduce catheter-related blood infections [46]. A study of residents' clinical skills in the insertion of a central venous catheter found improvement of junior residents' baseline scores in the simulation setting over a 3-year period. The authors speculated whether this was due to junior residents observing insertion of a central venous catheter in the clinical setting by more senior residents who have completed simulation-based training in that procedure and hence are better role models than before. This indicates that simulation-based training of residents may have an effect on others' clinical skills [47].

In a randomized controlled study, Wayne *et al.* [48] showed improved quality of care provided by residents during actual cardiac arrests. The simulator-trained residents showed significantly higher adherence to standards than traditionally trained residents. In a large study including almost 20 000 neonates, an improvement in perinatal outcome was shown after simulation-based team training [49]. The number of children with signs of distress after birth (Apgar scores 6 or lower) decreased significantly after the intervention. A recent systematic review on the effectiveness of multidisciplinary obstetric team training found this type of education to be potentially effective, but recommended new studies on its effectiveness and cost-effectiveness before wider implementation [50].

As described earlier, training with the 'real team' is considered to be important. Some writers have described a positive effect on outcome with this type of training [48,51], whereas others have failed to show an effect on outcome [52,53]. In the latter study, ward staff (doctors, nurses and nurse assistants) were trained in identifying the critically ill patient. An incidence of one out of five patients at risk was observed in both the pre- and post-intervention periods. No difference in staff awareness of patients at risk, 30-day mortality or 180-day mortality was found [53]. Approximately 70% of the staff members were trained. The authors speculate whether this might be one of the reasons for not finding an effect on mortality. It is clear that whole-team training in an entire organization can improve patient safety and health outcomes. For example, the association between implementation of a team training programme for doctors and surgical mortality has been demonstrated in a study involving 180 000 patients [54]. The training programme required briefings and debriefings in the operating theatre and introduced checklists as a part of the process. An 18% reduction in mortality was seen after the training programme compared with a 7% decrease in the facilities that had not undergone training. Studies of this type are necessary if an effect of simulation-based team training on patient safety is to be demonstrated.

Simulation used for high-stakes assessment

The simulated environment provides an opportunity to establish a standardized set up, in which all learners are exposed to the same scenario addressing the learning objectives in the curriculum. The challenge is to develop valid tools for the assessment and to train the raters in using these tools with an acceptable inter-rater agreement. Although it seems easy to establish a standard, it might be difficult for those playing the role of a team member to act exactly the same in all scenarios. When assessment takes place in the simulation environment, not only validity and reliability but also acceptability and cost are important. The importance of these factors varies depending on the situation. If used for high-stakes examination, it is important to have optimal validity and reliability and trained evaluators.

Following the Ottawa 2010 meeting, a consensus statement and recommendation regarding technology-enabled assessment of health professions' education was published [55]. The paper describes the role of technology in assessment, highlights challenges in using technology in assessment with a specific consideration of threats to the valid interpretation of assessment scores and associated outcomes, and points out further issues for research.

At present, simulation is incorporated in some of the Objective Structured Clinical Examinations (OSCEs) used in undergraduate education of nurses, medical students (USA, UK) and in specialist training programmes for anaesthesiologists (Royal College, UK). In Israel, the Board of Anaesthesiology Examination Committee has implemented simulation for high-stakes examination, and note positive experiences [56]. The American Board of Surgery requires completion of a fundamental laparoscopic surgery course for initial certification of residents [57]. Furthermore the Food and Drug administration (FDA) requires physicians to complete task training before they can use a stent in patients.

Moving forward – challenges and perspectives

Integration of simulation-based activities based on best practice

Simulation-based training enables health professionals to practice in a safe environment and to develop medical expertise and interprofessional skills making teamwork more efficient. Evidence is growing that this type of training facilitates and supplements clinical training. Patient safety data indicate a need for a change and several bodies have recommended the use of simulation-based training, first the Institute of Medicine [58] and later other bodies such as the National Institute of Health. European and American guidelines for resuscitation therefore recommend that team training and non-technical skills are included in the training programme [59]. The essential question is: *why aren't we there yet*? [60].

The sceptic will point out that the evidence is not good enough and that this training is too costly. This is a relevant criticism and simulation enthusiasts must carry out more robust studies to provide clearer evidence for the effective use of simulation-based training and how to use it most efficiently.

We may underestimate the need for training in using the evidence about medical education and simulation-based training and the necessity of supporting the implementation of simulation-based training, just as we do with new knowledge and with evidence-based medicine in general. Availability of a novel intervention does not necessarily ensure its implementation and effective use [61]. Studies looking at implementation in general have demonstrated a need for research on how to build up competence and facilitate implementation in order to see changes in practice.

We have to understand the barriers for using and implementing simulation-based training:
• Learners and faculty already using simulation-based training are enthusiastic about using this method, which might blind them to the difficulties in getting others familiar with the tool.
• Some staff members might not have been either a simulation learner or a facilitator or could have had a negative experience. They may be unfamiliar with the terminology, such as non-technical skills, with the simulated environment and the function of a facilitator.
• Some highly expert practitioners and academics might not accept and understand that they cannot just go and use simulation as a learning tool or simulators themselves without training and experience. Times are changing and we are now starting to gather more robust evidence about what makes simulation effective and when it is in appropriate to use it.

In the early days of medical simulation, enthusiasts explored the use of different simulation modalities, in different target groups and for a variety of topics. Simulation was used to train more or less everything in the curriculum, often without proper preparation and follow up. Overall, learners and facilitators were overwhelmed by the possibility of using an interactive learning method and, as no gold standard for how to do it was available, it ended up being a trial and error process. Based on building up these necessary and valuable 'hands on experiences' and becoming more aware of the available literature about simulation, education and psychology, we are now at a different stage. We know that we have to establish a multiprofessional team of educationalists, psychologists and clinicians to be able to use simulation-based training most cost efficiently. We are aware of the need to base activities on a conceptual framework and to existing knowledge of instructional design. Therefore, users of simulation are more familiar with the steps in developing an educational intervention which should be based on a proper needs analysis, selection of the right tool/method and taking context and evaluation into consideration.

The timing is right for integrating simulation-based training in clinical curricula. In order to do this, collaborative efforts are required from academics, clinicians, managers and policymakers alike. Although it can be a challenge to bring all these groups together, the process is necessary in order to obtain high level outputs in medical care, which will benefit all [60]. Establishment of national or regional workgroups that include all stakeholders is a way forward.

Research in simulation-based training

Simulation-based research is a new field, and studies that help us to better understand what works and why are needed to advance the field of simulation for the benefit of patients, health professionals and educators. The outcome of the Utstein-style meeting was a research agenda with research questions grouped within three main themes: instructional design, outcome measurements and translational research [4] (Table 3.2). The themes related to

translational research included how the principles of learning derived from simulation-based learning in standardized research projects translate into learning in other simulation centres or local training practices [4].

The ideas from the Utstein Style Meeting were brought forward to the 2011 Research Summit Meeting in relation to the International Meeting for Simulation in Health Care in New Orleans 2012. The publications from that meeting have provided further guidance to the simulation community [5]. Activities where people meet across disciplines such as these workshops and summits are necessary to advance research and hence the quality of training using simulation.

As mentioned previously, we have to improve research in simulation by linking theoretical frameworks, in both the preparation phase and in analysis of data, to a much greater extent than seen in already published papers. Some studies in this area should be based on a variety of research methods and could best be conducted by a multiprofessional team of experts. Ideas on how to conduct research in medical education can be found in a paper by Ringsted *et al.* [62]. Changes are not only necessary in the simulation community, but also in the medical education community. We need to move away from research that is intended to prove the effectiveness of our educational endeavours and towards research that aims to understand the complexity inherent in these activities [63].

SUMMARY

Owing to changes in the organization of health care, patient safety issues and challenges with clinical training, the necessity for simulation-based training in medical education of procedural and non technical skills can no longer be questioned.

Based on contemporary learning theories (including those of adult learning), simulation appears to be a very appropriate learning technique as it can be conducted in a safe learning environment and provides the opportunity for learners to receive feedback.

Complexity can be controlled and learners at different levels of education can train in relevant situations or cases. Furthermore, roles other than that of the medical expert can be emphasized using simulation and participants can work both as individuals and in teams of health professions. The activity can be planned according to the needs of the learner, prior to clinical encounters with a given type of patient or task. Important features for learning are feedback, repetitive and deliberate practice and curriculum integration.

Much literature about the effectiveness of simulation focuses on learners' satisfaction at the reaction level. There is overwhelming evidence that participants and facilitators value simulation based clinical education compared with traditional activities. Several reviews have shown simulation to be educationally effective and to complement clinical training [18,38]. Skills learned in the simulated environment have been shown to be transferable to the real clinical environment. Although the use of simulation technology is increasing, only a limited number of high-quality studies demonstrate positive effects on patient outcomes and safety. Many of the studies included in reviews, however, suffer from poor design. Robust studies of high-quality, based on a conceptual framework, including guidance on what to include in future studies are needed.

Faculty members familiar with the use of simulation-based medical education are more comfortable and confident in using the tools and the topics addressed here, and can work successfully in the simulated environment. This implies that professional development of clinical teachers and faculty members in university settings as well as in clinical contexts is paramount. The integration of simulation-based training into health professions' curricula during their specialist training and in training programmes for hospital-based teams is still a challenge. However, successful implementation can take place if all stakeholders are interested in change and collaboration between clinical staff, pedagogical experts and simulation interest groups is initiated.

✓ Key points

- Simulation-based training is needed due to changes in health-care organizations, patient safety issues and challenges with clinical training.
- Simulation-based training appears to be an appropriate learning technique for the training of clinical skills and non-technical skills.
- It enables deliberate and repetitive practice and encourages structured feedback.
- Simulation-based training is educationally effective and can complement clinical training, but needs to be embedded and integrated into curricula, not a bolt-on.
- Skills learned in the simulated environment are transferable to the real clinical environment.

REFERENCES

1. Issenberg SB, McGaghie WC, Petrusa ER *et al.* (2005) Features and uses of high-fidelity medical simulations that lead to effective learning: a BEME systematic review. *Medical Teacher* **27**: 10–28.

2. McGaghie WC, Issenberg SB, Petrusa ER, *et al.* (2010) A Critical review of simulation-based medical education research: 2003–2009. *Medical Education* **44**: 50–63.

3. Okuda Y, Bryson EO, DeMaria S, *et al.* (2009) The utility of simulation in medical education: What is the evidence? *Mount Sinai Journal of Medicine* **76**: 330–343.

4. Issenberg B, Ringsted C, Østergaard D, *et al.* (2011) Setting a research agenda for

simulation-based healthcare education. A synthesis of the outcome from an Utstein style meeting. *Simulation in Healthcare* **6:** 155–167.

5. Dieckmann P, Phero JC, Issenberg SB, *et al.* (2011) The first research consensus summit of the society for simulation in healthcare. Conduction and synthesis of the results. *Simulation in Healthcare* **6:** S1–S9.

6. Knowles M (1990) *The Adult Learner: A Neglected Species*, 4th edn. Houston: Gulf Publishing Company.

7. Østergaard D, Dieckmann P (In press) Simulation based medical education. In *A Practical Guide for Medical Teachers* (J Dent and RM Harden eds), 4th edn. Elsevier

8. Veloski J, Boex JR, Grasberger MJ, *et al.* (2006) Systematic review of the literature on assessment, feedback and physicians' clinical performance: BEME guide no.7. *Medical Teacher* **28:** 117–128.

9. Salvoldelli GL, Nail VN, Park J, *et al.* (2006). Value of debriefing during simulated crisis management. Oral versus video-assisted oral feedback. *Anesthesiology* **105:** 279–285.

10. Steinwachs B (1992) How to facilitate a debriefing. *Simulation and Gaming* **23:** 186–195.

11. Mezirow J (1990) *Fostering Critical Reflection in Adulthood*. San Francisco: Jossey-Bass.

12. Aronson L (2011) Twelve tips for teaching reflection at all levels of medical education. *Medical Teacher* **33:** 200–205.

13. Colthart I, Bagnall G, Evans A, *et al.* (2008) The effectiveness of self-assessment on the identification of learner needs, learner activity, and impact on clinical practice: BEME Guide no. 10. *Medical Teacher* **30:** 124–145.

14. Rudolph JW, Simon R, Raemer DB, *et al.* (2008) Debriefing as formative assessment: Closing the performance gaps in medical education. *Academic Emergency Medicine* **15:** 1–7.

15. Ericsson KA (2004) Deliberate practice and the acquisition and maintenance of expert performance in medicine and related domains. *Academic Medicine* **79** (Suppl)**:** S70–S81.

16. McGaghie WC, Siddall VJ, Mazmanian PE, *et al.* (2009) Lessons for continuing medical education from simulation research in undergraduate and graduate medical education: effectiveness of continuing medical education: American College of Chest physicians evidence-based educational guidelines. *Chest* **135** (Suppl)**:** 62S–68S.

17. Aggarwal R, Grantcharov TP, Eriksen JR, *et al.* (2006) An evidence-based virtual reality training program for novice laparoscopic surgeons. *Annals of Surgery* **244:** 310–314

18. Gurusamy KS, Aggarwal R, Palanivelu L, *et al.* (2009) Virtual reality training for surgical trainees in laparoscopic surgery. *Cochrane Database of Systematic Reviews* **21** (1)**:** CD006575.

19. Ahlberg G, Enochsson L, Gallagher AG, *et al.* (2007) Proficiency-based virtual reality training significantly reduces the error rate for residents during their first 10 laparoscopic cholecystectomies. *American Journal of Surgery* **193:** 797–804.

20. Larsen CR, Sørensen JL, Grantcharov T, *et al.* (2009) Impact of virtual reality training in laparoscopic surgery. A randomised controlled trial. *British Medical Journal* **338:** b1802. Erratum in *British Medical Journal* 2009; 338.

21. Nestel D, Groom J, Eikeland-Husebø S, *et al.* (2011) Simulation for learning and teaching procedural skills. *Simulation in Healthcare* **6:** S10–S13.

22. McGaghie WC, Issenberg SB, Cohen ER, *et al.* (2011) Does simulation-based medical education with deliberate practice yield better results than traditional clinical

education? A meta-analytic comparative review of the evidence. *Academic Medicine* **86:** 706–711.

23. Grantcharov TP, Kristiansen VB, Bendix J, Bardram L, Rosenberg J, Funch-Jensen P (2004) Randomized clinical trial of virtual reality simulation for laparoscopic skills training. *British Journal of Surgery* **91:** 146–150.

24. Sturm LP, Windsor JA, Cosman PH, *et al.* (2008) A systematic review of skills transfer after surgical simulation training. *Annals of Surgery* **248:** 166–179.

25. van Merrienboer J, Kirschner P (2007) *Ten Steps to Complex Learning: A Systematic Approach to Four Component Instructional Design.* Mahwah NJ: Lawrence Erlbaum Associates.

26. Gallagher AG, Ritter EM, Champion H, *et al.* (2005) Virtual reality simulation for the operating room. Proficiency-based training as a paradigm shift in surgical skills training. *Annals of Surgery* **241:** 364–372.

27. Nehring WM, Lashley FR (2009) Nursing simulation: A review of the past 40 years. *Simulation & Gaming* **40:** 528–552.

28. Passiment M, Sacks H, Huang G (2011) *Medical Simulation in Medical Education. Results of an Association of American Medical Colleges (AAMC) Survey.* Washington, DC: AAMC.

29. Schreuder HWR, Oei G, Maas M, *et al.* (2011) Implementation of simulation in surgical practice: Minimal invasive surgery has taken the lead: The Dutch experience. *Medical Teacher* **33:** 105–115.

30. Østergaard D (2004). The national medical simulation training program in Denmark. *Critical Care Medicine* **32** (Suppl): 58–60.

31. American Board of Anesthesiology. Maintenance of certification in anaesthesiology. Available from http// www.theaba.org/anaesthesiology_ maintenance (accessed 6 March 2013).

32. Sørensen JL, Løkkegaard E, Johansen M, *et al.* (2009) The implementation and evaluation of a mandatory multi-disciplinary obstetric skills training programme. *Acta Obstetricia et Gynecologia* **88:** 1107–1117.

33. Ayres-de-Campos D, Deering S, Siassakos D (2011) Sustaining simulation training programmes – experience from maternity care. *British Journal of Obstetrics and Gynaecology* **118** (Suppl 3)**:** 22–26.

34. Kirkpatrick DL (1998) *Evaluating Training Programs.* San Francisco: Berrett-Koehler Publishers, Inc.

35. Fletcher G, Flin R, McGeorge P, *et al.* (2003). Anaesthetists' Non Technical Skills (ANTS): evaluation of a behavioural marker system. *British Journal of Anaesthesia* **90:** 580–588.

36. Yule S, Flin R, Paterson-Browne S, *et al.* (2006) Development of a rating system for surgeon's non-technical skills for surgeons. *Medical Education* **40:** 1098–1104.

37. Undre S, Sevdalis N, Healey AN, *et al.* (2007) Observational teamwork assessment for surgery (OTAS): Refinement and application in urological surgery. *World Journal of Surgery* **31:** 1373–1381.

38. Cook DA, Hatala R, Brydges R, *et al.* (2011) Technology-enhanced simulation for health professions education. *Journal of the American Medical Association* **306:** 978–988.

39. Crofts JF, Ellis D, Draycott TJ, *et al.* (2007) Change in knowledge of midwives and obstetric emergency training: a randomized controlled trial of local hospital simulation centre and teamwork training. *British Journal of Obstetrics and Gynaecology* **114:** 1534–1541.

40. Birch L, Jones N, Doyle PM, *et al.* (2007) Obstetric skills drills: evaluation of teaching methods. *Nurse Education Today* **27:** 915–922.

41. Robertson B, Schumacher L, Gosman G, *et al.* (2009) Simulation-based crisis team training for multi-disciplinary obstetric providers. *Simulation in Healthcare* **4:** 77–83.

42. Mazlovitz S, Barkai G, Lessing JB, *et al.* (2007) Recurrent obstetric management mistakes identified by simulation. *Obstetrics and Gynecology* **109:** 1295–1300.

43. Ellis D, Crofts JF, Hunt LP, *et al.* (2008) Hospital, simulation center, and teamwork training for eclampsia management: a randomized controlled trial. *Obstetrics and Gynecology* **111:** 723–731.

44. Siassakos D, Draycott TJ, Montague I, *et al.* (2009). Content analysis of team communication in an obstetric emergency scenario. *Journal of Obstetrics and Gynaecology.* **29:** 499–503.

45. Siassakos D, Bristowe K, Draycott TJ, *et al.* (2011). Clinical efficiency in a simulated emergency and relationship to team behaviours: a multisite cross-sectional study. *British Journal of Obstetrics and Gynaecology* **118:** 596–607.

46. Barsuk JH, Cohen ER, Feinglass J, *et al.* (2009) Use of simulation-based education to reduce catheter related bloodstream infections. *Archives of Internal Medicine* **169:** 1420–1423.

47. Barsuk JH, Cohen ER, Feinglass J, *et al.* (2011) Unexpected collateral effects of simulation-based medical education. *Academic Medicine* **86:** 1513–1517.

48. Wayne D, Didwania A, Feinglass J, *et al.* (2008) Simulation-based education improves quality of care during cardiac arrest team responses at an academic teaching hospital. A case-control study. *Chest* **133:** 56–61.

49. Draycott T, Sibanda T, Owen L, *et al.* (2006) Does training in obstetric emergencies improve neonatal outcome? *British Journal of Obstetrics and Gynecology* **113:** 177–182.

50. Merién AER, Van de Ven J, Mol BW, *et al.* (2010) Multi-disciplinary team training in a simulation setting for acute obstetric emergencies. *Obstetrics and Gynecology* **115:** 1021–1027.

51. Morey JC, Simon R, Jay GD, *et al.* (2002). Error reduction and performance improvement in the emergency department through formal teamwork training: Evaluation results of the MedTeams Project. *Health Services Research* **37:** 1553–1581.

52. Nielsen PE, Goldman MB, Mann S, *et al.* (2007). Effects of teamwork training on adverse outcomes and process of care in labour and delivery: a randomized controlled trial. *Obstetrics and Gynecology* **109:** 48–55.

53. Fuhrmann L, Perner A, Clausen T, *et al.* (2009) The effect of multi-professional education on the recognition of patients at risk on general wards. *Resuscitation* **80:** 1357–1360.

54. Neily J, Mills PD, Young-Xu Y, *et al.* (2010) Association between implementation of a medical team training program and surgical mortality. *Journal of the American Medical Association* **304:** 1693–1700.

55. Amin Z, Boulet JR, Cook DA, *et al.* (2011) Technology-enabled assessment of health professions education: Consensus statement and recommendations from the Ottawa 2010 conference. *Medical Teacher* **33:** 364–369.

56. Ziv A, Rubin O, Sidi A, *et al.* (2007) Credentialing and certifying with simulation. *Anesthesiology Clinics* **25:** 261–269.

57. Holmboe E, Rizzolo MA, Rosenberg M, *et al.* (2011) Simulation-based assessment and the regulation of health care professionals. *Simulation in Healthcare* **6:** S58–S62.

58. Kohn LT, Corrigan JM, Donandson MS (1999) *To Error in Human – Building a*

Safer Health System. National Academy Press: Washington, DC.

59. Edwards S, Siassakos D (2012) Training teams and leaders to reduce resuscitation errors and improve patient outcome. *Resuscitation* **83:** 13–15.

60. Aggarwal R, Darzi A (2011) Simulation to enhance patient safety Why aren't we there yet. *Chest* **140:** 854–858.

61. McGaghie WC (2011) Implementation science: addressing complexity in medical education. *Medical Teacher* **33:** 97–98.

62. Ringsted C, Hodges B, Scherpbier A (2011) 'The research compass': An introduction to research in medical education: AMEE Guide no. 56. *Medical Teacher* **33:** 695–709.

63. Eva KW (2010) The value of paradoxical tensions in medical education research. *Medical Education* **44:** 3–4.

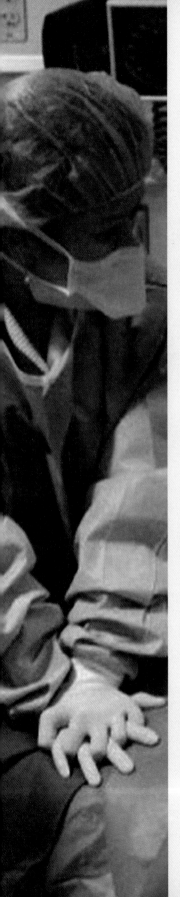

CHAPTER 4

Pedagogy in simulation-based training in healthcare

Peter Dieckmann[1] and Charlotte Ringsted[2]   [1]Herlev Hospital, Herlev, Denmark; [2]University of Copenhagen and Capital Region, Copenhagen, Denmark

Overview

The word 'pedagogy' originates from the Greek words 'paidos' (child) and 'agogus' (leader of) and initially referred to the art and science of educating children [1] but now refers to the art and science of teaching and education in general. There has been much debate about whether there is a need for a separate and parallel term, andragogy, referring to the art and science of helping adults to learn [2]. Some key differences highlighted between the way adults learn include self-directed learning and problem- or task-centred orientation rather than teacher-directed and subject-centred orientation. Although much simulation-based training refers to the application of adult learning theories, the issue of pedagogy versus andragogy is currently considered to be a matter of instructional principles tailored to levels and characteristics of learners and the task at hand, rather than the age of the learner. Hence, the term pedagogy is used in this chapter to discuss how different theories and concepts of learning and teaching relate to simulation-based training.

Simulation-based training is offered to a wide range of learners – from novices to experts,

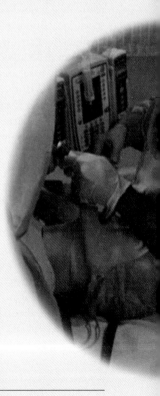

Essential Simulation in Clinical Education, First Edition. Edited by Kirsty Forrest, Judy McKimm, and Simon Edgar.

Overview (ctd)

representing a variety of health professions, targeting numerous sorts of skills and offering a diversity of contexts, i.e. simulation settings, technology and learning aids. The first section of this chapter presents an overview model of learning related to three interacting dimensions: the person, the task and the context.

The next four sections explore pedagogical theories and concepts grouped into four broad perspectives: behaviourism, cognitive psychological, humanistic and social learning. The key concepts of each perspective are described and related to a variety of principles and examples applied in simulation-based training. As the literature on theories on learning and teaching is so voluminous, only key principles and concepts will be reviewed.

The final section returns to the 'person–task–context' model and discusses how instructional strategies affect learning in the three dimensions.

Three related dimensions in skills learning

In simulation-based training the focus is primarily on skills learning which in the healthcare education context refers to performing a variety of tasks, i.e. cognitive, perceptual, procedural, technical, motor, reasoning, problem-solving, decision-making and social interaction in a team. Clinical skills learned in simulation settings often involve a composite of several of these aspects in addition to a biomedical knowledge base and some coordinated physical, cognitive and/or social activities.

Dreyfus and Dreyfus [3] suggest that as learners move from novice to expert, task performance develops from stepwise and rule-based actions to intuitive and situationally fluent actions. Lessons from motor skills learning indicate that strategies which novice learners apply to the learning of simple tasks are different from those applied to more complex tasks and used by more advanced learners [4]. Task performance is also dependent on contextual factors in which the task is performed, for example, the setting, the available support, and the complexity, stability or uncertainty of the environment. Figure 4.1 shows the interrelatedness of the person, the task and the context which facilitators need to take into account. Alongside this they need to analyse learning needs, translating them into aims and objectives of the session or course, and select appropriate content and methods of delivery. Also, adaptations during a simulation

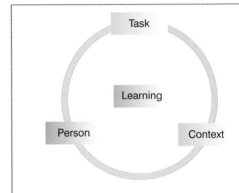

Figure 4.1 A person–task–context model of learning.

session depend on the interplay between those three factors and the interplay serves as the basis to define assessment criteria and select measurement methods.

The 'person' dimension relates to the learners' states and traits, e.g. prior knowledge, skills, attitudes and experience as well as the current state of motivation, alertness and involvement. The interplay between the different dimensions is seen from an individual learner's perspective. However, in many simulation sessions more than one learner is present at a time – either as a group of similar learners or as a mixed group of health professionals learning to work as a team on a common task (Figure 4.2). In this model, learner groups are seen as part of the 'context' dimension.

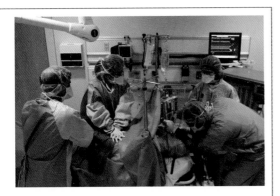

Figure 4.2 A mixed group of health professionals learning to work as a team on a common task. Photo by Laura Seul, copyright Northwestern Simulation.

The 'task' dimension relates to characteristics of the skill to be learned, whether simple, complicated or complex and relates to the context in which the skill has to be performed, e.g. available support, time and other resources. The task has also a personal perspective in that team members may have different roles and responsibilities to perform subtasks in the main task, for example during cardiopulmonary resuscitation.

The 'context' dimension relates to the physical, psychological and social dimensions of the simulation setting, i.e. the room layout, the technology and its authenticity, the aid and support given, concurrent feedback, encouragement or instruction, and the people acting and/or interacting. All this adds to the complexity, stability or uncertainty of the environment.

'Learning' (in the centre of the figure) indicates that learning is done by the participants themselves, but the simulation instructor(s) is responsible for creating the opportunities to learn and to make it easy for the participants to make use of them. In simulation-based training both task and context complexity can be manipulated, varied and graded to suit the level of learner and maximize learning.

Pedagogy and learning theory

Pedagogy is concerned with the planning, implementation and adaptation of the interplay between the task, person and context with the aim to create, recognize and use learning opportunities for the learners and focuses on the end point of learning and the processes to achieve it. Table 4.1 relates different educational theories to current practice and the future development of simulation-based training. These theories can be broadly categorized as behaviourism, cognitivist learning theories, the humanistic perspective, and social learning theories.

Behaviourism focuses on observable behaviours and how to influence them. Cognitivist theories are interested in the mental processes involved in learning. The humanistic perspective emphasizes learning as grounded in the potential for human growth, recognizing humans' responsibility and wish for self-realization and autonomy. Social learning theories emphasize that learning occurs in the interaction with other people and the environment. Social learning theories incorporate aspects of behaviourism, cognitivism and humanism, emphasizing issues of motivation, discussion and observational learning.

The core principles described are more clear-cut than current educational practice, where different types and approaches are mixed and boundaries blurred.

Instructional strategies

The different theoretical frameworks described earlier each imply that certain techniques and behaviours are most effective to aid learning. The key issue, in our view, is to see all that is happening in a simulation session as an educational intervention and to use those interventions to enable participants to maximize their learning. Theoretical frameworks help to explain why different interventions might work and help instructors select the right intervention to achieve certain learning outcomes. The next section presents a pragmatic selection of strategies that appear beneficial based on the literature and practical experience.

We distinguish between creating, recognizing and using learning opportunities. For all three aspects, pedagogical theories and concepts can and should guide the practical work.

Table 4.1 Overview of different learning theories

Theory	Core principles	Relation to current simulation practice
Behaviourism	Focus is on objective, observable behaviours. Internal processes in the mind such as knowing, thinking, and feeling are neglected. Learning is conceptualized as changes in the connections between stimuli and responses [5,6] based on rewards and punishment. Response is equated with feedback, learning occurs as a result of good feedback. Good instructional situations provide stimuli that are as close to the stimuli in the application situation as possible.	Clearly defined, competence based learning goals are of high priority. Highly standardized training-programmes. Assessment schemes that avoid any ambiguity about right or wrong. Reinforcement and 'punishment' of actions by the facilitators and other learners. Feedback can be given by teachers, actors/patients or through technology, e.g. haptic feedback. Standardized instruction formats, i.e. manuals and instructor training. Strive for high physical realism. [7]
Cognitive Learning Theory	The focus is on explaining how new knowledge or skills are perceived, encoded into the memory, stored, and retrieved. [8] Learning is seen as: the ability to improve short term memory by chunking meaningful pieces of information into larger units [9,10] and improving long-term memory by integrating new with prior information and optimizing the storing and retrieval of information. Deep, transferable learning is defined as a relatively permanent change in the capability to perform a task [11]. Measurement of learning requires a break or a change of context between training and measurement otherwise the results might reflect short-term memory effects and superficial learning [12,13].	Facilitation of the activation of prior knowledge in elaborations, discussions, comparisons, or seeking the boundaries of applicability of new information (e.g. during debriefing or workshops). The context in which the information is used is varied systematically, e.g. by discussing principles of good communication, then applying them in a scenario, then exploring them in a video example and finally discussing their scope of applicability.
Cognitive Load Theory	Focus on learning complex skills, by adjusting the complexity and 'cognitive load' to the level of the learner. The concept of 'Zone of Proximal Development' [14], described by Vygotsky, suggests that learning takes place when individuals are pushed out of their comfort zone and offered appropriate challenges.	Breaking tasks into smaller parts and using step-by-step instructional strategies. Providing structures (scaffolding) for the new information that facilitates processing. Instruction is based on examples and advanced organizers (i.e. an overview of the learning material in the beginning) [15,16].

Table 4.1 *(Continued)*

Theory	Core principles	Relation to current simulation practice
Motor skills learning	Focuses on the building and refinement of motor skills. Fitts and Posner [17], describe three stages of learning: In the initial (cognitive) stage the novice concentrates on understanding the task. Performance of the novice is typically characterized by substantial errors and large variation in quality of task performance. In the second (associative) stage the learner makes progress by the ability to associate knowledge of results and environmental cues with performance. There are fewer and less gross errors in the task performance. In the final (autonomous) stage, the performance becomes smoother and almost autonomous or habitual without conscious thinking about the movements. At this stage learners are capable of error detection and appropriate correction of performance.	Direction, guidance and frequent and immediate feedback for novice learners, e.g. to replicate a movement pattern. Chunking by breaking the movement into sub parts or by simplifying the movements. Development via reduction of help (e.g. instruction, feedback and scaffolding) and increasing the complexity of the task or environment. Use of different forms of feedback relevant to the skills being acquired.
Constructivist theories	Focus on the active nature of perception and learning and the 'reconstruction' of knowledge in each case it is applied. According to Jean Piaget (1896–1980) learners assimilate new information and accommodate it with existing knowledge through interpretation and the forming of individual and personal constructs. This helps to explain why every learner is different and learns differently even though the same information might be being conveyed. The instructor's role is to assist in this construction. [18].	Preparation needs to acknowledge that learners may have different perceptions and understandings of what might seem simple tasks or concepts. Discussion of the different meanings of complex constructs (e.g. leadership) and how they are seen by the individuals in the different contexts. Debriefs and deconstruction of events can help learners see why they performed or thought differently from others.
Experiential learning	Focuses on describing and using the active nature of learning by coordinating experiences with reflections. Learning is seen as better, more sustainable, deeper and more applicable, if more senses (e.g. haptics and vision) are involved in the learning situation and if knowledge, practise and reflection are meaningfully connected.	Tailoring the experience during scenarios and facilitate abstraction and generalization from the examples during debriefings [19]. Sharing observations, introducing, implying, deducing and explaining concepts.

(Continued)

Table 4.1 *(Continued)*

Theory	Core principles	Relation to current simulation practice
	Kolb's learning cycle relates the concrete experience, reflective observations of oneself and other learners, abstract conceptualizations, and active experimentation [13].	Generating insights and changes that go beyond the concrete scenario and have relevance for the actual work situation.
Observational learning	Bandura's social learning theory emphasized the function and value of role models and learning from observing others to fit into social groupings. Values, norms and believes are internalized.	The instructor (team) 'teaches' and demonstrate by the planned actions but also the (unplanned) way they interact. Role models may be inconsistent with their verbal messages, for example when a team teaching 'teamwork' does not work well together as a team. In the motor skills' domain, observational learning is emphasized as an important factor contributing to learning [11,20]. Observing a model which demonstrates erroneous performance and coping with the problems is more powerful than observing a faultless model [21].
Collaborative learning	Focuses on the possible learning relevant synergy effects of learning situations with more than one person. Learning with others includes an advantage of united memory and collaborative information processing and in particular when learning complex tasks this leads to reduction of cognitive load for the individual learner [22,23]. However, efforts required for collaboration with other learners may in turn increase the cognitive load [24]. The balance depends on the complexity of the task and becomes inadvertently negative when the task is simple [22] or the collaboration is malfunctioning [25].	During collaboration, individuals process information about the effectiveness of the partner's movement patterns and strategies applied. This additional information processing is often not possible during concomitant practice and hence having a group of learners taking turns in practicing while the others observe can be very powerful when training in complex tasks [12] Collaborative learning may help motivation due to competition or social enjoyment [11].

Creating learning opportunities

The *creation* of learning opportunities happens during the design and development of curricula, courses and scenarios. On the basis of analysing learning needs and defining learning outcomes, instructors select the content that best matches the needs and required outcomes. Then they pick methods which will best help participants to use the learning opportunities. The design might involve:
• surprises (e.g. to point to the impact of perception on errors)

• sequencing of events (e.g. theoretically explaining an issue and then providing time to practice it versus having people try the issue first and using theoretical explanations afterwards to help them fill the gaps of ability they have discovered)
• planned reduction of complexity (e.g. practising pieces of a whole task one by one and putting them together later versus practising all pieces at once in a simplified fashion).

Recognizing learning opportunities

Recognizing learning opportunities is related to being open to the processes in the 'here and now' of a training situation. Participants may follow the scenario as planned encountering the learning opportunities that the simulation team has laid out for them but they may also act unexpectedly reacting to the scenario in a way that was not foreseen by the simulation team or themselves. As the scenario plays out, 'scenario life savers' might be needed, to bring the scenario back on track, adjust it to the unexpected or stopping and restarting it [26]. If the scenario is too difficult, participants might require more time or a clearer presentation of the scenario to be able to solve it alone. If the scenario is too simple, participants might need to encounter additional challenges (to extend the zone of proximal development) [14]. The simulation team should be able to recognize the learning opportunities that evolve from such unexpected events. The goal is to find the right level of optimal difficulty for the learner, not necessarily to increase the difficulty of the scenario to the point where participants cannot cope any more.

During debriefings participants might say something that signals to the facilitator that they have a mental model of the situation that may be problematic for safety and quality of care. For example, if the team leader talks about their perception of needing to do all tasks alone in order to prove they are a good leader and if the team members support this by putting all responsibility onto the leader, the facilitator might recognize this dynamic as a learning opportunity, challenging some of the underlying assumptions and discussing the distribution of the workload.

Using a learning opportunity

Using a learning opportunity goes one step further than creating and recognizing it. In the example mentioned earlier, the facilitator might choose to describe her perception of the situation. The team would thus get an outside view on their functioning, a disturbing element, questioning their way of working and providing an 'imbalance' in their perceptions, thoughts and actions, unfreezing them. In the right context, this imbalance matches what the team can handle and if the team is willing to reflect and able to respond to this it can be a powerful trigger for change. If the imbalance does not match their perception of the situation, the team might not work with the facilitator in a constructive way and may instead try to defend their actions and possibly deny the value of simulation. For example, debriefing or using learning opportunities during scenarios depends on a sharp observation of what is happening in the 'here and now'. Facilitators need relevant content and educational and methodological abilities to see problems that participants are encountering and identify the reason for the problem (e.g. knowledge gap, stress-impaired perception, falling into old habits). They then can adjust the scenario in a way that helps participants get the best learning opportunity (e.g. providing the missing knowledge by a helping role player, reducing the complexity and thus stress in the scenario, reminding participants about the new approach that should be trained).

The design, recognition and use of learning opportunities can all be improved if facilitators draw on available theories and concepts. In the next section, we link some of the theoretical aspects to the person, task and context to the practice of simulation-based education.

Issues related to learners

Learning opportunities are experienced differently by different learners. Some of the dimensions along which learners differ are known and described: level of expertise in the task, learning style, perception preferences [27,28], current state, previous knowledge in terms of content of the course and previous experience of simulation.

For simulation-based education the implication of this is that we need to analyse a given group of learners or even individual learners in more detail. What is their starting point and in what way do they want to learn? This could be done through pre-course questionnaires or interviews, conversations at the beginning of a course or diagnostic test scenarios and debriefings. Based on the answers or performance of participants in the beginning of the course, the remaining and unfolding course would then, within the framework of the overall aims and objectives, be adjusted to learners [29].

For more advanced learners, the key issue is to diagnose their current state of ability and to negotiate with them what the next steps of their development should be. Using the zone of proximal development [14], facilitators should provide learning situations that are just out of the comfort zone of the participants, without stretching them too far. Here, a limited number of scenarios could be devised to allow the simulation team to form a frame of reference of performance. Once the team has observed a certain number of participants working through the scenario, they have a better foundation to assess a single team or person in a formative sense and to better anticipate the likely next steps. The debriefing is important here – especially the ending stages, when participants reflect on the next learning steps [30]. By listening closely to participants' views and feelings, facilitators get good information relating to the zone of proximal development and can then adjust subsequent scenarios.

Experts face different challenges. Expert perception and recognition patterns are qualitatively different from those of novices and intermediates. Their perception is more holistic and at times much more intuitive and less able to be articulated or observed, using rapid cognition and automated rules of thumb to analyse a situation and select the optimal course of action [31]. Much of their good performance stems from perceiving only those aspects of a situation relevant for its understanding and filtering out those they don't need. Simulation offers experts a safe environment to reassess their frames of reference and routines, benefiting from a coaching-oriented approach. For example an experienced physician might reconsider her way of leading a team, based on the feedback from and discussions with equally experienced other course participants and the instructor during a debriefing. They may not have received meaningful, structured feedback about their performance and actions for many years and a key challenge for some expert learners is to actively unlearn old habits. In order to do so, experts need a stimulus to 'unfreeze' [32] – seeing the need to change thoughts and actions that may have been unsuitable for a long time. New evidence needs to be convincing and presented in a way that allows adaptation. Simulation and video recordings, meaningful learning conversations during debriefings, or exchanges with other experts can achieve such an unfreezing. With guidance from the simulation team, taking the role of a sparring partner, experts can then develop their own motivation for change. The simulation team's task is to help develop realistic intentions and to provide learning opportunities that allow the testing of alternatives. Changing ingrained habits might be a challenge that cannot be managed in a single training event and the expert may need more time, support and maturation.

Issues related to task

The task that needs to be learned influences how the simulation is set up. One way of adjusting scenarios is to manipulate the complexity of the learning situation, taking into account that learners can only cognitively manipulate limited amounts of complexity [15]. As mentioned previously, the complexity can be reduced by breaking the task into sub-tasks that are practised independently or the task steps can be preserved in the whole task but the bar for doing the task is lowered. While the first approach seems intriguing, it has disadvantages, one of which is that key elements might be lost by breaking the task into the sub-tasks, because their relevance for the whole is underestimated. The context under which a person would actually perform a task should be carefully analysed and built into the scenario where needed. Is the equipment typically available in the clinical setting in the same way as in the simulation setting, or would it need to be found, prepared or used under difficult conditions? Can the learners in the clinical setting concentrate on the task only or do they also need to manage the interaction with team members, the patient or relatives?

Specific versus general tasks

Some tasks are specific, for example, diagnosing and managing a difficult airway; others are general (such as patient management or communication) to help participants learn on a more principle-oriented basis. For specific tasks, learning opportunities are established around (fine)tuning the perception and interpretation of symptoms and knowledge about treatment options for difficult airway management. For general tasks, the focus might be around principles of a complete investigation of a patient, using cognitive processes to establish a set of differential diagnoses and around implementing treatment with limited resources.

The advantage of the first approach is the specificity of the possible learning and the optimization of a concrete treatment situation, especially when taking real treatment context into account (e.g. with *in situ* training). The disadvantage is the potentially large numbers of situations that need to be trained. The advantage of the second approach is to potentially help participants develop more generic capabilities which can be used across a range of situations. The disadvantage is that each ability needs to be (re) translated into specific treatment options or clinical contexts and this transfer can be difficult. Combining approaches, where a variety of challenges that would be typical for a discipline are practiced, helps learners to make connections to underlying principles wherever possible [33].

In summary, one might ask whether learning about a specific situation should be the focus, or should learning be about learning and preparation for future learning? Ideally, simulation-based learning focuses on cognition *and* meta-cognition, for example know the signs relevant for recognizing the difficult airway but also know how you can best activate and use that knowledge in other future challenging situations.

Issues related to context

The experiential learning framework has its roots in the theory and thinking of Kurt Lewin [34] and writers such as Kolb [13] and Schön [19]. Human action unfolds in the interplay between the person and the environment. In Lewin's model, this interplay is conceptualized as a force field that contains physical, psychological and social forces. Actions are adapted to the present forces in a specific situation. One might assume that humans move in force fields according to the strongest positive force currently acting upon them. Lewin called the interplay between the force fields outside and inside the person 'life space'. Similar concepts are 'frames' and 'mental models'. This life space changes with learning, either by being more differentiated or reshaped. Humans use the life space to anticipate the future and guide their actions. The actual development of the state of the world will then provide feedback about the usefulness of the life space. Simulation can still aid learning, despite the fact that many (physical, semantic and phenomenal – see later on) elements of the simulation situation are different from the actual work situation. However, similar force patterns may actually underlie both situations. What looks different from the outside, might 'feel' similar from the inside. The appearance (phenotype) of a situation may be different, while the underlying structure (genotype) of the situation is similar or even identical (think of the falling apple and the moon circling the earth – both are moved by the same force: gravity). The key element of relevant learning is, however, to create situations that have impact on the life space during actual working situations – not only during the learning situation. People do not learn for simulation but for real work, which concerns the difference between 'shows how' and 'does' in Miller's pyramid [35].

When analysing learning in simulation, the life space or context is highly important. Context provides meaning to the interactions between people and between the people and the environment. As we work through the framework from the view of the learner, the facilitator and the other group members become part of the context. There are many different layers of context and many ways to address it. Starting from the larger to the smaller views upon context, one might distinguish:

• the basic traits of a society and its ideas about health care learning influence expectations for teacher and learner roles

• professional fields and specialities develop their own norms, values and beliefs around the way to do business as well as teaching and learning

• organizations commissioning or providing education provide (limited) resources to the educational event and require a certain return of investment

• a specific simulation training team has certain expertise and preferences for goals, contents and methods

• a specific group of learners develops patterns of interactions, taboo topics, and a certain depth of discussion.

In terms of learning objectives, simulation teams often need to find a balance between the different stakeholders involved: individual learning needs and wishes of a person, the prescription by curricula and personal preferences.

For example, a chief of a department may hire a simulation team to do *in situ* trainings in his/her hospital. Imagine that the chief of the department asked the simulation team to focus on 'unproductive communication patterns' in his/her teams. During the course, however, it may become clear that the 'real problem' is not communication, but long shifts and fatigue. It may happen that the commissioner of the learning event misjudges the actual goals and needs. Simulation teams then have the challenge to balance the different needs and wishes, which may impact the educational interactions.

Looking at a specific simulation course, the different phases within provide the context for its single elements [36]. For example, does the scenario depend on a good simulator briefing, where the learners get familiar with using the simulator as a technical tool? Scenarios provide the input for debriefings. If the scenario is not 'run' well by the simulation team (e.g. giving inconsistent vital signs), the debriefing will suffer.

Simulation fidelity

Simulation fidelity, the 'similarity' between the simulation and the simulated system has been a prime argument for simulation for a long time; however, the value of simulation fidelity has been challenged [37] and it should be a means to optimize learning opportunities not a goal in itself

[38,39,40]. Fidelity is conceptualized as having several sub-dimensions. One conceptualization addresses three modes of thinking about fidelity [40,41]:

1. Physical – all aspects and only those that can be measured in centimetres, grams or seconds (e.g. the weight of a manikin in pounds, the lengths of the screen diagonal of a screen-based simulator).

2. Semantic – all aspects and only those that can be expressed as concepts and their relation (e.g. the representation of the electrocardiogram trace by the computer on a monitor, the verbal announcement of the patient developing a rash on the thorax).

3. Phenomenal – all aspects and only those that can be expressed as direct experience of being in the world (e.g. the tension felt by the participants, when they hear the changing tone of the pulse oxymeter or the joy of getting relevant feedback).

Simulators are often highly unrealistic in physical terms but allow users to construct consistent meanings of the situation and experience it as relevant (Figure 4.3).

Consider, for example, an infusion arm on which participants learn to place an intravenous line. The physical properties are unrealistic in terms of the material used (plastic instead of flesh) but realistic in the resistance force properties against needle penetration. The colour and material differences within the arm allow participants to interpret

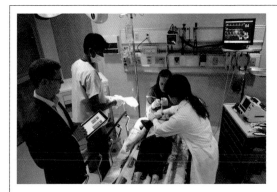

Figure 4.3 Simulated patients allow users to construct a meaning of the situation and experience it as relevant. Photo by Laura Seul, copyright Northwestern Simulation.

those differences as vessels in the arm – the arm is semantically realistic. Users will try to insert the needle in the vessels that are visible and palpable, not in other parts of the arm. Users will also experience the simulation situation in a certain way. The participants might feel a mix of joy to practice and a fear to get the manoeuvre wrong and be nervous because the instructor and their fellow learners are observing them. The situation is partly phenomenally realistic, as some elements of the experience correspond to what would be expected in a clinical setting, working with a real patient arm. Some other elements, however, would not be expected in the typical healthcare setting (e.g. the direct observation and feedback). Any simulation thus combines aspects of different levels of fidelity. The different elements within a simulation scenario may well have different degrees of fidelity along all three modes [42,43].

Optimizing simulation fidelity relates to the educational value of simulation and explicitly does not mean maximizing. In many circumstances, departing from realism might provide the most effective training [37]. For example, it might be good to slow down the physiological deterioration of the patient to give a learner more time to react. The key is to understand the salient characteristics of the task and how much realism of what type is needed to create the learning opportunities for participants [37,40,44]. In general, more physical realism is needed for simulators aiming at developing or testing psychomotor abilities, more semantic realism for scenarios that help people to optimize their diagnostic skills and more phenomenal realism where teamwork is the focus. However, all forms are needed to a certain extent for all scenarios. How much realism of what type will become clearer over time as we learn from research on the different combinations of forms of realism and achievement of learning goals. Reducing the realism might enable the learner to act in the scenario, because she or he might be overwhelmed by too much realism. Purposefully changing aspects of the realistic scenario to unrealistic ones on the other hand might be a trigger for reflections and also to better understand the impact of certain elements of a situation. For example, learners might benefit from systematically changing their leadership style (acting in an unreal-

istic way) to experience the consequences within one or across several scenarios. Likewise, it might be interesting to reflect about the boundaries of communication strategies, when they are – unrealistically – taken to the extreme, for example by closing *every* communication loop during a scenario or discussing *each* decision. These aspects are discussed in more depth in Chapter 11 in the section on simulation fidelity and selective abstraction.

The as-if as a learning tool

The purpose of the educational use of simulation is to provide learning opportunities for the participants. The 'as-if' during simulation is a (cognitive) tool for learning, not the goal. Hans Vaihinger's philosophy on as-if processes is applicable to simulation [36,45]. According to this line of thinking, some as-if processes help people to learn, orient oneself in the world and construct meaning – Vaihinger calls these 'fictions'. The question as to whether they are 'true' or 'false' does not matter as their relevance is to provide orientation in the world. Similarly, simulation scenarios need to be relevant for the aims and objectives of the session and not necessarily realistic. One extreme example of this might be in the large-scale simulation of major crises such as a nuclear incident where people are expected to suspend disbelief for the purposes of the simulation.

Relevance for the learning opportunities needs to be negotiated between the different stakeholders involved and is only influenced in parts by the realism of the simulator and simulation. If both parties agree, then they can use relevant learning opportunities by simulating with a few pieces of wood, on paper or even in the mind. In this perspective the actual scenario and its form is not the key issue. Missing pieces, alienated elements, overemphasized aspects, etc., can open the eyes and minds for relevant learning in the real world – they are unrealistic but help learning. Comparing what we take for granted with different ways of perceiving and interpreting facilitates the assessment of knowledge and actions. In this sense, deliberately changing the simulation in certain aspects can be the learning-relevant 'unfreezing' that users need to progress. Clear and augmented feedback during and after simulation is what helps participants to learn. Consider the example of simulating in roles that participants usually do not have: the consultant plays a medical student, the nurse plays the physician, etc. Both could argue about the low realism of this set up and negate any relevance for running the scenario in this way, as it will not happen in real life. They can, however, also agree to engage into such an experiment and accept its results as relevant for their learning and work. By radically changing the tasks and responsibilities one has and by looking at routines from such different angles, frames and assumptions might become obvious that would have otherwise remained unexplored. The consultant can learn about what a student might require to feel secure in a learning situation whereas the nurse might appreciate the pressure of the physician's responsibilities. Another example could be to agree to find the boundaries of the application scope of techniques and actions. What would happen if a leader never discusses a decision – or always does? What would be the effects on the leader, the team or the patient? It can be relevant to explore these unrealistic extreme actions, but the relevance needs to be explained and participants need to agree otherwise they might simply disengage or be resistant.

One of the inherent dangers (or fears) of unrealistic, or potentially alienating scenarios and using low fidelity is that of negative learning. Consideration of realism and the awareness that unrealistic elements may strongly influence learning help to detect potential areas of negative learning. This is why careful observation of the processes during scenarios is important as well as the reflection during debriefing. No matter how different the as-if during simulation was, compared with the so of actual work – during debriefing what participants can learn from the as-if in simulation for their actual work can be explored.

Facilitators, learners and their interaction

The different phases of the simulation setting imply different roles for the facilitators. During the intro- duction to the simulation, facilitators might instruct, during the debriefing, they might facilitate (Figure 4.3). During scenarios it might be necessary for the instructor to leave the educational role and become a 'protector' if participants engage in dangerous activities (e.g. unsafe handling of the defibrillator). During a debriefing, a facilitator might oscillate between different roles like 'facilitator', 'coach', 'devil's advocate', etc., and the most effective facilitators need to have the skills to move seamlessly into different, appropriate roles and to develop meaningful learning relationships with learners. However, some facilitators do not always act according to the ideals they formulate for their role [46].

The social nature of learning implies that the interaction between those involved impacts on learning and learners need to feel motivated, engaged in the fiction contract and open to learning [36], feeling being tricked and exposed during simulation inhibits learners' engagement [43]. For experienced participants in particular, whose role is to observe and give feedback to others rather than receive feedback on their practice there can be much at stake and simulation events can feel like a big step out of their comfort zone.

Feedback

One of the advantages of simulation settings is that they offer possibilities for augmented feedback. During scenarios, some simulators or the instructors may offer data about the performance in real time, such as measurement values (e.g. movements in laparoscopic simulators) and verbal feedback. Feedback can be an in-built part of the simulation (e.g. vital signs that change, providing feedback about treatment options) or via comments from role players. It can also specifically be part of an augmentation of simulation, where special monitors or displays provide the additional information, or where role players are introduced in their 'augmented role' (e.g. 'the role-played nurse will help you in treating this patient'). Strategies to stop and restart the scenario or leave the framework of the simulation completely (having time out) can help participants develop specific abilities.

During debriefing, the video recording and log files of the simulator can be analysed and used as a data source that would not be available in other settings. There is little empirical evidence about the advantages and disadvantages of, for example, video use in debriefing [47,48], yet the face validity is high.

Defining what is emphasized as the major advantage of simulation is very difficult [49,50]. As humans we have great protective strategies for assuring that we do not need to change – as change can be unpleasant, fear-inducing and challenging. From a conceptual basis, it is necessary to refine simulation-based learning and the way that facilitators help learners to learn from errors, such as:
• Acknowledge that change can be challenging. Questions can be: what exactly can you apply to your day-to-day practice? What would be the next step for you to avoid a similar error? How can you reduce the chance for systematic recurrence?
• Establish an error-friendly atmosphere [51]. Error friendliness means to address errors as errors, avoid euphemisms, do not treat them as a taboo topic and as a concept that cannot be named. The facilitator must find the right tone and mindset to lead the discussion on errors. Learners' errors should not be seen as a personal victory in scenario design and implementation and participants should not be used to boost facilitators' egos.
• Provide time and opportunity to change. Although insight might be the first step to change, implementing change may comprise many steps. Helping participants to acknowledge this, taking the necessary time to change and not giving up in the face of challenges seems to be an important element of supporting people to learn from errors.

SUMMARY

For those developing future simulation pedagogy, the implication of understanding learning theories is that a much more rigorous analysis of situations that form the basis for simulation scenarios should be undertaken. Often the starting point for scenario design is the phenotypical description of a clinical situation or challenge, such as simulating a myocardial infarction or the placing of an intravenous line. However, cases that look very different on the surface might actually have many structural elements in common – and vice versa. As we have seen, the starting point of scenario design is around defining the learning goals and objectives, to understand the structural characteristics of the task and define which context elements will create the best learning opportunities around those elements. The perspective of 'What is important to learn when you deal with a myocardial infarction?' could be supplemented with: 'What are the underlying challenges, when you treat myocardial infarction and which situations allow best to create learning opportunities for around those challenges?'

Once the learning goals are defined and the necessary content is selected, all the theories and strategies in the literature and this chapter can help facilitators to select the most relevant methods that create learning opportunities for the participants and to help them make use of them. Further research is needed to identify which theoretical and practical ingredients would best be combined to help learners make the most of simulation-based training. The important thing about the theories from our perspective is to use them to understand why – or why not – certain methods and approaches work. Evaluation of the effectiveness of certain methods has not provided clear evidence but learning theories help our understanding under which conditions and with whom, specific effects and learning can be expected. In this light, as Kurt Lewin reminds us: 'Nothing is so practical as a good theory' [34, p. 169, 52]

✓ Key points

- Understanding learning theories helps instructors design run and evaluate effective simulation-based training.
- The context of simulation-based learning contributes significantly to create, recognize and use learning opportunities.
- Different theoretical aspects apply to different practical teaching and learning strategies.
- The starting point is always to define the required learning outcomes and learners' needs, then design the simulation session to include activities to help learners achieve the outcomes.
- Building in time for ongoing feedback and debriefing is essential to optimize learning.
- High fidelity is not necessarily vital as long as participants are willing to suspend their disbelief.

REFERENCES

1. Holmes G, Abington-Cooper M (2000) Pedagogy vs. andragogy: a false dichotomy? *Journal of Technology Studies* **26:** 50–55.

2. Knowles MS (1990) *The Adult Learner: A Neglected Species*. Houston: Gulf Publishing Company.

3. Dreyfus H, Dreyfus S (1986) *Mind Over Machine: The Power of Human Intuition and Expertise in the Era of the Computer*. Oxford: Basil Blackwell.

4. Wulf G, Shea CH (2002) Principles derived from the study of simple skills do not generalize to complex skill learning. *Psychonomic Bulletin & Review* **9:** 185–211.

5. Watson JB (1913) Psychology as the behaviorist views it. *Psychological Review* **20:** 158–177.

6. Skinner BF (1974) *About Behaviorism*, 1st edn. New York: Knopf.

7. Caro PW (1988) Flight training and simulation. In: *Human Factors in Aviation* (EL Wiener and DC Nagel, eds). San Diego: Academic Press: 229–261.

8. Miller GA (1956) The magical number seven, plus or minus two: Some limits in our capacity for processing information. *Psychological Review* **64:** 81–87.

9. Chase WG, Simon HA (1973) Perception in chess. *Cognitive Psychology* **4:** 55–81.

10. Ericsson KA, Kintsch W (1995) Long-term working memory. *Cognitive Psychology* **102:** 211–245.

11. Wulf G, Shea CH, Lewthwaite R (2010) Motor skill learning and performance: a review of influential factors. *Medical Education* **44:** 75–84.

12. Magill RA (2007) *Learning and Control: Concepts and Applications*. New York: McGraw-Hill.

13. Moulton AC, Dubrowski A, MacRae H, *et al.* (2006) Teaching surgical skills: what kind of practice makes perfect? A randomized, controlled trial. *Annals of Surgery* **244:** 66–75.

14. Vygotsky LS (1978) *Mind in Society*. Cambridge, MA: Harvard University Press.

15. Van Merriënboer JJG, Sweller J (2005) Cognitive load theory and complex learning: recent developments and future directions. *Educational Psychology Review* **17:** 147–177.

16. Van Merriënboer JJG, Sweller J (2010) Cognitive load theory in health professional education: design principles and strategies. *Medical Education* **44:** 85–93.

17. Fitts PM, Posner MI (1967) *Human Performance*. Belmont: Brooks Cole.

18. Brydges R, Carnahan H, Rose D, Dubrowski A (2001) Comparing self-guided learning and educator-guided learning formats for simulation-based training. *Journal of Advanced Nursing* **66:** 1832–1844.

19. Schön D (1987) *Educating the Reflective Practitioner.* San Francisco: Jossey-Bass.

20. Mattar AAG, Gribble PL (2005) Motor learning by observing. *Neuron* **46:** 153–180.

21. van Gog T, Rummel N (2010) Example-based learning: integrating cognitive and social-cognitive research perspectives. *Educational Psychology Review* **22:** 155–174.

22. Kirschner F, Paas F, Kirschner PA (2009) A cognitive load approach to collaborative learning: united brains for complex tasks. *Educational Psychology Review* **21:** 31–42.

23. Kirschner F, Paas F, Kirschner PA (2011)Task complexity as a driver for collaborative learning efficiency: the collective working-memory effect. *Applied Cognitive Psychology* **25:** 615–624.

24. Crook AE, Bier ME (2010) When training with a partner is inferior to training alone: The importance of dyad type and interaction quality. *Journal of Experimental Psychology. Applied* **16:** 335–348.

25. Pass F, Tuovinen JE, van Merriënboer JJG, Darabi AA (2005) A motivational perspective on the relation between mental effort and performance: optimizing learner involvement in instruction. *Educational Technology Research and Development* **53:** 25–34.

26. Dieckmann P, Lippert A, Rall M, Glavin R (2010) When things do not go as expected: Scenario Life Savers. *Simulation in Health Care* **5:** 219–225.

27. Hukki K, Norros L (1993) Diagnostic orientation in control of disturbance situations. *Ergonomics* **36:** 1317–1327.

28. Hukki K, Norros L (1998) Subject-centred and systematic conceptualisation as a tool of simulator training. *Le Travail Humain* **61:** 313–31.

29. Mehl K (2009) Simulation as a tool for training and analysis. In: U*sing Simulations for Education, Training and Research* (P Dieckmann, ed.). Lengerich: Pabst: 157–179.

30. Steinwachs B (1992) How to facilitate a debriefing. *Simulation & Gaming* **23:** 186–192.

31. Gigerenzer G, Todd PM, ABC Research Group (1999) *Simple Heuristics that Make Us Smart.* New York: Oxford University Press.

32. Lewin K (1947) Frontiers in group dynamics. *Human Relations* **1:** 5–41.

33. Gaba DM, Fish KJ, Howard SK (1994) *Crisis Management in Anesthesiology.* Philadelphia: Churchill Livingstone.

34. Lewin K (1951) Field theory and learning. In: *Field Theory in Social Science* (Cartwright D, ed.). New York: Harper & Brothers: 60–86.

35. Miller G (1990) The assessment of clinical skills/competence/performance. *Academic Medicine* **65**(Suppl)**:** S63–67.

36. Dieckmann P (2009) Simulation settings for learning in acute medical care. In: *Using Simulations for Education, Training and Research* (Dieckmann P, ed.). Lengerich: Pabst: 40–138.

37. Hays RT, Singer MJ (1989) *Simulation Fidelity in Training System Design: Bridging the Gap Between Reality and Training.* New York: Springer.

38. Curran I (2008) Creating effective learning environments – key educational concepts applied to simulation training. In: *Clinical Simulation: Operations, Engineering, and Management* (Kyle R, Murray BW, eds). Burlington: Academic Press: 153–161.

39. Kneebone R, Arora S, King D, *et al.* (2010) Distributed simulation – accessible

immersive training. *Medical Teacher* **32:** 65–70.

40. Dieckmann P, Gaba D, Rall M (2007) Deepening the theoretical foundations of patient simulation as social practice. *Simulation in Health Care* **2:** 183–193.

41. Laucken U (2003) *Theoretische Psychologie* [Theoretical Psychology]. Oldenburg: Bibliotheks- und Informationssystem der Universität Oldenburg.

42. Rettedal A (2000) When reality is difficult to simulate. *European Journal of Anaesthesiology* **8:** 518.

43. Dieckmann P, Manser T, Wehner T, Rall M (2007) Reality and fiction cues in medical patient simulation. an interview study with anesthesiologists. *Journal of Cognitive Engineering and Decision Making* **1:** 148–68.

44. Scerbo M, Dawson S (2007) High fidelity, high performance? *Simulation in Healthcare* **2:** 224–230.

45. Vaihinger H. *The Philosophy of As If.* [Translated reprint of the original book 'Die Phiolosophie des Als-Ob' from 1927.] Abingdon: Routledge, 2000.

46. Dieckmann P, Molin Friis S, Lippert A, Ostergaard D (2009) The art and science of debriefing in simulation: Ideal and practice. *Medical Teacher* **31:** e287–294.

47. Raemer D, Anderson M, Cheng A, *et al.* (2011) Research regarding debriefing as part of the learning process. *Simulation in Health Care* **6**(Suppl)**:** 553–557.

48. Salvodelli G, Naik VN, Park J, *et al.* (2006) Value of debriefing during simulated crisis management: oral versus video-assisted oral feedack. *Anesthesiology* **105:** 279–295.

49. Edmondson AC (2011) Strategies of learning from failure. *Harvard Business Review* **89:** 48–55, 137.

50. Wehner T, Stadler M (1994) The Cognitive organisation of humans errors: a gestalt theory perspective. *Applied Psychology: An International Review* **43:** 565–584.

51. von Weizsäcker C, von Weizsäcker U. Fehlerfreundlichkeit [Error friendliness]. In: *Offenheit – Zeitlichkeit – Komplexität: Zur Theorie der offenen Systeme* [Openness – Timeliness – Complexity: On the Theory of Open Systems] (K. Kornwachs, ed.). Frankfurt: Campus; 1984, 167–201.

52. Lewin, K (1951) *Field Theory in Social Science: Selected Theoretical Papers.* (Cartwright, D, ed.). New York: Harper & Row.

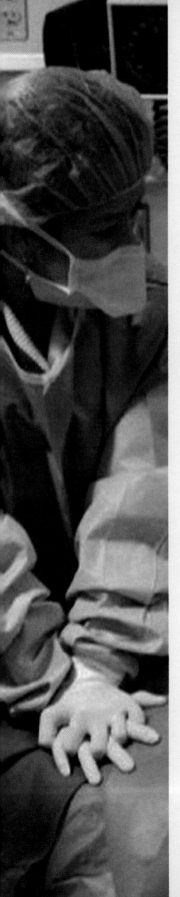

CHAPTER 5
Assessment

Thomas Gale and Martin Roberts   Peninsula Schools of Medicine and Dentistry, Plymouth, UK

Overview

Simulation provides a vast array of opportunities to carry out assessment of participants. A recent critical review of simulation-based literature has outlined the importance of good quality assessment when using simulation as a training modality [1]. McGaghie *et al*.'s comprehensive critical review of simulation-based research (from 2003 to 2009) identified '12 features and best practices, which every simulation based medical education teacher should know in order to use medical simulation to maximum educational benefit' [1, p. 50]. The review highlighted that assessment (in the broadest sense) is integral to at least seven of the elements of best practice:

- ensure opportunities for *feedback* (both formative and summative) are utilized appropriately
- provide facilities for *deliberate practice* involving focused repetitive practice and evaluation
- ensure *curriculum integration* so that simulation is incorporated into the wider curriculum to complement clinical education
- define *outcome measurements* from educational interventions to establish reliability and validity of those interventions
- provide opportunities/programmes for *mastery learning* (deliberate practice with clearly defined learning objectives with set minimal standards required before progression to further stages)
- establish use for *high-stakes testing* procedures including undergraduate/postgraduate examinations, and licensing of professionals
- ensure simulation training is used in the correct *educational and professional context*.

Simulation-based educational programmes can require relatively heavy resources in terms of faculty/

Essential Simulation in Clinical Education, First Edition. Edited by Kirsty Forrest, Judy McKimm, and Simon Edgar.

Overview (ctd)

participant ratio and capital costs to set up. However, simulation provides excellent opportunities to create authentic scenarios and observe skills which may be difficult to assess using other assessment tools [2].

Simulation can be used for both the assessment of procedural/examination skills and the assessment of behaviours or non-cognitive skills within immersive team-based scenarios. The potential advantages of simulation include the highly reproducible nature of scenarios and activities plus the ability to observe how individuals actually perform. In this way simulation can demonstrate competence of a doctor who 'shows how' rather than just 'knows how' in Miller's hierarchy of clinical assessment [3]. In addition, in response to recent attempts to define what professionalism is and how to measure it, behaviours and attitudes can be assessed which can elicit aspects of professionalism in participants [4]. Figure 5.1 shows where assessment fits into levels of competence in Miller's pyramid. Simulation, including the use of clinical skills assessments, simulated patients, objective structured clinical examinations (OSCE) and immersive simulation can be used alongside workplace-based assessment (WPBA) methods to assess a trainee's ability at the performance levels of 'shows how' and 'does'.

Simulation may also have an increasing part to play in performance-based assessment to complement WPBA methods which are utilized to measure clinical skills and behaviour [5]. WPBA instruments which measure observed behaviour and competence of trainees performing procedural skills and clinical exercises have shown low inter-rater reliability (i.e. between assessors) despite rigorous efforts to train observers and the use of a nationally administered electronic rating mechanism for input of assessments. A national study evaluating performance of anaesthesia trainees using the Mini-Clinical Evaluation Exercise (Mini-CEX) found more variation in scores due to raters and case specificity rather than between trainees [6]. Using simulations to measure performance and competence of trainees may help standardization of assessments with key index cases and the ability to use the same observers for particular cases. The potential to use simulation for standardizing the assessment of procedural skills has been highlighted in the medical education literature in parallel with the need for development of appropriate metrics with adequate reliability and validity [1].

This chapter outlines the fundamental principles of educational assessment in general and then covers the aspects involved in establishing a quality assessment programme using simulation. Case examples have been chosen to share best practice and future areas for development and research are identified along with particular challenges.

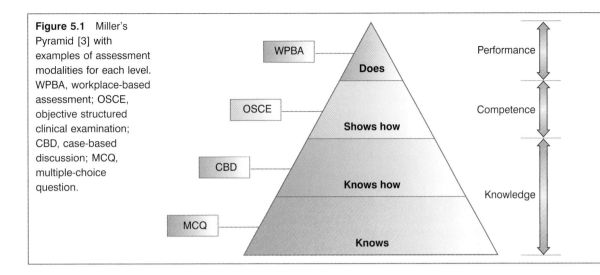

Figure 5.1 Miller's Pyramid [3] with examples of assessment modalities for each level. WPBA, workplace-based assessment; OSCE, objective structured clinical examination; CBD, case-based discussion; MCQ, multiple-choice question.

Purposes of assessment in education

Epstein [7] suggests that the three main goals of assessment in medical education are to:

1. identify learning needs including knowledge, skills and professionalism in order to drive future learning
2. set professional standards of competence and performance to safeguard the public
3. rank applicants for recruitment to postgraduate training posts.

The first of these goals encapsulates the formative purpose of assessment, sometimes referred to as *assessment for learning*, while the last two describe the summative purpose of assessment, or *assessment of learning*, in making judgements about the standards that learners have achieved. In high-fidelity simulation, formative assessment commonly takes the form of the post-scenario debrief and covers both technical and non-technical aspects of performance. The importance of the debrief has been widely highlighted by educationalists as a powerful tool where reflective practice can increase the value of the educational experience (see also Chapters 4 and 12).

Tools have been developed for structuring feedback and providing a framework for the assessment of non-technical skills in various healthcare groups [8,9,10]. Most commonly, these assessments are undertaken with the intention to provide constructive feedback to the participants rather than make a pass/fail judgement as a part of a summative assessment. Educators who are involved in assessment should be clear in the differentiation of formative assessment (which is used to help drive learning and provide feedback on performance against learning goals) and summative assessment (which uses assessment tools with appropriate reliability/validity to pass, fail or rank participants in high-stakes assessments) [11] (Table 5.1).

Principles of assessment

The Consensus Statement from the 2010 Ottawa (Assessment in Medicine) Conference published criteria for good assessment in 2011 [12]. The report highlights the wide range of assessment tools which have been developed for the assessment of competency in medicine, and the breadth of teaching and learning strategies employed. The Statement acknowledges the increasing use of advanced psychometrics to test reliability and validity of assessments, together with the need to take into account other factors which determine the utility of an assessment.

Cees van der Vleuten [13] describes a utility index to consider with any assessment tool. The index variables include educational impact, cost-efficiency and acceptability along with reliability

Table 5.1 Characteristics of formative and summative assessment

Formative assessment	Designed to help direct future learning and professional development Provides opportunities for individual feedback Uses multiple forms to elicit patterns of performance/behaviour Validity of assessment is more important than reliability Engagement of learners is paramount in order for them to understand their strengths and weaknesses
Summative assessment	Timed to relate to achievement of standards at particular stages of course/career Prerequisite for progression to further stages Requires high reliability for high-stakes assessments Robust quality assurance required Should collate all sources of data/evidence relevant to performance criteria

and validity. Recently, feasibility and catalytic effect (whether the assessment drives future learning forward) have been added to this index by national and international policy makers on assessment in medical education [5,12,14] The ideal assessment methods would score highly in all elements of the utility index but efforts to increase reliability and validity of certain assessment methods may do so at the expense of others, e.g. cost-efficiency and feasibility of large-scale national processes.

Principles which have been highlighted as important in the process of assessment in education include [7]:

• Use multiple methods and a variety of contexts to assess different aspects of performance.
• Align assessments to learning outcomes within defined curricula.

• Organize repeated and ongoing assessments which are set at the appropriate level for each stage of the curriculum.
• Use a developmental programme which builds on competences and learning outcomes that have already been assessed (e.g. as part of a spiral curriculum).
• Combine focused assessments in controlled environments with more complex and contextual assessments in real life environments.
• Use appropriate assessors (raters) including experts to assess specific domains.
• Combine formative assessment with summative assessment to allow personal feedback and practice but also ensure standards at the appropriate level are met.
• Provide timely and constructive feedback.

Advances in technology

Innovations in the development of part task trainers and manikins are rapidly expanding, providing increased fidelity in an ever-widening range of clinical situations and hence greater opportunity for refining assessment processes [15]. Furthermore, there is increasing evidence supporting the use of simulation for assessment; a recent systematic review by Van Nortwick and colleagues [16] yielded 942 articles which evaluated the reliability or validity of using simulation for the assessment of technical skills in surgery.

Simulation is no longer confined to the simulation centre due to the advent of the *wireless manikin*; simulations can now be set up in the clinical environment where teams that work together can be assessed in their own working environment using *in situ simulation*, which enhances both the educational and professional context of the assessments [17]. *In situ simulation* also provides the opportunity to identify latent threats which exist in the clinical environment by replicating challenging scenarios in the workplace; this other dimension allows the facilities, equipment, protocols and processes in place, to be tested [17].

Hybrid simulation [18] is a term coined by Roger Kneebone to describe the process of attaching part-task trainers to simulated patients so that assessment of clinical skills can include added complexity to measure aspects of the doctor–patient interaction. Aspects of communication skills, empathy and professionalism can then be assessed during the simulation which can take place in either the simulation centre or more realistic ward-based areas. *Distributed simulation* uses mobile simulated environments to increase the fidelity of simulations outside of the clinical environment which can also enhance the realism of assessment of clinical skills (see Chapter 11).

The use of virtual patients using web-based resources is expanding, especially in the field of undergraduate education [19] Opportunities exist here for standardized learning and assessment which can incorporate interprofessional learning to improve the educational experience. There are many challenges to establishing interprofessional learning programmes including coordination of faculty, resources and timetabling involving multiple specialties. The use of virtual patients, wards and communities may provide a vehicle to overcome some of these barriers.

Innovations in technology allow educational providers the chance to assess a wider range of medical competences [20]; however, the 2010 OTTAWA Consensus Statement on technology-enabled assessment of health professions education [21] emphasized:

One should ensure that the measures of assessment are well linked to the practical context rather than what the 'simulator' can effectively model and measure.

Choosing the appropriate level of fidelity for each assessment is important and the blind use of the highest fidelity available is a principle which should be avoided. The following sections of this chapter outline how assessments can be appropriately integrated into simulation training programmes.

Assessment: the practicalities

This section describes the practicalities of designing, implementing and evaluating an assessment of individual or team performance using simulation. How can participant behaviours and events that are observed during carefully designed scenarios be meaningfully measured?

An important first step in the process is to define the aims and significance of the assessment, typically to appraise the competence (e.g. in knowledge, technical skills or interpersonal skills) of the individuals or teams involved. The purpose of this appraisal may be formative, in which case the results can be fed back to participants with the aim of facilitating their ongoing professional development, or may be summative, in which case the results have consequences for the learners such as certification of achievement, remediation against potential failure in a course, licensing, gaining employment or acquisition of insurance cover.

Simulation may also be used to evaluate the performance of non-human entities such as medical equipment, emergency protocols, workplace environments, educational interventions, curricula [22] and even types of simulator [23]. In such circumstances, while participant behaviour in the simulated scenario will still be measured, the assessment scores attached to particular individuals are not the focus. The focus is on group level outcomes enabling questions such as 'Did the doctors who used emergency protocol A perform differently from those using protocol B?' to be answered.

Defining the domains of assessment

Having defined the overarching aim of an assessment, the aspects of behaviour in the simulated clinical scenario that are to be measured must be identified. These might come under domains of technical skills, non-technical skills, medical knowledge, personal attributes, teamwork, clinical reasoning, patient management skills and confidence. Where the assessment forms part of a wider educational or training programme then the domains to be assessed should be carefully *blueprinted* onto defined curricula [24].

The choice of what to assess will be both guided and limited by the technical capabilities of the simulation facilities available, though the temptation to assess something just because it can be done with the latest gadgetry should be avoided. Some aspects of clinical performance are more appropriate than others to assess via simulation. Medical knowledge for instance is generally better tested by written examinations, which are less expensive to conduct than simulations, whereas skills such as teamwork and situational awareness are difficult (if not impossible) to test via written examinations. Nevertheless, assessment of knowledge specific to a particular scenario could form a minor part of a simulation-based assessment.

Another consideration in defining the domains to be assessed is the balance between assessing process (the actions that learners take) and outcomes (the results of those actions). The choice of assessment domains may also be limited by feasibility. Within a simulated scenario of restricted duration there is a limit to what may be reliably observed and assessed even by highly trained assessors. Overloading the assessors by asking them to rate too many different domains of performance may simply lead to omissions and errors in the ratings that they make.

Scoring metrics

The creation and evaluation of robust metrics for the assessment of performance under simulation is a major challenge. The simulator may incorporate equipment that can capture a range of technical measures (for example depth and rate of chest compression in cardiopulmonary resuscitation) but educators are frequently interested in aspects of performance that can only be observed and assessed by human examiners using carefully constructed assessment instruments. It is easy to underestimate the difficulty of developing such instruments and before embarking on this potentially long and complex process it is best to consider the use of those that have been previously validated.

Examples of established instruments include:
• the Anaesthetists Non-Technical Skills (ANTS) taxonomy [8,25]
• Non-Technical Skills for Surgeons (NOTSS) [9,26]
• Scrub Practitioners' List of Intra-operative Non-Technical Skills (SPLINTS) [10]
• the Objective Structured Assessment of Technical Skills (OSATS) [27]

• the Imperial College Evaluation of Procedure-Specific Skill (ICEPS) [28]
• the McGill Inanimate System for Training and Evaluation of Laparoscopic Skills (MISTELS) [29]
• Rescuing A Patient In Deteriorating Situations (RAPIDS) [30]
• the Rochester Communication Rating Scale (RCRS) [31].

If an existing instrument cannot be used or adapted for a particular assessment then a new one will need to be developed. On the basis that many heads are better than one, it is common to gather input into the development process from multiple experts using a Delphi process or similar approach (see, for instance, the studies by Scavone et al. [32] and Morgan et al. [33]). An important choice in instrument development is the decision to adopt checklist scores or global ('holistic') rating scales (see sections Checklist scores, Global rating scales and Checklists versus global rating scales), though the two are not mutually exclusive: it is perfectly possible to combine both in a single assessment tool (see, for instance, the RAPIDS instrument developed by Liaw and colleagues [30] for scoring student nurses' simulation performance in a clinical deterioration scenario). Any new instrument will also require careful piloting, followed by participant feedback, psychometric evaluation and possible refinement, before being used for real. Having decided on appropriate scales for assessing different aspects of the simulation performance, the expert group may also need to decide how to weight the separate scores and combine them into either a single score, or possibly a small number of summary scores.

Technical measures

Technical equipment in the simulation environment such as digital timers, motion sensors, pressure sensors, cardiopulmonary resuscitation sensors and instrument trackers can be used to automatically record aspects of performance. Such data, which Pugh and Youngblood [34] have termed 'internal metrics', may then be converted to measures of performance such as task completion time, palpation pressure, number of areas touched, frequency of touch [34], finger movement [35], compression depth, ventilation rate [36], path length and smoothness [37].

Of course, not all instrumentation is automated. For example, Hislop and colleagues [38] recorded task completion times and Hunt and colleagues [39] measured times to critical actions by equipping observers with stopwatches. Although the potential might arise for human error in the measurements, video recording can assist in obtaining accurate timings during simulation: see Berkenstadt and colleagues [40] for example.

Checklist scores

A checklist scoring system comprises a list of observable actions and/or outcomes, appropriate to the presented scenario, which are important for the learner to complete in order to exhibit their proficiency in managing the situation. Generic guidelines for checklist development are available [41] and have been used in creating simulation-based assessments [42]. Items in a checklist are usually scored on a yes/no basis (a 'binary' checklist) though ordered categories of completion, such as not done/adequately done/well done, can also be adopted. Checklists of errors or undesirable actions can also be used: Pugh and colleagues [43] for instance counted decision-making errors made during simulated laparoscopic surgery. Checklists can be used for the measurement of both technical and non-technical skills, for example the RAPIDS tool [30] uses binary checklist items to assess both clinical actions and interprofessional communication.

Expert consensus should be used to determine which actions to include in a checklist, although gaining agreement on which actions are important or critical is not always straightforward and checklist content can be subjective [44]. The learner's final score is commonly just a simple count of the number of actions that were performed or a sum of the item scores if ordered completion categories are employed. Where some actions are deemed more important than others the item scores can be weighted, although again determination of appropriate weights is a matter of subjective judgement. Scavone and colleagues [32] for example used the expertise of six nationally recognized obstetric anaesthetists in a modified Delphi

process to weight the actions in a checklist for performance of general anaesthesia for emergency caesarean delivery. Shortening of checklists to crucial key actions is an alternative approach which effectively weights the critical tasks.

Global rating scales

A global (or 'holistic') rating scale comprises an ordered list of levels of performance to which numerical scores are attributed (Figure 5.2). The wording of the scale may be highly generic, for example 1 = very poor; 2 = poor; 3 = satisfactory; 4 = good; 5 = very good, or can be made more specific by anchoring to observed behaviours. For instance we might rate examinees' ability to remain calm during a stressful situation using the scale:
0 = tense and agitated most of the time
1 = became tense or agitated under pressure
2 = remained calm most of the time
3 = appeared relaxed and comfortable throughout.
Performance in a number of dimensions of teamwork is identified on the grid and used to inform a single overall score. ANTS, NOTSS, SPLINTS, ICEPS and the RCRS all use global rating scales. As with checklists, the development of global rating scales can involve a good deal of subjective choice: the number of scale points, the wording used to anchor them, whether to attach numbers to them, etc. Developing global rating scales is complex, and Streiner and Norman [46, pp. 37–54] give a helpful summary of these matters.

Checklists versus global rating scales

Checklists have a number of limitations. They may not differentiate between levels of performance [47] and may fail to detect incompetence [48]. It is easier to identify the actions that constitute appropriate behaviour in a scenario than to anticipate all of the mistakes that participants are liable to make. Checklists may therefore fail to adequately account for erroneous or irrelevant actions and their use may lead learners to adopt rote behaviours or perform unnecessary tasks [15]. It can also be difficult to construct checklists that take into account the sequence and timing of actions performed. This problem may sometimes be circumvented by using 'time to key actions' as an outcome

Personal Attribute: Team Working				
Capacity to work effectively with others and demonstrate appropriate leadership				
Please circle one indicator for each applicable row				
1. Unsatisfactory	2. Weak	3. Typical	4. Very good	5. Outstanding
Lacked awareness of performance of team members	⟺	Showed awareness of the level of competence of team members	⟺	Ensured that the capabilities of whole team match tasks
Showed no evidence of understanding others needs or concerns	⟺	Negotiated and compromised appropriately with team members	⟺	Always confirmed understanding and instructions, communicated plans clearly
Was rude or offhand to other team members	⟺	Built rapport with other team members	⟺	Remained very sympathetic and considerate to all other team members
Failed to delegate and demonstrate leadership	⟺	Delegated effectively	⟺	Demonstrated leadership with authority and justification
Pursued complex tasks with no additional support	⟺	Called for help when needed	⟺	Called for appropriate help with clear instructions
Was confrontational and critical of other team members	⟺	Maintained a non-confrontational approach	⟺	Maintained a very participative non-confrontational approach
Overall rating : Teamworking				
Please circle a single score for this attribute				
1	2	3	4	5

Figure 5.2 Behavioural marker grid and global rating scale (from work of Gale *et al.*). Assessee performance is identified on six dimensions of team working (the rows of the grid) and used to inform an overall global rating score.

measure, particularly where accurate observation of timings can be facilitated by use of video recordings. Examples include Hunt and colleagues [39], who assessed the times taken to initiate important resuscitation manoeuvres in simulated paediatric medical emergencies and Girzadas and colleagues [49], who showed that time to critical actions in anaphylactic shock scenarios distinguished novice and experienced emergency medicine residents. Finally, checklists that record technical actions are likely to be scenario-specific whereas global ratings tend to assess generic aspects of performance and are therefore more widely applicable, reducing the need to develop new score sheets for every new scenario.

The principal problem in using global ratings is that they are more prone than checklists to rater subjectivity, both in interpreting the wording of anchor points on the scale and in harshness or leniency of judgements. These problems may be countered however by rigorous rater training [50] and it has been shown that global ratings can be more appropriate and reliable than checklists for use in performance-based examinations [51,52]. Global ratings are also regarded as being more suitable than checklists for rating non-technical skills such as teamwork and situational awareness that are complex and multidimensional in nature [15].

The decision to use either checklists or global rating scales can also affect learners' behaviour during the assessment tasks. McIlroy and colleagues [52], for instance, showed that medical students undergoing an OSCE adapted their behaviours according to their perception of the scoring system being used. One solution to the problem of choosing between checklists and global rating scales is to incorporate both as Martin and colleagues did in developing the OSATS [27]. Similarly, Liaw's RAPIDS tool [30], while primarily checklist based, also incorporates two global rating items (Figure 5.3). Combined scoring systems of this nature have been recommended by some reviewers [53].

Example 1 Multiple metrics in a single assessment

The study conducted by Hayter and colleagues [54] in Toronto illustrates the use of all three types of score in assessing performance of epidural anaesthesia. A hand motion analysis device, the Imperial College Surgical Assessment Device (ICSAD), was used to produce technical measures of manual dexterity: total distance moved by each hand, number of movements, and total time. A 27-item checklist score (Figure 5.4) was used to identify which important actions were performed well, poorly or not at all. Global rating scales (Figure 5.5) were used to assess six important anaesthetic skills together with a score for overall performance.

Assessors

How should assessors be chosen? Those responsible for scoring candidate performance will frequently have a wide range of experience and clinical expertise, beyond that of the individuals being assessed. However experts are an expensive resource and it is possible, depending on the domains of assessment, to use non-expert raters such as patients, standardized patients, trainee doctors, nurses, medical students or lay people. Boulet and colleagues for instance, have shown that standardized patients (see Chapter 6) are reliable assessors of both clinical skills and spoken language proficiency in simulated consultations [55,56] but there is no clear evidence to prefer them over other rater groups [50]. Checklists scored on a yes/no basis may be more feasible for non-expert raters than global rating scales which call on knowledge and experience to accurately judge levels of performance.

Peer rating can also be useful in formative situations where subjects train in small groups and then observe each other undertaking scenarios, however there may be potential conflicts of interest in using peers as assessors in summative assessments. Self-assessment is another possibility. While several studies have shown that self-assessment can be accurate in simulation settings [57,58,59] others have provided less positive results [60] and the wider medical education literature suggests that doctors' assessment of their own performance does not generally agree with those of other observers [61].

Training of assessors, through observation of pilot assessments or videoed performances, is essential if consistent judgments are to be made. This can be both difficult and time consuming however. Graham and colleagues found that levels of inter-rater reliability in use of the ANTS system remained unacceptably low even after eight hours of training [62]. For a newly devised assessment, it is good

Date: _____ Candidate: _____ Assessor: _____

ABCDE: Assessment and Management of Clinical Deterioration			
CHECKLIST: Please rate each item by ticking in the box (1 = performed; 0 = not performed; NA = not applicable)			
		1	**0**	**NA**

		1	0	NA
AIRWAY	Assess airway (look/listen/feel)			
	Perform head tilt, chin lift or jaw thrust			
	Insert oropharyngeal airway			
	Place patient on the side			
	Perform oropharyngeal or tracheal suctioning			
BREATHING	Assess breathing (rates/patterns/depth)			
	Measure oxygen saturation level			
	Auscultate chest for breath sound			
	Place patient in a head-up position			
	Initiate oxygen			
	Titrate oxygen (keep SpO_2 > 94% or SpO_2 at 90–92% for patients with COPD)			
CIRCULATION	Palpate pulses			
	Measure heart rates			
	Measure blood pressure			
	Observe skin colour			
	Feel skin temperature			
	Measure body temperature			
	Check urine output			
	Measure capillary refill time			
	Lower patient head of bed position			
	Establish intravenous (IV) access			
	Prepare an IV infusion line with normal saline 0.9%			
	Attach a cardiac monitor			
	Perform 12-lead ECG			
DISABILITY	Assess level of consciousness using AVPU or GCS			
	Examine pupillary reaction and size			
	Monitor blood glucose level			
EXPOSE/ EXAMINE	Expose body to examine			
	Examine dressing site or drainage system			
	Examine pain using PQRST			
	Examine patient's chart or document			

GLOBAL RATING SCALE

Please make a mark on the scale below to rate the participant's overall performance in assessing and managing deteriorating patient

1	2	3	4	5	6	7	8	9	10
Unsatisfactory									Outstanding

Total ABCDE score:_____

Figure 5.3 Example of a checklist combined with a global rating scale: part of the RAPIDS instrument. COPD, AVPU, GCS, ECG, PQRST. Reproduced from Rescuing A Patient In Deteriorating Situations (RAPIDS): An evaluation tool for assessing simulation performance on clinical deterioration, Liaw *et al*. Resuscitation 82(11) with permission from Elsevier.

Stages performed	Not performed	Performed poorly	Performed well
1 Ensures patient is positioned comfortably and safely in the middle of the bed			
2 Adjusts height of bed appropriately			
3 Carefully prepares a sterile work surface			
4 Pours antiseptic solution (or has nurse pour it) without contaminating the epidural set			
5 Washes hands and puts on gloves in a sterile fashion			
6 Optimally positions him/herself for the procedure			
7 Prepares the skin at the back widely and aseptically (skin prep ×3)			
8 Allows solution to dry			
9 Neatly lays out and prepares all necessary equipment (needles, syringes, local anesthetic)			
10 Asks patient to arch her back			
11 Places drape over patient's back in a sterile fashion			
12 Landmarks site of injection after palpating iliac crests			
13 Warns patient of needle insertion			
14 Infiltrates subcutaneous layers with local anesthetic			
15 Places epidural needle with correct positioning of bevel			
16 Inserts epidural needle through skin, subcutaneous tissue and into ligament before attaching the syringe			
17 Attaches air/saline filled syringe to the needle hub with needle well controlled			

Figure 5.4 Part of the examiners task-specific checklist for assessing performance of epidural anaesthesia. Reproduced from Validation of the Imperial College Surgical Assessment Device (ICSAD) for labour epidural placement, Hayter *et al*. Canadian *Journal of Anesthesia* 56(6) with permission from Springer.

practice for each performance to be scored by two or more raters in order to establish the extent of inter-rater agreement. Consistent use of a scoring tool is likely to improve with practice so in assessing large numbers of individuals it is desirable to maximize the number of performances rated by each assessor while guarding against potential rater fatigue.

Live versus video rating

Assessment may take place in real time or can take place post-simulation, provided it is practicable to accurately score videoed performances. Live and video-based ratings have been shown to be equally reliable whether technical or non-technical skills are being assessed [63] For live assessments it can be feasible for participants in the scenario such as nurses or standardized patients to act as assessors. This has the advantage that they may be better placed than external observers to detect the subtleties of activity and interpersonal communication during the scenario but risks the possibility that assessee behaviour towards participants may alter if they are known to be assessors. The use of video has both ethical and legal implications: consent to being filmed must be obtained from all concerned and videos must be securely stored. A particular advantage of video-based rating is that assessors can be blinded to aspects of the performance, such as assessee identity, that might otherwise engender bias in the ratings.

Preparation for procedure				
1	2	3	4	5
Did not organize equipment well. Has to stop procedure frequently to prepare equipment		Equipment generally organized. Occasionally has to stop and prepare items		All equipment neatly organized prepared and ready for use
Respect for tissue				
1	2	3	4	5
Frequently used unnecessary force on tissue or caused damage		Careful handling of tissue but occasionally caused inadvertent damage		Consistently handled tissues appropriately with minimal damage
Time and motion				
1	2	3	4	5
Many unnecessary moves		Efficient time/motion but some unnecessary moves		Clear economy of movement and maximum efficiency
Instrument handling				
1	2	3	4	5
Repeatedly makes tentative or awkward moves with instruments		Competent use of instruments but occasionally appeared stiff or awkward		Fluid moves with instruments and no awkwardness
Flow of procedure				
1	2	3	4	5
Frequently stopped procedure and seemed unsure of next move		Demonstrated some forward planning with reasonable progression of of procedure		Obviously planned course of procedure with effortless flow from one move to the next
Knowledge of procedure				
1	2	3	4	5
Deficient knowledge		Knew all important steps of procedure		Demonstrated familiarity with all aspects of procedure
Overall performance				
1	2	3	4	5
Very poor		Competent		Clearly superior
Overall, should the candidate:	Pass		Fail	

Figure 5.5 Global rating scales for assessing performance of epidural anaesthesia. Reproduced from Validation of the Imperial College Surgical Assessment Device (ICSAD) for labour epidural placement, Hayter *et al. Canadian Journal of Anesthesia* 56(6). Reproduced with permission from Springer.

Piloting the assessment

For summative assessments, it is essential that some form of piloting takes place before the assessment goes live. This allows the timing and realism of the scenario, the difficulty level of the tasks, the ade- quacy of the participant instructions and the appro- priateness and feasibility of the scoring system to be checked. Feedback from participants in a pilot study can be invaluable in identifying unanticipated problems and shortcomings with both the simu- lated clinical material and the assessment instruments. It is important therefore to use scenarios, assessors and 'trial' assessees closely resembling those to be used when the assessment goes live. It is also desirable to evaluate, as far as possible in a small-scale pilot, the reliability and validity of the assessment (see section Quality assurance). Thus two or more raters might be employed to score each performance in a pilot study in order to establish the degree of inter-rater reliability, even though it might be intended to use only one rater in the live assessment.

Organizing and running the assessment

Once an assessment has been satisfactorily piloted, the logistics of running it for real must be planned. Efficient organization and attention to the minutiae of conducting an assessment will help to ensure its acceptability to participants. A skeleton outline of the necessary steps is provided here:

Well ahead of the assessment:
• Draw up a timetable encompassing the availability of suitable facilities, equipment, paperwork, assessors, assessees, standardized patients and/or other scenario participants, technical and administrative support personnel. Attention will also need to be given to catering arrangements and the comfort of participants.
• Compile contact details for all participants.
• Consider contingency plans for the 'failure' of any of the components: what to do if an assessor fails to turn up on the day or a video camera decides not to work?
• Prepare and print paperwork, including score sheets, information and guidance for all those involved. Remember to give clear directions for where to go, when to arrive, what to expect, how long the assessment will take and when the results will be available.
A day or two in advance
• Double check that facilities are functioning, paperwork is organized and equipment is available. If possible set up and test all equipment before the day of the assessment.
On the day:
• If possible conduct short verbal briefings for assessees, assessors, technicians and administrative assistants to remind them of what to expect

and to impart any last-minute information that may not have been included in the advance information.

Post assessment (on the day or soon after):
• Transfer checklist scores and ratings from paper sheets to a computer database, by hand or electronic scanning if possible, as promptly as possible after the assessment in order to facilitate timely feedback to assessees. For high-stakes assessment double-entering of all marks is recommended.
• Deliver results and feedback to the assessees regarding their performance in the assessment. Debriefings for all other participants are desirable.

Quality assurance

According to Van der Vleuten's 'utility index' (described earlier) [13] good assessments should combine five properties: reliability, validity, educational impact, cost efficiency and acceptability – a sixth attribute, feasibility, has latterly been added to this list [5,14]. These six properties are not independent and improving one will likely result in detriment to another: greater cost efficiency for example, might only be possible at the expense of poorer reliability. The relative importance given to each of these properties may depend on the goals of the assessment and the setting in which it is being conducted. Given that simulation is less cost-effective than many other forms of assessment we must ensure that our simulation-based assessments possess greater strength in the remaining five attributes that contribute to their utility.

Reliability

A reliable assessment must produce measurements of individual performance that are reproducible in similar circumstances such as on other occasions (test–retest reliability) or using other raters (inter-rater reliability). Reliable assessments also help differentiation between individual learners. Given the potentially high cost of running simulation-based assessments, it is important to avoid wasting resources by employing unreliable measures. Reliability is not, however, solely a property of the assessment instrument itself but of that instrument when used in a particular population of individuals. For instance a test of the ability to perform a simple clinical procedure such as venepuncture might differentiate well between newly qualified doctors but not among experienced consultants, even though the scores obtained could be equally reproducible in both groups.

Reliability is measured by a coefficient that expresses the between-individual variance in scores as a proportion of the total variance (between-individual variance + error variance). Thus an assessment with no error variance is 'perfectly reliable' and has a reliability coefficient of one. Coefficient values between zero and one represent less-than-perfect reliability and represent the proportion of total variability in scores that is attributable to genuine differences in performance between the individuals being assessed. Numerous authors have suggested cut-off points for what we might regard as poor, satisfactory and good reliability. A threshold of 0.80 is generally regarded as a minimum for high-stakes assessments.

There are many forms of reliability coefficient, for example intraclass correlation coefficients, Cohen's kappa (and related kappa-type statistics) and Cronbach's alpha, that are used in different circumstances. The choice of which measure to use depends partly on the source of error being investigated, for example:
• variation in scores awarded by a single rater at two viewings of the same performance (intra-rater reliability)
• variation between multiple raters scoring the same performance (inter-rater reliability)
• variation in scores awarded on two different performance occasions (test–retest reliability)
• variation in scores across different scale items (internal consistency reliability)

Choice of reliability coefficient also depends on the format of the data and whether individuals are being assessed to rank them in order or to compare their scores with a fixed criterion such as a pass/fail threshold.

As an alternative to reliability coefficients the standard error of measurement (SEM) can be used as a measure of reliability. The SEM is a statistic which indicates the likely error in an individual score. The multiplicity of available reliability measures for use in different circumstances can be somewhat bewildering and the inexperienced clinician is strongly advised to seek advice from a suitably qualified psychometrician or statistician.

The assessment of performance in a simulated scenario is often based on the judgement of human observers and inter-rater reliability is therefore of particular concern. Unless all examinees can be assessed by the same observers then variable rater stringency (the 'hawk-dove' effect) is likely to be a source of extraneous error in the awarded scores, though if sufficient data is available this can be corrected for using statistical methods such as Rasch analysis [64]. It has long been recognized however that rater subjectivity is a lesser threat to the reliability of simulation-based performance assessments than the effect of 'case specificity' [13,65]. This is variation in scores caused by the tendency of individuals to perform inconsistently from one simulated clinical encounter to another, so that the final rank order of assessees will depend to some extent on the particular simulations used in the assessment. Both of these problematic sources of unwanted score variance can be ameliorated by increasing their numbers, i.e. assessee scores averaged across more raters and more scenarios will generally contain less unwanted error and better reflect true differences between individuals (see Example box 2). However, such an approach to increasing reliability would have adverse implications for cost efficiency.

Where assessment scores are subject to two or more sources of error (e.g. raters, scenarios, etc.) the use of separate reliability coefficients (inter-rater reliability, interscenario reliability, etc.) can be less than helpful. An alternative is to use generalizability theory, an approach that is becoming more widespread in the analysis of performance-based assessments in medical education [53,66,67]. Generalizability theory produces a single measure of reliability, the G coefficient, which takes account of multiple sources of error simultaneously. Using analysis of variance (ANOVA) techniques, overall score variance is partitioned into components attributable to the various sources of error. This allows assessors to see which sources contribute most error to the assessment scores and to investigate the most (cost) efficient methods of reducing that error.

> ### Example 2 Case specificity and the application of generalizability theory
>
> Paskins and colleagues analysed a two-scenario manikin-based assessment of skills in emergency medicine amongst third and final year medical students and FY2 (Foundation year 2) doctors. Using generalizability theory they found that, in each group, examinee-scenario interaction (i.e. case specificity) was the greatest single source of error variance, accounting for 34–50% of the overall variation in scores. In contrast, the proportion of variation in scores due to inconsistent rater stringency was less than 2% while that due to true differences in examinee ability was between 42% and 52%. The high proportion of variation due to examinee-scenario interaction means that the final rank ordering of examinees depends to a large extent on the particular scenarios that are used. The investigators showed that increasing the number of scenarios rather than the number of raters would be more effective in improving the overall reliability and furthermore that an average score across four scenarios would provide an acceptably reliable assessment of final year students [68].

Approaches to reliability analysis using item response theory have also been advocated in medical education and can provide methods that adjust scores for rater variability [69]. Robust statistical analysis using item response theory does however require large sample sizes making the methods less useful for some simulation-based assessments. As with generalizability theory and other approaches to reliability analysis, seeking statistical advice on the implementation of item response theory is strongly advised.

Validity

Validity refers to the confidence that can be placed in any judgements that are made on the basis of the assessment scores about what the assessment is purporting to measure (e.g. a clinical skill, knowledge, etc.). Thus validity is not solely a property of the assessment instrument; rather, it is a property of the interpretations that are based on it such as being a 'good doctor', passing or failing a course, gaining a licence to practise, obtaining a job. Validation is a process of gathering evidence, from multiple sources, to show that such interpretations are sound and sensible.

The concepts of face and content validity embody the idea that an assessment looks to be a reasonable way to assess what is being assessed. Face validity indicates whether the assessment appears to be realistically measuring the desired attributes, while content validity indicates whether it effectively assesses the relevant or important domains at a level appropriate to the intended examinees. Both face and content validity are established on the basis of subjective judgements of the assessment tool made by stakeholders in the process. These stakeholders may include subject-matter experts, programme directors, institutional regulators, trainers, assessors and even assessees. While the methods used to develop an assessment (e.g. a Delphi process) can provide some evidence of face and content validity, such evidence may also take the form of questionnaires asking stakeholders to rate the assessment for qualities such as relevance, appropriateness, and thoroughness. Evidence in support of face and content validity can, and generally should, be gathered before an assessment is implemented. Evidence for other forms of validity, such as criterion and construct validity, is based on post hoc analyses of the scores obtained in one or more trials of the assessment.

Criterion validation involves correlating the results of an assessment with those of a second assessment (on the same group of individuals) that captures some of the same dimensions of performance. The second assessment should, ideally, have been previously used and accepted in the field, thereby providing some sort of 'gold standard'. It can be conducted simultaneously or close in time to the first assessment (concurrent validation) or at some point in the future (predictive validation). An important aspect of predictive validation in relation to simulation-based training is research into whether or not such training translates into practice. Bruppacher and colleagues [70] for instance, showed that simulation training was superior to an interactive seminar in improving the performance of senior anaesthesia trainees in weaning real patients from cardiopulmonary bypass. Recruitment processes are another situation where predictive validation is important: Gale and colleagues [45] showed that performance in a selection process incorporating medium-fidelity simulation correlated with subsequent workplace-based assessments of trainee anaesthetists.

Some attributes that we wish to assess are more readily observable than others. The ability to draw a precise 10 ml dose of substance X into a syringe for instance, can be objectively measured and is thus easier to assess than say, the ability to work well in a team. Attributes such as teamwork ability, communication skills, decision-making capacity, empathy and so on are regarded as 'constructs', or latent variables, that cannot be measured directly but only through subjective observation of behaviours that we believe are connected to them. Behavioural markers have been developed to increase the reliability of these measurements but they are still constructs which are devised to estimate how a person actually (for example) communicates in real life. So, we can measure specific behaviours directly, such as whether a doctor says good morning to a patient at the start of a consultation, but 'communication' cannot be tackled so easily as it is a thread that runs through all interactions between people. Therefore we must first try to define what behaviours are indicative of good or bad communication and use these as partial measures of communication. It is this impossibility of pinning down exactly what defines good or bad communication that makes it a 'construct'

Construct validation is the process of gathering evidence that our assessment does indeed measure the constructs that we intended it to measure. A common approach to construct validation is to show that two or more groups, who we would expect to differ in terms of the construct being measured, do indeed differ in the way that we would expect. Devitt and colleagues [71], for example, showed that faculty anaesthesiologists scored higher than residents in scenarios based on anaesthetic problems, while Wilson and colleagues [72] demonstrated that eye gaze measures differentiated experienced surgeons from novices. Correlational approaches to construct validation are also common. Adrales and colleagues [73], for example, validated a measure of competence in laparoscopic surgery by showing that scores were positively correlated with years of surgical experience.

It is important to note that validity is dependent on reliability: an unreliable instrument cannot be used to establish evidence in support of validity. Despite this, validation studies are often lax in reporting the reliability of the assessment tools employed [16] and we should be aware of this when reviewing existing 'validated' tools for use in our own assessments. Finally, we reiterate our earlier advice to the inexperienced clinician to seek assistance from a suitably qualified statistician before embarking on a validation study.

Educational impact

A formative assessment, accompanied by comprehensive feedback, can inform learners about their current levels of performance, highlight their individual strengths and weaknesses, and point the way towards future learning and development. The educational impact of such an assessment can be strong and positive. At the other extreme, a summative assessment that reports no more than a simple pass/fail decision for each examinee gives those who fail little idea how they might pass next time and therefore has little effect on learning. The nature and extent of feedback, often delivered in simulation settings as part of the debrief, is thus an important factor in the educational impact of any assessment (see Chapters 3 and 4)The use of immediate feedback is seen as particularly beneficial in simulation settings [2,74]. Not all feedback is good feedback however, and assessor skills in constructing high-quality feedback, structured methods for delivering that feedback, and supportive environments for receiving it, all need careful consideration and development [75].

A second factor in the educational impact of assessment is the well-known dictum that assessment drives learning [76]. This refers to the tendency of learners to 'learn to the test': to focus their learning on whatever aspects of the curriculum are to be assessed and to ignore those which are not. It is imperative therefore to assess the domains of competence that are regarded as essential or important for clinical practice and to make it clear in advance to learners exactly what they will be tested on.

Acceptability

Assessment in the simulated setting is more likely to be acceptable to all of those involved, where careful scenario design has been used to construct a realistic simulation of real-world clinical practice. Surveys that gather stakeholder perceptions of whether the assessment is fair, is set at an appropriate level of difficulty and affords adequate opportunity for learners to display their abilities can provide evidence in support of acceptability. In addition to collecting stakeholder perceptions of the acceptability of an assessment it may also be desirable, where numbers permit, to analyse the outcome scores for possible discrimination against certain assessee subgroups on the basis of age, gender, ethnicity or disability.

Feasibility and cost-effectiveness

Simulation is both time and resource intensive. Assessing large numbers of individuals within limited time frames can therefore be challenging and realistic piloting of the assessment will be crucial in determining its feasibility ('ease of use').

The cost of simulation-based assessment, including both the technological and human resources involved, tends to rise as the fidelity of the simulation increases. High fidelity is not however necessary or even desirable in achieving all of our assessment objectives. Thus it behoves us to use resources wisely by matching the fidelity of the simulation to the constructs being measured and to the level of expertise and clinical specialty of the learners [21]. Other possible ways of reducing costs include collaboration in scenario development and the use of already-validated assessment instruments, distributed simulation or non-expert raters where possible. Attempts to improve cost efficiency will often however, involve a trade-off against the other desirable properties of an assessment. Money might be saved by using fewer raters or scenarios but this will usually be at the expense of reduced reliability. Similarly, shortening the length of scenarios will improve cost efficiency but risks diminishing the authenticity and validity of the assessment.

Standard setting

For summative assessments that result in pass/fail decisions for the participants a choice of standard setting methods is available for deciding on the pass mark or 'cutpoint'. Methods can be classified as either relative (norm-referenced), absolute (criterion-referenced) or a combination of the two. All use some form of expert judgement to reach a consensus on professional standards. For example:
• The *fixed percentage method* is a relative method whereby the proportion of examinees who will pass is predetermined for each cohort. Thus the pass mark is determined by the quality of the examinees and the clinical competence of passing candidates will vary from one cohort to the next.
• The *modified Angoff process* asks a panel of expert judges to determine a score that would be achieved by a borderline ('just passing') candidate. The average of these scores is then the final pass mark.

The *Hofstee method* creates a cutpoint by combining the Angoff and fixed percentage methods. The panel of expert judges is asked to set minimum and maximum pass scores and minimum and maximum acceptable failure rates. A graphical method is then used to identify a cutpoint that falls between these extremes.
• In the *contrasting groups method* judges are asked to examine the overall performance of a sample of candidates and award each one a pass or fail, regardless of the actual scores awarded. The score distribution within the pass group is then compared with that for the fail group and used to establish a cutpoint where the distributions overlap.
• The *borderline groups method* uses clinician-assessors rather than independent judges. After

scoring each candidate, assessors grade them as pass, fail or borderline and the pass score is the average score obtained by those in the borderline group The aforementioned methods are described in greater detail by Norcini and by Boursicot and colleagues [24,77]. For OSCEs, the borderline groups method has become regarded as the standard setting method of choice [24] and is therefore eminently suitable for use in simulation-based assessments. In relation to learning clinical procedures, Michelson and Manning [74] have argued that because of the growing evidence linking skills learned in simulation with clinical performance, it is desirable to set standards for acceptable performance by using expert performance in the simulator to establish benchmarks.

Challenges and future directions

Criticisms remain with regard to the use of simulation for high-stakes assessment including: limited realism of medical simulators, inability to control for simulator related behaviours such as *hypervigilance* and *cavalier attitudes* (see the Glossary), plus the use of complicated scoring methods [78,79]. Further work is needed to address these criticisms including refinement of scoring methods and the development of feasible models of assessment which utilize adequate numbers of scenarios and raters to demonstrate acceptable reliability for high-stakes assessment. These models should be evaluated in high-stakes settings with criterion-related measures incorporated, so that comparisons can be made with current standards of assessment in these situations.

Simulation takes many different forms, all of which may be appropriate for assessment in a variety of contexts. An important focus for future progress will be to identify those forms of simulation which are proven to have high utility in specific contexts. Simulation providers have an important role to play in embedding simulation within overarching assessment programmes and helping to evaluate the future role of simulation for assessment.

SUMMARY

The use of simulation for assessment encompasses various modalities including part task trainers, simulated patients, virtual patients, OSCEs, immersive simulation and equipment containing 'internal metrics' to measure performance. Best practice in simulation based medical education should aim to incorporate both formative and summative assessment so that *assessment for learning* can be combined with *assessment of learning*. Simulation can be used for both the assessment of procedural/examination skills and the assessment of behaviours or non-cognitive skills within immersive team based scenarios. Advantages compared to other methods of assessment include the highly reproducible nature of scenarios and activities, plus the ability to observe how individuals actually perform.

Assessments in simulation are commonly undertaken with the intention to provide constructive feedback to the participants rather than make a pass/fail judgement as a part of a summative assessment. However, much work has already been done in developing metrics with appropriate reliability and validity to pass, fail or rank participants in high-stakes assessments using simulation.

Metrics include both checklist and global rating scales with some assessments using a combination of the two scoring methods. Checklists are commonly used for assessment of technical skills whereas global rating scales are more appropriate for evaluation of non-cognitive domains and higher levels of performance observed during immersive simulation.

Simulation should be part of an overall approach to assessment and should focus on specific learning outcomes identified within the curriculum. Appropriate fidelity should be chosen for each assessment so that methods are chosen from a practical context rather than from how a simulation can actually perform. Careful consideration should be given to the choice of domains to be tested, the type and number of assessors, and measures to ensure adequate reliability/validity of the assessment. Figure 5.6 describes the development of simulation-based assessment in a flow chart Constant innovations in technology used for simulation, plus research around good quality assessment methods, are sure to pave the way for future progress in the use of simulation for assessment.

✓ Key points

- Simulation can be used to provide a combination of formative and summative assessments for specific learning outcomes within a curriculum.
- A significant amount of evidence supports the use of simulation for assessment of technical skills as well as non-technical skills.
- Appropriate levels of fidelity should be chosen for each assessment based on the practical context.
- Assessments utilizing simulation should be integrated with other methods within an overall assessment programme.
- Assessments should ideally possess the attributes of reliability, validity, feasibility, cost-effectiveness, acceptability and educational impact.

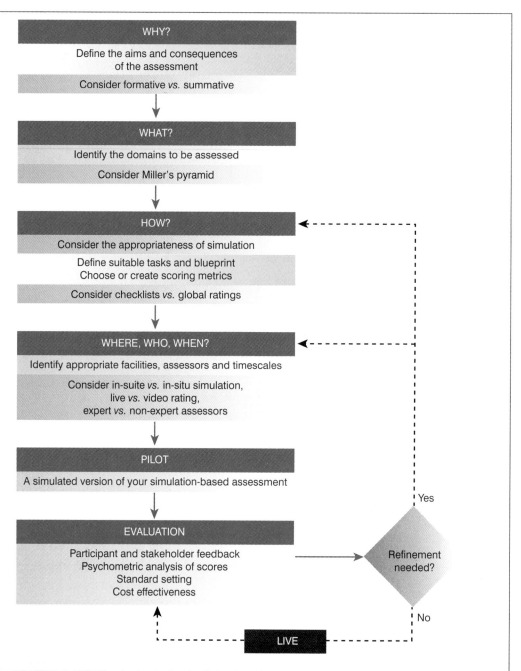

Figure 5.6 Flowchart for development of a simulation-based assessment.

Case study   Development and evaluation of a multi-station selection centre for recruiting junior doctors

Gale and colleagues [45] developed a selection centre structure to assess applicants for entry to anaesthesia training posts. The domains to be assessed were identified from job analysis research [80,81] as attributes/non-technical skills which were defined by experts as desirable for junior anaesthetists. Multiple stations were designed to test these attributes and a selection centre blueprint (Table 5.2) was designed which matched the relevant national person specification [82]. Traditional interview style methods were combined with evaluations of work-related tasks using simulated stations. The simulated stations included 'role play' using a standardized patient, 'telephone communication' with assessors talking on the role of professional colleagues and a 'medium fidelity simulation station'. The medium fidelity simulation station incorporated two nurses in role play and a wireless manikin to simulate acute medical emergencies. Situation awareness and teamwork could then be assessed which is difficult using traditional interview methods. Linear programming was used to standardize scenarios for all participants. Behavioural markers from existing tools such as the ANTS taxonomy [8] were incorporated into behaviourally anchored scoring grids (Figure 5.2). These scoring grids were designed specifically for assessment of non-technical skills in a short (10-minute) simulation station utilizing pre-programmed scenarios and nurses in role play.

All applicants are given detailed information regarding the overall selection centre prior to the interviews plus specific details regarding the simulation station and manikin utilized (Figure 5.7). Further familiarization regarding the conduct of the simulation station and the way in which the applicants are assessed, is given on the day of the interviews.

The simulation station has been run in a variety of settings from high-fidelity simulation suites to hotel function rooms depending on the availability of facilities (Figure 5.8). The set-up does not necessarily require a dedicated clinical skills facility and will be dependent on other factors influencing the choice of venue.

Reliability and validity of the selection centre was measured by:
- Internal consistency/overall reliability: Cronbach's alpha and generalizability.
- Inter-rater agreement: Kappa coefficients
- Face and content validity: candidate/assessor feedback questionnaires
- Predictive validity: correlation of selection centre scores with subsequent workplace based assessment scores once appointed, plus marks awarded in professional examinations.

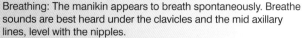

South West Peninsula Deanery Interviews The Laerdal 'SimMan3G' Medical Stimulator

Airway: Is anatomically normal. You may use airway adjuncts, perform bag valve mask (BVM) ventilation and intubation in the normal way. Assisted ventilation must be effective. Though it can be difficult to get a good seal with a BVM, a two person technique is recommended. Needle cricothyroid puncture can be performed in the usual way.

Breathing: The manikin appears to breath spontaneously. Breathe sounds are best heard under the clavicles and the mid axillary lines, level with the nipples. Respiratory rate and breath sounds can be changed to simulate physiological derangement and pathology (wheeze, crackles, etc.) If suspected tension pneumothorax can be decompressed in the usual manner with a cannula.

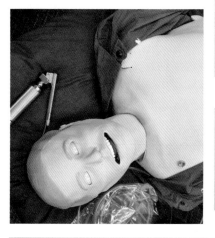

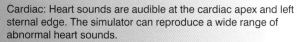

Cardiac: Heart sounds are audible at the cardiac apex and left sternal edge. The simulator can reproduce a wide range of abnormal heart sounds. Defibrillation leads must be plugged into the 2 larger metal sockets on the manikin's chest. There are also three smaller electrode points for a standard 3 lead ECG configuration.

Circulation: Pulses can be found in both carotid, femoral and radial arteries. To activate a pulse in this manikin, press firmly, release and then palpate again. The right arm will have a cannula in place through which infusions and drug boluses may be given. Blood pressure measurement is simulated via an attached brachial cuff or by a simulated arterial line.

Neurology: The manikin cannot move its limbs, but it can respond verbally. The eyes can open, close and his pupils will react to light (direct and indirect reflexes). You should assess level of consciousness and perform a neurological examination in the normal way, you will be informed of any important clinical signs.

Monitoring: The manikin has its own monitoring. It must be applied as in real life. There is a cuff for BP measurement. ECG electrode points can be found under little flaps on the chest, for defibrillation use the two larger chest studs. The S_pO_2 monitor can automatically recognise if it is in place, it is important to note that if the finger probe becomes displaced, if the systolic BP is too low OR if the simulated patient's blood S_pO_2 is very low, the saturation monitor will stop to read.

Try to behave in the simulation scenario as you would in real life. There will be nursing assistance for you. All the information you need can be found within the scenario. An invigilator will meet you outside the station and will introduce you to your assessors, nurses and the equipment in the room. GOOD LUCK!

Dr Ian Anderson, Dr Tom Gale, Dr Paul Sice

Figure 5.7 Information sheet for candidates in the anaesthesia selection centre (from work of Gale *et al.*).

Table 5.2 Blueprint for assessment of candidate attributes in the anaesthesia selection centre (from the work of Gale *et al.*)

	Selection centre stations					
	Interview	Portfolio	Presentation	Role Play	Simulation	Telephone
Personal skills/attributes — Communication	✓	–	✓	✓	–	✓
Empathy and sensitivity	–	–	–	✓	–	–
Organization	–	✓	✓	–	–	✓
Working under pressure	✓	–	✓	–	✓	✓
Situation awareness and decision-making	–	–	–	✓	✓	–
Team working	✓	–	–	–	✓	–
Content of professional portfolio	–	✓	–	–	–	–
Overall performance rating	✓	✓	✓	✓	✓	✓

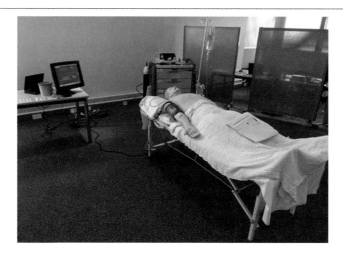

Figure 5.8 Simulation station set-up in a non-dedicated simulation facility (from work of Gale *et al.*).

REFERENCES

1. McGaghie WC, Issenberg SB, Petrusa ER, Scalese RJ (2010) A critical review of simulation-based medical education research: 2003–2009. *Medical Education* **44:** 50–63.

2. Issenberg SB, Mcgaghie WC, Petrusa ER, *et al.* (2005) Features and uses of high-fidelity medical simulations that lead to effective learning: a BEME systematic review. *Medical Teacher* **27:** 10–29.

3. Miller GE (1990) The assessment of clinical skills / competence / performance. *Academic Medicine* **65:** S63–S67.

4. Smith AF, Greaves JD (2010) Beyond competence: defining and promoting excellence in anaesthesia. *Anaesthesia* **65:** 184–191.

5. Postgraduate Medical Education and Training Board (2007) *Developing and Maintaining an Assessment System – a PMETB Guide to Good Practice*. London: PMETB.

6. Weller JM, Jolly B, Misur MP, *et al.* (2009) Mini-clinical evaluation exercise in anaesthesia training. *British Journal of Anaesthesia* **102:** 633–641.

7. Epstein RM (2007) Assessment in medical education. *New England Journal of Medicine* **356:** 387–396.

8. Fletcher GCL, Flin RH, McGeorge P, *et al.* (2003) Anaesthetists' Non-Technical Skills (ANTS): evaluation of a behavioural marker system. *British Journal of Anaesthesia* **90:** 580–588.

9. Yule S, Flin R, Paterson-Brown S, *et al.* (2006) Development of a rating system for surgeons' non-technical skills. *Medical Education* **40:** 1098–1104.

10. Mitchell L, Flin R, Yule S, *et al.* (2010) Thinking ahead of the surgeon: developing a behavioural rating system for scrub practitioners non-technical skills (SPLINTS). *Human Factors and Ergonomics Society Annual Meeting Proceedings* **54:** 862–866.

11. Harlen W, James M (1997) Assessment and learning: differences and relationships between formative and summative assessment. *Assessment in Education: Principles, Policy & Practice* **4:** 365–379.

12. Norcini J, Anderson B, Bollela V, *et al.* (2011) Criteria for good assessment: consensus statement and recommendations from the Ottawa 2010 conference. *Medical Teacher* **33:** 206–214.

13. van der Vleuten CPM (1996) The assessment of professional competence: developments, research and practical implications. *Advances in Health Sciences Education* **1:** 41–67.

14. General Medical Council (2010) *Standards for curricula and assessment systems*. London: GMC.

15. Boulet JR, Murray DJ (2010) Simulation-based assessment in anesthesiology. *Anesthesiology* **112:** 1041–1052.

16. Van Nortwick SS, Lendvay TS, Jensen AR, *et al.* (2010) Methodologies for establishing validity in surgical simulation studies. *Surgery* **147:** 622–630.

17. Riley W, Davis S, Miller KM, *et al.* (2010) Detecting breaches in defensive barriers using in situ simulation for obstetric emergencies. *Quality & Safety in Health Care* **19**(Suppl 3)**:** i53–i56.

18. Kneebone R, Kidd J, Nestel D, *et al.* (2002) An innovative model for teaching and learning clinical procedures. *Medical Education* **36:** 628–634.

19. Round J, Conradi E, Poulton T (2009) Improving assessment with virtual patients. *Medical Teacher* **31:** 759–763.

20. Dev P, Youngblood P, Heinrichs WL, Kusumoto L (2007) Virtual worlds and team training. *Anesthesiology Clinics* **25:** 321–336.

21. Amin Z, Boulet JR, Cook DA, *et al.* (2011) Technology-enabled assessment of health professions education: consensus statement and recommendations from the Ottawa 2010 conference. *Medical Teacher* **33:** 364–369.

22. Chipman JG, Schmitz CC (2009) Using objective structured assessment of technical skills to evaluate a basic skills simulation curriculum for first-year surgical residents. *Journal of the American College of Surgeons* **209:** 364–370.e2.

23. Youngblood PL, Srivastava S, Curet M, *et al.* (2005) Comparison of training on two laparoscopic simulators and assessment of skills transfer to surgical performance. *Journal of the American College of Surgeons* **200:** 546–551.

24. Boursicot KAM, Roberts TE, Burdick WP (2010) Structured assessments of clinical competence. In: *Understanding Medical Education* (Swanwick T, ed.). London: Wiley-Blackwell.

25. Flin RH, Patey R (2011) Non-technical skills for anaesthetists: developing and applying ANTS. best practice & research: *Clinical Anaesthesiology* **25:** 215–227.

26. Flin R, Yule S, Paterson-Brown S, *et al.* (2007) Teaching surgeons about non-technical skills. *The Surgeon* **5:** 86–89.

27. Martin JA, Regehr G, Reznick R, *et al.* (1997) Objective structured assessment of technical skill (OSATS) for surgical residents. *British Journal of Surgery* **84:** 273–278.

28. Pandey V, Wolfe JHN, Moorthy K, *et al.* (2006) Technical skills continue to improve beyond surgical training. *Journal of Vascular Surgery* **43:** 539–545.

29. Vassiliou M, Ghitulescu G, Feldman L, *et al.* (2006) The MISTELS program to measure technical skill in laparoscopic surgery. *Surgical Endoscopy* **20:** 744–747.

30. Liaw SY, Scherpbier A, Klainin-Yobas P, Rethans J-J (2011) Rescuing A Patient In Deteriorating Situations (RAPIDS): an evaluation tool for assessing simulation performance on clinical deterioration. *Resuscitation* **82:** 1434–1439.

31. Epstein RM, Dannefer EF, Nofziger AC, *et al.* (2004) Comprehensive Assessment of professional competence: the Rochester experiment. *Teaching and Learning in Medicine* **16:** 186–196.

32. Scavone BM, Sproviero MT, McCarthy RJ, *et al.* (2006) Development of an objective scoring system for measurement of resident performance on the human patient simulator. *Anesthesiology* **105:** 260–266.

33. Morgan P, Lam-McCulloch J, Herold-McIlroy J, Tarshis J (2007) Simulation performance checklist generation using the Delphi technique. *Canadian Journal of Anesthesia/Journal canadien d'anesthesie* **54:** 992–997.

34. Pugh CM, Youngblood P (2002) Development and validation of assessment measures for a newly developed physical examination simulator. *Journal of the American Medical Informatics Association* **9:** 448–460.

35. Wang N, Gerling GJ, Krupski TL, *et al.* (2010) Using a prostate exam simulator to decipher palpation techniques that facilitate the detection of abnormalities near clinical limits. simulation in healthcare. *Journal of the Society for Simulation in Healthcare* **5:** 152–160.

36. Weidman EK, Bell G, Walsh D, *et al.* (2010) Assessing the impact of immersive simulation on clinical performance during actual in-hospital cardiac arrest with CPR-sensing technology: A randomized feasibility study. *Resuscitation* **81:** 1556–1561.

37. Ritter E, Kindelan T, Michael C, *et al.* (2007) Concurrent validity of augmented reality metrics applied to the fundamentals of laparoscopic surgery (FLS). *Surgical Endoscopy* **21:** 1441–1445.

38. Hislop SJ, Hsu JH, Narins CR, *et al.* (2006) Simulator assessment of innate endovascular aptitude versus empirically correct performance. *Journal of Vascular Surgery* **43**: 47–55.

39. Hunt EA, Walker AR, Shaffner DH, *et al.* (2008) Simulation of in-hospital pediatric medical emergencies and cardiopulmonary arrests: highlighting the importance of the first 5 minutes. *Pediatrics* **121**: e34–e43.

40. Berkenstadt H, Yusim Y, Ziv A, *et al.* (2006) An assessment of a point-of-care information system for the anesthesia provider in simulated malignant hyperthermia crisis. *Anesthesia and Analgesia* **102**: 530–532.

41. Stufflebeam DL. Guidelines for developing evaluation checklists: the checklists development checklist (CDC) 2000. Available from http://www.wmich.edu/evalctr/archive_checklists/guidelines_cdc.pdf (accessed 6 March 2013).

42. Adler MD, Vozenilek JA, Trainor JL, *et al.* (2009) Development and evaluation of a simulation-based pediatric emergency medicine curriculum. *Academic Medicine* **84**: 935–941.

43. Pugh C, Plachta S, Auyang E, *et al.* (2010) Outcome measures for surgical simulators: Is the focus on technical skills the best approach? *Surgery* **147**: 646–654.

44. Boulet JR, van Zanten M, de Champlain A, *et al.* (2008) Checklist Content on a Standardized Patient Assessment: An Ex Post Facto Review. *Advances in Health Sciences Education* **13**: 59–69.

45. Gale TCE, Roberts MJ, Sice PJ, *et al.* (2010) Predictive validity of a new selection centre testing non-technical skills for recruitment to training in anaesthesia. *British Journal of Anaesthesiology* **105**: 603–609.

46. Streiner DL, Norman GR. *Health Measurement Scales*. 4th ed. Oxford: Oxford University Press; 2008.

47. Hodges B, Regehr G, McNaughton N, *et al.* (1999) OSCE checklists do not capture increasing levels of expertise. *Academic Medicine* **74**: 1129–1134.

48. Ma I, Zalunardo N, Pachev G, *et al.* (2012) Comparing the use of global rating scale with checklists for the assessment of central venous catheterization skills using simulation. *Advances in Health Sciences Education* **17**: 457–470.

49. Girzadas DV, Clay L, Caris J, *et al.* (2007) High fidelity simulation can discriminate between novice and experienced residents when assessing competency in patient care. *Medical Teacher* **29**: 472–476.

50. Whelan GP, Boulet JR, McKinley DW, *et al.* (2005) Scoring standardized patient examinations: lessons learned from the development and administration of the ECFMG Clinical Skills Assessment (CSA). *Medical Teacher* **27**: 200–206.

51. Regehr G, MacRae H, Reznick RK, Szalay D (1998) Comparing the psychometric properties of checklists and global rating scales for assessing performance on an OSCE-format examination. *Academic Medicine* **73**: 993–997.

52. McIlroy JH, Hodges B, McNaughton N, Regehr G (2002) The effect of candidates' perceptions of the evaluation method on reliability of checklist and global rating scores in an objective structured clinical examination. *Academic Medicine* **77**: 725–728.

53. Edler AA, Fanning RG, Chen MI, *et al.* (2009) Patient Simulation: a literary synthesis of assessment tools in anesthesiology. *Journal of Educational Evaluation for Health Professions* **6**: 3.

54. Hayter M, Friedman Z, Bould M, *et al.* (2009) Validation of the Imperial College Surgical Assessment Device (ICSAD) for labour epidural placement. *Canadian Journal of Anesthesia/Journal canadien d'anesthesie* **56**: 419–426.

55. Boulet J, McKinley D, Norcini J, Whelan G (2002) Assessing the Comparability of Standardized Patient and Physician Evaluations of Clinical Skills. *Advances in Health Sciences Education* **7**: 85–97.

56. Boulet JR, Van Zanten M, McKinley DW, Gary NE (2001) Evaluating the spoken English proficiency of graduates of foreign medical schools. *Medical Education* **35**: 767–773.

57. MacDonald J, Williams RG, Rogers DA (2003) Self-assessment in simulation-based surgical skills training. *American Journal of Surgery* **185**: 319–322.

58. Moorthy K, Munz Y, Adams S, *et al.* (2006) Self-assessment of performance among surgical trainees during simulated procedures in a simulated operating theater. *American Journal of Surgery* **192**: 114–118.

59. Sadosty AT, Bellolio MF, Laack TA, *et al.* (2011) Simulation-based emergency medicine resident self-assessment. *Journal of Emergency Medicine* **41**: 679–685.

60. Weller JM, Robinson BJ, Jolly B, *et al.* (2005) Psychometric characteristics of simulation-based assessment in anaesthesia and accuracy of self-assessed scores. *Anaesthesia* **60**: 245–250.

61. Davis DA, Mazmanian PE, Fordis M, *et al.* (2006) Accuracy of physician self-assessment compared with observed measures of competence. *Journal of the American Medical Association* **296**: 1094–1102.

62. Graham J, Hocking G, Giles E (2010) Anaesthesia non-technical skills: can anaesthetists be trained to reliably use this behavioural marker system in 1 day? *British Journal of Anaesthesia* **104**: 440–445.

63. Williams JB, McDonough MA, *et al.* (2009) Intermethod reliability of real-time versus delayed videotaped evaluation of a high-fidelity medical simulation septic shock scenario. *Academic Emergency Medicine* **16**: 887–893.

64. McManus IC, Thompson M, Mollon J (2006) Assessment of examiner leniency and stringency ('hawk-dove effect') in the MRCP(UK) clinical examination (PACES) using multi-facet Rasch modelling. *BMC Medical Education* **6**: 42.

65. Schuwirth LWT, van der Vleuten CPM (2003) The use of clinical simulations in assessment. *Medical Education* **37**(Suppl. 1): 65–71.

66. Downing SM. Reliability: on the reproducibility of assessment data (2004) *Medical Education* **38**: 1006–1012.

67. Crossley J, Davies H, Humphris G, Jolly B (2002) Generalisability: a key to unlock professional assessment. *Medical Education* **36**: 972–978.

68. Paskins Z, Kirkcaldy J, Allen M, *et al.* (2010) Design, validation and dissemination of an undergraduate assessment tool using SimMan® in simulated medical emergencies. *Medical Teacher* **32**: e12–e7.

69. Downing SM (2003) Item response theory: applications of modern test theory in medical education. *Medical Education* **37**: 739–745.

70. Bruppacher HR, Alam SK, LeBlanc VR, *et al.* (2010) Simulation-based training improves physicians' performance in patient care in high-stakes clinical setting of cardiac surgery. *Anesthesiology* **112**: 985–992.

71. Devitt JH, Kurrek MM, Cohen MM, *et al.* (1998) Testing internal consistency and construct validity during evaluation of performance in a patient simulator. *Anesthesia and Analgesia* **86**: 1160–1164.

72. Wilson MR, McGrath JS, Vine SJ, *et al.* (2011) Perceptual impairment and psychomotor control in virtual laparoscopic surgery. *Surgical Endoscopy* **25**: 2268–2274.

73. Adrales GL, Park AE, Chu UB, *et al.* (2003) A valid method of laparoscopic simulation training and competence

assessment. *Journal of Surgical Research* **114:** 156–162.

74. Michelson JD, Manning L (2008) Competency assessment in simulation-based procedural education. *American Journal of Surgery* **196:** 609–615.

75. Wood DF (2010) Formative assessment. In: (Swanwick T, ed.) *Understanding Medical Education*. London: Wiley-Blackwell.

76. Newble DI, Jaeger K (1983) The effect of assessments and examinations on the learning of medical students. *Medical Education* **17:** 165–171.

77. Norcini JJ (2003) Setting standards on educational tests. *Medical Education* **37:** 464–469.

78. Weller JM, Bloch M, Young S, *et al.* (2003) Evaluation of high fidelity patient simulator in assessment of performance of anaesthetists. *British Journal of Anaesthesia* **90:** 43–47.

79. Johnson KB, Syroid ND, Drews FA, *et al.* (2008) Part task and variable priority training in first-year anesthesia resident education: a combined didactic and simulation-based approach to improve management of adverse airway and respiratory events. *Anesthesiology* **108:** 831–840.

80. Patterson F, Ferguson E, Thomas S (2008) Using job analysis to identify core and specific competencies: implications for selection and recruitment. *Medical Education* **42:** 1195–1204.

81. Kearney RA (2005) Defining professionalism in anaesthesiology. *Medical Education* **39:** 769–776.

82. MMC (2012) Medical Specialty Training (England): Person Specifications 2012. Available from http://www.mmc.nhs.uk/pdf/PS%202012%20ST1%20Public%20Health.pdf (accessed 6 march 2013).

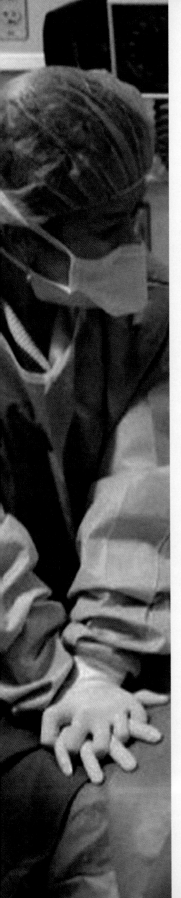

CHAPTER 6

The roles of faculty and simulated patients in simulation

Bryn Baxendale, Frank Coffey and Andrew Buttery   Nottingham University Hospitals NHS Trust, Nottingham, UK

Overview

Equipment and facilities often monopolize the discussion when talking about simulation-based education (SBE). However, effective learning using simulation as a methodology usually involves facilitators; be they faculty or simulated patients (SPs). This chapter will consider the roles of these important groups, and for both will address relevant definitions and standards of practice, and current issues in relation to ongoing professional development. Chapters 6 and 12 explore in more depth some of the techniques faculty and SPs might use when working with individuals and teams.

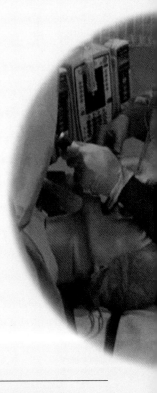

Essential Simulation in Clinical Education, First Edition. Edited by Kirsty Forrest, Judy McKimm, and Simon Edgar.
© 2013 John Wiley & Sons, Ltd. Published 2013 by John Wiley & Sons, Ltd.

Faculty

'Faculty' is a term which has different interpretations among educational and clinical practice communities in healthcare. The term 'faculty' is often used interchangeably with descriptors such as 'simulation-based educator', 'healthcare simulation educator', 'clinical educator', 'teacher' or other terminology to describe those individuals who interact with learners to facilitate experiential learning through some form of simulated event or process. For the purposes of this chapter we shall use the term simulation-based (SB) educator.

Ethical and professional values

Certain values and behaviours are core to anyone seeking to develop their role as an educator in healthcare, regardless of the educational resources they use. The UK Higher Education Academy (HEA) articulates these values within its Professional Standards Framework [1]:
• respecting individual learners and diverse learning communities
• promoting participation in higher education and equality of opportunity for learners
• using evidence-informed approaches and the outcomes from research, scholarship and continuing professional development
• acknowledging the wider context in which higher education operates recognizing the implications for professional practice.

These values are also described within the Professional Standards for medical educators in the UK (Academy of Medical Educators, 2012) [2] and endorsed by the General Medical Council's recommendations on recognizing and approving trainers (GMC, 2012) [3], which describe the need to demonstrate professional integrity, educational scholarship, equality of opportunity and diversity, and respect for public, patients, learners and colleagues.

SBE can produce unique circumstances where such values need to be exhibited more explicitly than in other educational settings. The nature of well-designed SB experiential learning can expose behaviours previously hidden by the learners concerned. Alternatively, debriefing after complex or challenging scenarios can highlight features of clinical performance or interpersonal behaviour about which the learner was previously unaware but which has now been revealed. Facilitating feedback and constructive discussion about such episodes of emotional cognitive dissonance needs skills that require specific development, and cannot be assured simply by being an 'enthusiastic teacher' in other types of educational encounter.

Educational context

The SB educator is required to adopt different styles of interaction with learners according to the purpose of the educational interaction, the relationship between educator and learner, and the nature of the educational session. The spectrum of ways in which simulation is applied to healthcare (Table 6.1) as described by Gaba [4] helps determine the ideal relationship between the faculty educator and participants. The range of styles of interaction (or educator role) that arise are summarized in Table 6.2.

When simulation is used for novices, for example learning new psychomotor skills (such as inserting a central venous cannula) or rehearsing patterns of responses to specific situations (e.g. basic and advanced life support skills, obstetric major haemorrhage drills), the faculty member will often adopt a more directive instructional style (Figure 6.1). This acknowledges their role as more 'expert' in the content of the task being taught, and will involve giving specific instructions to the learner(s) about following prescribed actions or sequences which culminate in completing the overall goal. Similarly the feedback during or following task performance will be more direct and didactic in nature, perhaps even demonstrating to the learner how their performance can be improved to meet a defined standard. For more advanced learners who may be on a level with or senior to the trainers, a supportive coaching or mentoring style may be more appropriate.

When using simulation to support assessment, interactions may be limited while the assessor observes and measures performance against a defined standard or marking scheme. Feedback, if provided at all by the faculty member, is either for the purpose of clarification of actions (or inactions) to inform the assessment outcome, or to inform the

Table 6.1 Spectrum of applications of simulation in healthcare (adapted from Gaba [4])

The different applications and factors influencing the nature of the simulation-based learning activity will have an impact on the role of the faculty member and their interaction with those participating. It is acknowledged that this list is not exhaustive.

Purpose and aims	Education Training Assessment	Clinical rehearsal Research Quality improvement
Level of learning	Individual Peer group learning Multiprofessional team	Clinical service or pathway Institutional
Participant's experience	School/pre-college/university Undergraduate students Early postgraduate development	Specialty postgraduate training Career-based continuing professional development
Domain of application	Community Practice (e.g. Primary Care, Mental Health, Dental, Nursing Care Homes) Pre-Hospital Emergency Care Major Emergency Planning	Hospital – acute care admissions environments Hospital – in-patient ward care Hospital – complex high hazard environments (e.g. critical care, Labour suite, interventional suites and operating theatres)
Participant disciplines and responsibilities	Staff without professional registration (e.g. Clerical, Porters, Care Assistants) Allied Health Professionals (e.g. Physiotherapy, Occupational Therapy, Operating Department Practitioner)	Nurses Midwives Medical Practitioners Managers and Organizational Leaders Non-healthcare emergency services (e.g. Police, Fire Department) Regulators
Intended outcomes	Conceptual understanding Technical/procedural skills Non-technical skills Critical thinking	Team working and leadership skills Team/crew resource management Systems improvement and preparation
Degree of interaction	Remote viewing only Remote viewing with live link verbal interaction Local viewing with immediate direct interaction	Direct engagement by immersive participation and involvement in feedback (some surgical procedure haptic simulators can provide automatic feedback which is software driven)
Style of feedback	None Automated analysis by simulator technology Critique from simulated patient (either 'in role' or 'out of role')	Instructor led based on performance against predefined goals/standards Facilitator-led debrief with open discussion and self critique Peer-led discussion with self critique Video-enhanced feedback (either immediately or post hoc)

Table 6.2 Styles of interaction between faculty and learners during simulation-based educational activities

Styles of interaction	Comments
Instructor	The terms imply the different manner in which the faculty member might interact with the learner both during the active educational experience as well as during the feedback process where reflection-on-action is encouraged.
Coach	The 'instructor-coach' end of this spectrum tends to imply more didactic tuition, including demonstration of procedures or behaviours, and providing more direct feedback with explicit guidance about improving performance.
Mentor Supervisor Facilitator	The 'mentor-supervisor-facilitator' grouping has a more questioning and probing type of approach, encouraging learners to question their own reasoning and evaluate their decision-making, actions and behaviours critically. Feedback is framed through open questioning to enable learners in recognizing and articulating aspects of their performance which might be improved and how this could be achieved, either through development of individual skills and behaviours or by being more critically aware of external factors and contexts that might influence individual or team performance.
Assessor/examiner Researcher	Faculty engaging in the assessor/examiner or researcher role are likely to manage their interaction with the learner in such a way to optimize observation of key actions actively and objectively, with little immediate feedback or discussion on the analysis of performance with the learner at that time. However, this relies on the design of the simulated encounter being sufficiently robust to obviate unplanned interjections, aided by a focused brief for participants.
Quality improvement lead Patient safety/governance lead Clinical service lead	The final three roles relating to quality improvement, patient safety and governance, or leading a clinical service imply an emphasis on improving the quality and safety of care and service through design of safe, reliable clinical systems, or assuring appropriate values and behaviours amongst clinical colleagues in terms of their engagement with local or professional standards of practice. The nature of the interaction between them individually and those participating in the simulated practice activity will be determined by its purpose.

learner about the outcome. It is likely to be descriptive rather than analytical with the key features being the accuracy of observation and the metrics used.

Roles and skills required

The roles 'instructor' and 'assessor' are well established within healthcare educational contexts, and professional practitioners know of the styles of interaction involved with each. Some educators may be less familiar with adopting a more explicit facilitator style, where the aim of the interaction is to elicit active reflection by learners 'in action', 'on action' or 'for action' depending on the timing of the feedback process [5]. The ability to support reflection by the facilitator requires the following skills:

• accurate observation and non-judgmental description of actions and behaviours

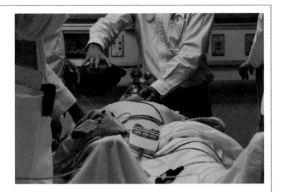

Figure 6.1 When teaching new psychomotor skills the instructor will often adopt a more direct style. Photo by Laura Seul, copyright Northwestern Simulation.

• active listening to the verbal communication skills used by learners during educational exercises, feedback or debriefing conversations
• use of effective open questions, with techniques such as advocacy and inquiry, when probing to explore the mental processing and reasoning that underpins the decisions and actions made by learners.

These skills are especially appropriate when facilitating SB exercises for multiprofessional groups or teams which can be applied to support both debriefing and improving team performance in clinical practice. Skilful and adept debriefing helps to bridge the gap in translating learning from the simulated context into relevant lessons applicable in clinical practice. The SB educator will be expected to display a balance of subject credibility and mastery of the educational approach being applied. This situation can, however, pose some interesting issues within SB learning:

• The subject credibility may not always be held by those with significant experience as clinical educators, for example the emergence of patient safety as a core theme within curricula requires educators to draw on concepts and materials from a wide range of academic disciplines such as psychology, social sciences, business and industry.
• The design and delivery of effective education using different forms of simulation requires educators to learn about these new techniques in order to

apply them optimally. This is true for technology-based simulators (computer based, part task, haptic, or full body manikins) as well as activities using SPs, who may have their own expertise in subject content and in facilitating the learning activity.
• The style of interaction with the learner in SBE can be different from that normally employed by educators. In particular, the techniques required when debriefing a group of participants or a team following a simulation scenario is quite specialized and often underestimated by faculty who are used to teaching in different ways, even if on the same topic.

Harden and Crosby [6] described the roles of the medical teacher, ranging from content expert to role model, and this can be applied to the SB educator. Each of these roles has a different emphasis depending on the extent to which the educator is directly involved with the learner (in terms of delivering versus developing educational materials) and whether the educator is a 'subject expert' or is more facilitative, focussing on the learning process:
• facilitator – mentor, learning facilitator
• role model – 'on the job' or teaching
• information provider – lecturer, clinical or practical skills teacher
• resource developer – study guide, learning resources, cognitive aids
• planner – curriculum planning, course design and organization
• assessor – individual or team assessment, course or curriculum evaluation

However, in any one encounter, an educator might adopt any one or more of these roles depending on the activity, the learners' needs and stage of training. These attributes can be mapped against evidence from systematic reviews that have addressed the educational effectiveness of simulation in healthcare. Issenberg [7] and subsequently McGaghie et al. [8] identified a number of features that contributed to educational effectiveness including:
• nature and timeliness of effective feedback
• adaptability of simulation to support individualized learning
• need for defined outcomes and metrics for their measurement
• ability to vary levels of difficulty of challenge for learners

- opportunity to repeat practice
- alignment with clinical variations in the workplace
- importance of creating and maintaining a non-threatening environment (physically and psychologically)
- integration of the learning into a curriculum rather than existing in isolation.

Faculty training

The subject of instructor training was addressed in McGaghie *et al.*'s [8] review, where it was noted that there is no uniform model by which SB educators are prepared and assessed as competent. This is partly due to the diversity of simulation activities. The review also commented that the process of effective SBE is not easy or intuitive, clinical experience does not act as a proxy for effectiveness as a SB educator, and that it is not necessary for the educators and learners to be from the same profes-

sional backgrounds. Although many different faculty development courses have been described, limited evidence exists about their effectiveness or longer term utility. However, the themes of standards for educators, quality assurance, recognition and certification are becoming more prevalent, and the international Society for Simulation in Healthcare (www.ssih.org) has recently begun to explore the feasibility and utility of certification programmes for SB educators.

The key 'competencies' of the SB educator are described in Table 6.3.

Each of these can be subject to particular development programmes, some of which have broader relevance to clinical educators, whereas others are more focused on SB educational techniques.

One of the strengths of simulation is engagement with students individually and in small groups, which provides opportunities for learner-centred education. However, maintaining a high teacher-to-learner ratio is not always sustainable

Table 6.3 Competencies of the simulation-based educator

Orientation and familiarization with different simulation modalities	This includes addressing knowledge and skills in using the various forms of technology, understanding limitations in its use, and being able to select most appropriate technologies for the educational purpose Increasingly this aspect of development requires familiarity with the hardware and an ability to use relevant software aspects of these technologies
Developing and sustaining a safe learning environment	This pertains to whatever environment is going to be the location for simulation-based learning, whether in a dedicated centre or skills training area or in the workplace itself Safety relates to physical and psychological aspects of learning, and this must be paramount in the attitudes and behaviours of the SBE throughout the planning and delivery phases
Designing effective simulation-based learning	This feature relates to broader aspects of curriculum integration (i.e. where does this learning exercise 'fit' into the education and professional development of those participating). Design also relates to the actual learning episode itself, which must be properly structured and prepared from the perspectives of the specified outcomes for the intended learners, the faculty involved in its delivery, and any technical staff involved 'behind the scenes' to ensure it will run properly The final component of effective design is the inclusion of criteria by which outcomes can be measured and reviewed to evaluate success of the learning episode

Table 6.3 *(Continued)*	
Facilitation skills	The educator plays a crucial role in managing the expectations and experiences of the learners when engaging in simulation-based learning. This involves rapidly developing a relationship with individual learners or in a small group setting, and this is paramount in supporting the development of a safe leaning environment. This relationship is dynamic during any encounter, and the educator must be sensitive to the experiences and emotions being elicited for individuals within any setting The educator also has a role in acknowledging or managing the 'fidelity' of the simulation encounter. This is a crucial element of achieving agreement with the learner(s) that there is value in the activities they are about to experience. This fidelity has several facets to be considered: • psychological • physical • environmental • temporal
Effective feedback and debriefing skills	The process of 'dismantling' the simulated experience and translating it into learning that can be applied in practice is a complex process, and in a small group setting needs to be handled sensitively. Many new faculty find this the most challenging component of their development, yet it is probably the skill set that will be most beneficial to their wider professional development as an educator or clinician. There are different guides described about the debriefing process, many of which involve some form of chronological description of events followed by non-judgemental analysis of the behaviours and actions (or inactions) observed, concluded by discussion about application of any learning points identified.
Use of video-enhanced debriefing	The use of mobile video recording equipment and sophisticated software packages to allow timely event recording and playback is becoming increasingly available and used. This can enhance the feedback process significantly if used in a discriminating fashion. Some programmes allow 'anonymous' marking of events by faculty or peers observing the simulation to encourage honest feedback subsequently. Provision of a 'hard copy' for learners also allows subsequent review and reflection, but only if faculty help provide focus for this process. Videos of the debriefing activity also allows new and experienced faculty to review their own skills and others at facilitating the process, with attention to the language and non-verbal cues used as well as identifying missed opportunities to highlight learning points.

because the educational faculty may not have the time, enthusiasm or skill set to take part or the institution may not provide appropriate or sufficient resources. The release of clinical staff to act as faculty is a major limiting factor faced by many institutions and centres attempting to establish and sustain SB educational activities. It is essential to consider at the outset what expectations or demands might be placed on potential faculty in terms of their participation in SBE activities. It is also important to identify funding streams to support faculty development (see Chapter 10). If being a SB educator is a properly commissioned and valued activity, the credibility of the role to individuals and institutions is much more easily established.

Recruitment tends to come from one of two prime routes: existing staff educators wishing to develop new skills (professional development), or more novice educators following up their experience of SBE as a learner and wishing to develop skills of a teacher by supporting similar learning opportunities for junior colleagues.

The principles of a faculty development programme

A successful SB educator faculty development programme should:
• Provide leadership to identify clear outcomes for individuals and the organization.
• Acknowledge the diversity of participants, and encourage multiprofessional engagement.
• Mirror the experiential interactive learning used in SBE by designing training on sound educational principles, emphasizing concepts of reflection, adult lifelong learning and techniques to support feedback and debriefing.
• Provide opportunities to observe and discuss performance of experienced faculty, and have additional resources and materials available for reference, e.g. educational texts, published literature and reports, feedback and commentary from learners, video archive of relevant educational activities.
• Provide a development pathway over a period of time, with planned opportunities to record and practise new techniques, receive timely feedback, and demonstrate improved performance.
• Reinforce this pathway by establishing collaborative peer/colleague relationships with a mentoring scheme, identifying role models, and encouraging peer observation and feedback. New and existing faculty should be encouraged to translate feedback into actionable development plans with feasible timelines and opportunities to address these actions stated.
• Incorporate educational scholarship and leadership for those who wish to pursue more academic or strategic roles and responsibilities.
• Identify opportunities to initiate and support collaborative activity within and between different institutions. Many educational and professional networks are already established, and faculty development in SBE should build on prior experience and expertise.
• Link the faculty development pathway for SB educators with existing or emerging standards for educators described by professional bodies and reinforced by requests for evidence from regulatory bodies.

These principles align with the models describing the 'excellent teacher' developed by Hesketh *et al.* [9] and Harden and Crosby [6] based on:
• Tasks – 'Doing the right thing' – performing the activities of the teacher according to the requirements at the time, including 'best use' of the simulation modality for the intended outcomes and applying the most appropriate feedback style.
• Attitudes – 'Doing the thing right' – applying appropriate intellectual, emotional and analytical intelligences to the SB educational process and its intentions.
• Professionalism – 'The right person doing it' – having a broader understanding of the educational spectrum within which simulation exists, pursuing personal development and maintaining an awareness or ability to influence organizational or institutional goals and learning strategies.

Standards, quality assurance and recognition

Organizations are paying increased attention to the need to formally recognize educators and accredit educational programmes which make use of simulation. The principles and content of such processes are useful when considering the strategic development and quality assurance of SBE in national or regional educational contexts. The professional standards frameworks described earlier in the chapter (Table 6.4) and their international equivalents can help with this process.

The key components of the goal of professionalizing clinical educators include:
• A clear description of the standards to be met by educators and the programmes making use of simulation.
• A framework and process which supports the measurement of performance and professional

Table 6.4 Comparative professional standards frameworks published by the Higher Education Academy (HEA) and the Academy of Medical Educators (AoME)

	Academy of Medical Educators		Higher Education Academy	
Framework structure	Core values and five domains		Three dimensions	
Levels of accreditation	Accreditation described at three levels of recognition • Associate, Membership, Fellowship Achieved through evidencing core values and different levels of educational activity or responsibility across each of the domains, each of which has descriptors to guide expectations for each level of recognition		Four levels of accreditation • Associate, Fellow, Senior Fellow and Principal Fellow Achieved through evidencing different levels of educational activity and responsibility across all three dimensions	
Framework details	Core values	• Professional integrity • Educational scholarship • Equality of opportunity and diversity • Respect for public, patients, learners and colleagues	Dimension one – Areas of Activity	• Design and planning of learning activities • Teach/support learning • Assess/give feedback • Learning environments and support • CPD
	Five domains	• Design and planning of learning activities • Teaching and supporting learners • Assessment and feedback to learners • Educational research and evidence-based practice • Educational management and leadership	Dimension two – Core knowledge	• Subject material • Teaching and learning methods • How students learn • Learning technology • Evaluation of effectiveness • QA processes
			Dimension three – Professional values	• Respect for learners & communities • Participation and equality • Evidence informed approaches • Wider context of HE recognized
Application	Designed to recognize standards for both clinical and non clinical medical educators. Standards used to develop and support CPD of medical educators and provide formal recognition of role.		Supports CPD of all types of educators working in HE. Generic standards which can be applied across all subjects. Allows formal recognition of teaching and supporting learning.	

development against specified educational standards. This involves collecting a 'portfolio' of evidence: self reflection statements, peer evaluation, learner feedback, videos, scholarly activities such as research, curricular evaluation and other work related to educational leadership/management.

• Regular educational appraisal to review portfolios and other evidence, set development goals and identify training and development needs.

• Recognition of the role of the educator within organizations through job planning, promotion and career development pathways.

For education and learning to be effective it must be supported strategically and valued by organizations. This might take the form of protected time within individual job plans supported by a robust and meaningful appraisal process linked to continuing professional development as an educator. Those responsible for commissioning simulation activities must have processes in place by which they can monitor and evaluate its implementation, with appropriate accountability via relevant regulatory frameworks. It is essential that individual educators are capable of using these resources wisely and similarly that their institutions value and recognize these abilities explicitly.

Educational leadership

Within teams and clinical services, educators can provide an important leadership role in helping to provide a supportive learning environment and culture among clinical and managerial colleagues. A significant component of learning for healthcare professionals takes place in the clinical context, either as planned learning opportunities or integrated into participation in service delivery under varying degrees of supervision. This creates a degree of tension within the clinical workplace when attempting to create an appropriate balance of learning and service provision.

Educational faculty must be cognisant of these issues and help facilitate this balance as part of their role providing educational supervision in practice. Creating a culture within clinical teams that supports learning is an extremely positive goal, not just for learners but also for team dynamics and morale. This can be enhanced by supporting educational

research in practice, either exploring how simulation accelerates or enhances learning and performance in the clinical setting, or by applying simulation to explore and improve clinical systems and technologies to improve patient care.

At the broader organizational level, educational leaders should help create, support and make visible a learning culture among the whole workforce. An important concept for faculty attempting to influence such matters requires them to develop and support learning strategies that can be mapped to short- and longer term organizational goals, which will include performance against a patient safety and care quality agenda.

Simulated patients

The use of SPs has grown over the past 50 years in the context of training and assessment of clinical skills in healthcare professionals. This has been driven by a growing recognition of the educational advantages offered by this methodology, as well as responding to the changing landscape and constraints being faced in clinical education including workforce development, healthcare delivery and the expectations of patients and the public regarding the safety and quality of care.

This section considers the origins, definitions and nomenclature of simulated patients in a wide range of educational contexts in which they can enhance or provide a unique addition to the learning experience. The qualities, professionalism and expertise of SPs, their recruitment and training are discussed, as well as how clinical educators can make the best use of SPs and can assure quality and standards, especially of high-stakes assessments.

Definitions and nomenclature

The terms 'simulated patient' and 'standardized patient' are often used interchangeably, the latter being more commonly used in the North American literature. Other terms used include 'role player', 'medical actor', 'simulator', 'clinical teaching associate', patient educator (instructor) or 'patient expert'.

Barrows [10] defined the terms as:

• **Simulated patient:** someone who has been coached or trained to portray actively a specific patient when given a history and physical examination, incorporating a display of relevant symptoms, signs, emotions and behaviour.

• **Standardized patient:** this incorporates simulated patients but also includes real patients who have been coached to present *their own* illness in a standardized way.

One of the dilemmas surrounding nomenclature is that as well as portraying patients, simulated or standardized patients are also being used to simulate relatives, carers and other healthcare workers, amongst others. The term 'confederate' has been applied to such roles in North America but this term has not met with universal support. Increasingly the generic term 'SP' is being used to describe a person undertaking the diverse range of roles in this sphere of simulation education. The Association of Standardized Patient Educators (ASPE) [11] definition is shown in Box 6.1.

Collins and Harden [12] consider the various contributions of SPs to the educational encounter:

• Minimal interaction between the learner and SP, e.g. in a physical examination, where the SP has only basic background information or intended responses.

• More significant interaction based on scripted briefing information, detailed narrative or storyline, in which the SP must stick to certain details but has flexibility in other responses depending on the learner's questions, actions and behaviours.

• Closely considered scripted, standardized SP interactions/responses, based on detailed specification of role and condition.

The SP's feedback might be purely 'in role' during the encounter and based on genuine human interaction, carefully given to support specific learning outcomes or given to the learner post encounter, which might be given in or out of role. Some trained SPs can facilitate the feedback and reflective process themselves, providing independent reliable summative assessments of student performance.

Patient educators (or instructors) and patient experts can present personal and specific aspects of clinical conditions alongside genuine display of emotional and psychological components. Other SP roles include Gynaecology Teaching Associates who are trained to undergo intimate or internal physical examinations and provide guided feedback to students. The diversity of those involved as an SP or Patient Expert highlights that the educational context and intended learning outcomes of the exercise is paramount, and should influence the type of 'simulator' selected and the level of preparation given (Figure 6.2).

Box 6.1 The Association for Standardized Patient Educators (ASPE) definition of a Standardized/Simulated Patient (Source: ASPE, 2011)

A standardized/simulated patient (SP) is an individual who is trained to portray a patient with a specific condition in a realistic, standardized and repeatable way (where portrayal/presentation varies based only on learner performance). The SP can be used for teaching and assessment of learners including but not limited to history/ consultation, physical examination and other clinical skills in simulated clinical environments. SPs can also be used to give feedback and evaluate student performance.

A brief history of SPs

Howard Barrows (an American neurologist and academic) pioneered the concept of simulated patients in the 1960s [13] based on several sentinel experiences in his career:

• Observing medical students 'carrying out their professional tasks', addressing errors and improving their history taking, physical examination and 'thinking' skills, as well as overcoming the time-consuming nature of learning.

• Discovering that a patient selected for specialty training summative exams in neurology deliberately altered presentation of his physical signs to one learner who he had felt was 'hostile and performing a very uncomfortable examination', thus influencing the outcome of this assessment.

• Training a lay person to simulate a range of physical neurological signs, anxieties and concerns based

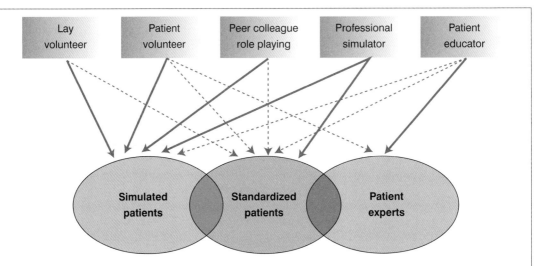

Figure 6.2 Sources of SP's and their potential contribution to the educational encounter. Bold lines indicate main opportunities for contribution, whilst dashed lines indicate potential contributions depending on attributes of the individual and suitable training.

on the emotional component of the disease process. Using a checklist, the SP provided feedback following all encounters, including some unique insights into 'interpersonal skills' and 'thinking skills'.

The popularity of SPs grew slowly, held back in part by the level of assurance and acceptance required from medical education communities. However, the widespread uptake of the objective structured clinical examination (OSCE) from the 1970s [14] led to a dramatic increase in demand for SPs who were trained to support OSCEs, particularly at the undergraduate level.

The formal development of and research into 'Standardized Patient Programmes' within US Medical Schools expanded significantly during the next two decades. Landmark papers addressed questions about the validity and reliability of SPs [15] and their wider integration into the teaching and evaluation of clinical skills [16]. The requirement to enhance clinical skills teaching led many UK Schools of Nursing, and subsequently Medical Schools, to develop devoted teaching areas for SPs [17].

Another significant landmark was SP's use in 'high-stakes' examinations, first used in a licensure

examination in 1993 in Canada. In 1998 the Education Commission for Foreign Medical Graduates (ECFMG) in the USA implemented the Clinical Skills Assessment (CSA) using standardized patients within a performance-based examination to assess international medical graduates. In the UK, SPs are used in postgraduate examinations, selection processes for specialty training schemes and in assessment schemes for international graduates to demonstrate achievement of professional and linguistic capabilities.

More recently, SPs have been used in the innovative teaching and assessment of practical skills, in particular the integrated teaching of technical and communications skills in performing specific clinical procedures [18,19]. Other novel applications have explored the use of SPs in the UK to compare the quality of care in Walk-in-Centres with General Practice and NHS Direct facilities [21] and the use of SPs to assess clinical practice in the workplace from the USA and the Netherlands [21,22]. Specialized examples of SP practice emerged such as female SPs specifically trained to help teach undergraduate medical students, GP trainees, nurses and other health professionals procedures such as internal examinations [23] and using SPs as educators in their own right [24].

The most recent developments focus on developing standards and quality assurance processes, including whether accreditation and certification are necessary in relation to the professionalization of SPs.

Educational contexts

SPs are used extensively in the training of undergraduate and postgraduate medical professionals and increasingly for the allied health professions, mainly involving the SP acting as a proxy for the patient or a carer/immediate family member. Less frequently SPs may portray a healthcare colleague or professional. SPs can also provide assessment of clinical services, like a 'mystery shopper'. SPs are primarily used for teaching and assessing communications skills and/or physical examination skills. As in the Collins and Harden [12] description the SP role can be:

• as a 'prop' to enable teaching led by clinical educators
• more interactive where the SP has opportunity to contribute to feedback and group discussions
• leading and facilitating the learning experience
• to provide formal formative feedback on the performance of the learner or undertake summative assessment.

Some examples of typical activities are listed in Box 6.2.

The advantages of SPs for teaching and assessing these skills include:

• **Availability and planning:** SPs overcome the uncertainty of relying on the availability of suitable patients.
• **Consistency:** the SP can be used for several students consecutively without presentations altering.
• **'Safe Teaching Environment':** SPs allow students to practise dealing with problems which, if handled inexpertly, could be very distressing or damaging for real patients, e.g. bereavement or breaking bad news.
• **Direct feedback:** SPs can provide timely, constructive and honest feedback to the student from the patient's perspective, either 'in role' or 'out of

---

> ### Box 6.2 Examples of educational or other activity where SPs have been used successfully
>
> **Communication skills**
> Taking a patient history
> • Gaining consent for procedures or surgery
> • Handling difficult conversations, such as breaking bad news, being open about an error, discussing wishes about end of life
> • Developing advanced consultation skills
> • Undertaking telephone interviews
> • Using structured communication tools, e.g. for escalating care in acute emergencies
> • As part of a hybrid simulation exercise in order to explore the influence of context on ability to communicate effectively
> Physical examinations
> • Teaching physical examination skills with normal signs
> • Developing ability to display (simulate) abnormal signs
> • Portraying patients with acutely abnormal physiology (usually aided by moulage)
> • Performing as a specialist Teaching Associate to help teach intimate examinations
> Evaluating clinical services
> • Acting as a 'mystery shopper' to assess performance of community or hospital based patient services and clinics

---

role', during a 'time out' period mid-scenario or at the end of the exercise.

• **Deliberate practice:** the opportunity to repeat consultations or examinations and try different approaches offers learners a unique opportunity to refine skills and competences or apply skills under increasingly complex contexts, e.g. hybrid practical simulations combining a part-task trainer and a SP.

• **Reducing clinical educator requirements:** some SPs are trained in high level facilitation skills and act as clinical educators within well-rehearsed educational activities or summative assessments.

Integrated teaching of technical skills and communication ('hybrid simulation')

Communication is a vital component of safe practice but it is not often considered an important integrated part of procedural or technical skills training. Poor communication between patient and doctor prior to or during intervention risks inadequate understanding of the intended benefits versus risks and potential patient dissatisfaction and complaints. Kneebone *et al.* [18] introduced SPs into teaching sessions with medical students which combined technical and communication skills teaching. Two common clinical scenarios were chosen, wound closure and urinary catheterization, with latex models attached to SPs who displayed the behaviours and emotions that a patient being catheterized or sutured would exhibit. The procedures were observed, recorded and assessed by tutors. Students received immediate feedback from tutors and SPs, and were encouraged to pursue individual feedback through private review of their own video recordings.

Students found the opportunity to integrate communication and technical skills valuable, challenging and an appropriate learning experience. Immediate feedback, including that from the SPs, was highly valued. Kneebone concluded that the integrated model for clinical skills and communication teaching was feasible and was perceived to be a valuable enhancement to existing teaching methods when performed within a safe learning environment. Similar integrated approaches using SPs and part task trainers have been used to teach intimate examinations [19], which has been complemented further by engaging SPs versed in their ability to portray physical signs or be subject to intimate physical examinations (see later).

Reviewing videos of an SP encounter can help learners develop clinical reasoning skills and scenarios can be designed to test specific areas of clinical reasoning (Figure 6.3). The clinician is carefully interviewed while watching a replay of the video to elicit their thinking during the encounter. This permits non-judgemental debriefing while providing the learner with specific triggers to help recall their thinking at particular points during a consul-

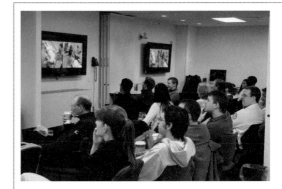

Figure 6.3 Review of a video encounter can help learners develop clinical reasoning skills. Photo by Laura Seul, copyright Northwestern Simulation.

tation. The SP can help stimulate recollection as well as explaining how they felt in response to the approach and actions of the learner at critical moments. Videos can be archived to demonstrate improvements in time, for appraisal or assessment purposes.

SPs as teachers

Using expert patients to teach medical students about their illnesses is long established, but the use of SPs as teachers is much less frequent. In the 1970s, Stillman *et al.* [25] developed the concept of SPs as 'patient instructors' (PIs). PIs are non-medical people taught to simulate an actual patient encounter and who function in the multiple roles of patient, teacher and evaluator. Careful preparation of the PIs demonstrated their ability to support effective teaching and assessment of interview skills [26]. In addition to communication and straightforward physical examination skills, some individuals now train to be Simulated Teaching Associates, with more precise titles describing the type of physical examination involved, e.g. Gynaecology Teaching Associates (GTAs) are trained women who support undergraduate medical students, postgraduate level nurses, midwives, GP trainees and others to perform speculum and bimanual examinations by acting both as an SP and teacher. Male Urogenital Teaching Associates (MUTAs) and Breast Teaching Associates (BTAs) are other examples of this concept.

SPs as assessors

Trained SPs are most commonly used to support formative assessment processes. Learners can receive instant feedback, which can mould their future behaviour and performance. Use of SPs demonstrates validity, reproducibility, reliability, and feasibility, providing they are properly trained and integrated into a well-designed scheme of assessment. The psychometric qualities of these assessments are less important especially when the SP is working under supervision of a clinical educator. However, the SP must have undergone appropriate preparation and training in feedback skills.

The use of SPs to evaluate clinical competence has also become commonplace in summative assessments, selection processes, and the examination of specific skills, particularly in multi-station OSCE examinations. SPs are accurate and consistent recorders of students' performances in clinical encounters [27]. SPs can portray the patient problem and record accurately on a checklist the precise actions performed by the examinee in the encounter, offering a valid and cost-effective method for recording information. SPs record items of history and the process of patient education more accurately than those of physical examination. Extra care is needed when developing checklists and training SPs specifically as recorders of information or as assessors who make judgements about a candidate's competence [12]. Although issues remain about using SPs instead of experienced clinicians, SPs can help to decrease the requirement for large numbers of senior clinicians to be present at multiple assessment stations in large institutions with complex assessment logistics. This use of SPs as assessors is more prevalent in North America than in the UK and other countries.

Collins and Harden [12] outlined several advantages of the use of SPs in assessment. Many of these advantages echo the benefits of their use for teaching:
• SPs may be more readily available than real patients and can be relied upon to be present.

• SPs can be trained to respond more consistently than real patients. Stations using SPs can be duplicated allowing multiple examinations to be administered. Using an SP can allow an examination to be standardized and used in different centres.
• The complexity of the presentation can be more easily controlled and matched to the stage of training of the examinee.
• SPs can be used in situations where the use of a real patient would be inappropriate e.g. counselling a patient with HIV or cancer.
• SPs may be more tolerant of multiple student exposures in an examination such as an OSCE than real patients.
• SPs offer an alternative method to help assess the learner's ability to evaluate and respond to some acute care conditions, often not possible in the clinical workplace
• SPs can be trained to assess the students' performance and provide feedback in both formative and summative assessments.
• Recruitment of SPs from the community contributes to the development of working partnerships and good relationships.
Disadvantages regarding the use of SPs in assessments include:
• It is time-consuming to recruit, train and organize SPs.
• SPs cannot completely duplicate the 'real patient'.
• There are some conditions are not easily assessed through simulation, e.g. the physical signs of goitre or oedema.

Using SPs to assess clinical practice and healthcare systems

SPs are also involved in remedial training and high-stakes assessment of fitness to practise for poorly performing practitioners where the requirement for face validity is high. If the assessment takes place in an environment similar to the workplace or in the workplace itself e.g. simulated surgeries [28,29] the face validity is even more impressive. Quality assurance and training is important to ensure the input of the SP is robust and sensitive enough to judge a clinician's ability to perform in the workplace on the basis of his/her performance in a simulated situation.

Rethans and van Boven [30] found that SPs produce reliable, valid and relevant data about the performance of GPs during patient consultations, discovering gaps or deficiencies in practice compared with national standards that otherwise would not have been identified [22]. Similar studies have demonstrated the feasibility of using SPs in this way in hospital clinics and community-based practices with extremely low recognition by practising clinicians that they were consulting with an SP. Elman *et al.* [31] studied the effectiveness of unannounced standardized patients in the clinical setting as a teaching intervention for medical students. During their family medicine rotation, in addition to the traditional method of teaching domestic violence in a seminar, one group of students encountered an unannounced SP portraying a scenario which stimulated exploring the possibility of domestic violence. Students received immediate feedback about their performance. Students who had undergone the SP intervention performed 'dramatically' better in a subsequent assessment on the subject of domestic violence than those who had only participated in the seminar.

The covert use of SPs may only be justified under certain conditions, i.e. a specific question is posed that can be answered by a limited number of SP cases, blinding is maintained, the patient's presentation is standardized, the SP accurately records relevant details of the visit and the aspect of the performance to be assessed can be evaluated during the first visit [32,33]. However, covert use of SPs may be perceived as unethical; therefore, any such exercises need to be carefully planned with proper consideration of the ethical, professional and practical issues. Research involving dental practitioners revealed the majority of clinicians recognized the value of covert SPs in considering how the outcome would improve future care in their practice [22].

Recruitment and selection of SPs

The criteria and processes for selecting SPs has received relatively little attention compared with studies exploring their use in educational and clinical contexts [34]. Barrows' early premise was that almost anybody could be trained as an SP provided they possessed the interest, intelligence, motivation

---

> **Box 6.3   Characteristics and attributes sought when selecting suitable SPs**
>
> - Intelligence and good recall
> - Good communication and interpersonal skills
> - Reliability and punctuality
> - Ability to work with others in a respectful manner
> - Ability to follow directions
> - Commitment to the education of health professionals
> - Lack of bias towards the healthcare system

and a flair for acting [10]. Others have added comments about the desire to enhance the education of health care professionals and improve the quality of healthcare delivery, but also highlight the benefits of availability and stamina.

Educational institutions use local advertisement campaigns [12], word of mouth, the internet and SP agencies to recruit and select SP's. Selection criteria should include the requirement for the SP to perform under varying conditions and contexts, and with different levels of responsibility for contributing actively to feedback (Box 6.3).

Criteria should also include broader professional behaviours, and attitudes and perspectives of the prospective SP toward health care, the system(s) in which it is organized and delivered, and toward the professionals (or students) who they will meet as part of their role. Negative attitudes or deeply held beliefs in any of these fields should preclude selection. SPs should be representative of the patient population they are asked to embody. Particular difficulties arise in recruiting for some cultural, age-related (i.e. paediatric) groups and those with learning or physical disabilities.

Some institutions use professional actors as SPs, especially where patient portrayals might require simulation of physical findings or be highly emotionally charged but for less complex scenarios willing, 'healthy' volunteers from many walks of life (including medical students) are used. Using medical students can provide a unique insight into the patients' perspectives on consultations which may help them become better doctors, develop their teaching skills and act as positive role models. As with all SPs, training and preparation is important as student SPs are more likely to overestimate performance of peers, tending to give the benefit of the doubt when experiencing ambiguous statements or questions and overlooking the use of technical language. Student SPs can however identify marginal students who need to improve significantly in the skill being assessed.

Being an SP

Few papers focus on how being an SP affects personal health and wellbeing but there is no evidence to suggest being an SP has any significant detrimental effect on physical or emotional health. Naftulin and Andrew [35] investigated the effects on a cohort of professional actors of simulating patients with 'a variety of physical and emotional disorders'. Many indicated that the most difficult aspect was repeating encounters frequently within two to three hours for several groups of medical students. They compared it with repeating 'takes' of a scene and that their energy and irritability increased with frequently repeated portrayals. Bokken *et al.* [36] found that 73% of SPs questioned had suffered (relatively mild) stress symptoms due to performing patient roles and suggest that more measures should be taken to prevent and treat these symptoms.

Woodward and Gliva-McConvey [37] studied SPs' perspectives of health professionals. They described a more balanced view of health professionals, better communication skills and becoming more tolerant of others. They became more critical and assertive consumers, more able to elicit higher quality, relevant information from physicians because they learned to ask good questions and were willing to change their doctors if they were unhappy. Regarding high-stakes examinations, the SPs recognized the value of experienced SPs providing well-rehearsed simulations, commenting that these were 'demanding, exhausting and exhilarating'.

Training and assessment of SPs

SP recruitment and training is the cornerstone of successful educational programming, although the

duration, content and quality of training varies considerably and there are no widely accepted training standards. These differences may persist due to a lack of clarity about the key competences or capabilities of an SP. In the USA, a movement towards standardizing training is supported through the creation of institutional consortia and the development of expert consensus with organizations such as ASPE. This emphasizes issues of quality assurance and standards, and introduces the concept of certification of SPs or their training programmes (see later). Other countries (such as the UK) are at an earlier stage of this journey. One driver in the US is that some SP educators (who train SPs) are not health professionals and thus must learn to take a clinical history and conduct physical examinations themselves in order to help facilitate SP training.

Box 6.4 sets out key factors to consider in training SPs.

Barrows [10] originally structured his training of the SP around the history, the physical findings, and the 'dress rehearsal' with a doctor which is observed by the SP Trainer. Clearly the experience of the SP in different types of educational encounter is a significant feature influencing the training process for these different exercises. Building on the

---

Box 6.4   Factors influencing the training requirements of the SP

Relating to the SP
- Experience as an SP
- Previous medical or health care knowledge
- Previous employment and frequency of work as an SP
- Familiarity with the patient or role characteristics from previous work or learning from scratch
- Presence of long term medical conditions

Relating to the educational context
- Complexity of the case to be simulated
- Requirement to recount history alone or simulate physical signs
- Planned involvement of the SP in any feedback elements
- Requirement of the SP to evaluate or assess performance of the learner

experiences and sharing the reflections of other SPs is valuable but requires time from SPs. Educators and faculty also need training in designing and supporting the delivery of educational encounters involving SPs.

Training SPs in the history and consultation

The method of coaching Barrows employed for developing SPs, using their own background and experience, is a recognizable adaptation of 'method acting'. In the UK, the 'Leicester Method' (introduced by the Simulated Patient Service at Leicester Medical School) is one well-described and replicated approach to help prepare SPs for consultation encounters with students or qualified practitioners [38]. Based on videotapes of actual general practice consultations, Collins and Harden [12] describe its structure as follows:

1. Consultations are recorded during a normal surgery where the patient characteristics appear to match the age and sex of the simulator.
2. The video recording is first seen by the simulator who decides whether it is possible to identify sufficiently with the patient.
3. The consultation is then discussed exhaustively at a mutual viewing with the doctor who recorded the consultation (the originating doctor). The simulator is encouraged to enquire from the patient's perspective about issues relevant to the consultation. Factual information about the patient not known by the trainer can be hypothesized by the simulator as long as this is then incorporated into the patient's character, a process described as 'creative consistency'. Such additions, which are never medical, are only made to sustain credibility.
4. The simulator decides how to present the patient. For some cases the symptoms, body language and voice are telling enough. In others, credibility is helped by attention to hair style, dress or distinctive items such as spectacles or a handbag. Personal effects help the simulator become the patient.
5. The patient simulator has 'first time' consultations with at least four other trainer doctors.
6. The SP and the originating doctor decide which issues are to be assessed in the training consultation, which are then incorporated into a checklist.

One study exploring the use of SPs to assess clinicians in practice [20] collected data on the accuracy of portrayal and the reliability of assessment during the day of training of the SPs. Across all scenarios, 1038 of 1164 (89%) clinical features were portrayed correctly and this consistency of portrayal was helped by the SPs watching a video of their planned performance before each consultation. This reinforces the Leicester method and offers some direction for those managing an SP service about archiving performances captured on video for future viewing and preparation. SPs can reflect on their performance through self- and peer evaluation which can be helped through access to live or archived video resources, although this has cost and logistical implications.

Training SPs to portray physical signs

McDowell [39] evaluated clinical performance in nurse practitioners using SPs and noted 'the limited range of physical signs which can be replicated' however Barrows [10] lists a wide range of physical findings which can be simulated by SPs, even including pneumothoraces (collapsed lung) or thyroid bruits. Training SPs to exhibit complex signs requires specific expertise and good actors. For example, to simulate a pneumothorax the SP manipulates their body so that asymmetric breathing is apparent during gross observation and when the doctor listens with a stethoscope. Many other physical signs such as limb weakness or sensory changes are obviously much easier to simulate. With good make-up, signs such as cyanosis, sweating, pallor and jaundice can be simulated.

Hybrid simulation refers to the combination of an SP with other simulation techniques to address some of the limitations of SPs and enhance the reality of encounters. It is becoming increasingly sophisticated. Examples of hybrid simulation are the combination of an intravenous access task trainer with an SP or the use of a sound generating stethoscope to produce abnormal cardiorespiratory abnormalities such as wheezes, crackles or murmurs when the chest is auscultated. Hybrid simulation should be distinguished from multimodal simulation which is the use of two or more simulation techniques within a simulation, e.g. an SP acting as a relative to a manikin patient.

Training SPs to provide feedback and facilitate a small group

Stillman [25,26] recognized the potential of SPs as teachers, but commented that this level of capability takes time to develop and should not be assumed to be desired or within the reach of all. However, SPs should be available and skilled in giving feedback to the learners immediately after the encounter, bringing their perspective through the 'lens' of the patient or another role. Various authors have described the method and language for the feedback process (Box 6.5 for one useful model used at Maastricht Medical School), although a recent systematic review described this process as heterogeneous in preparation and practice [40].

One important facet is whether this feedback is provided 'in role' (i.e. still portraying the feelings, emotions and perspective of the actual person portrayed) or 'out of role' where the SP can articulate these same emotions and reactions but from a third-party position and hence facilitate reflection in the learner with different types of question.

Some SPs receive training to facilitate the teaching session themselves, either alongside a clinical educator or unsupervised. This requires deeper engagement with the design of the session and its learning outcomes, and a clearer picture of how this integrates with other educational activities and the real-world experiences of the learners. In common with any educator involved in SBE, these SPs need to develop and demonstrate skills of small group facilitation, and ideally have some degree of knowledge regarding theories of adult learning.

Training the trainers and clinical educators

Trainers of SPs should have some background in clinical medicine or work very closely with someone who does. Clinical educators and faculty (as 'users' of the SP as an educational resource) need to be well prepared when they are either designing the learning encounter in which the SP will feature, or when they are facilitating the actual session itself. The SP

> **Box 6.5** Rules of feedback developed for use by SPs, based on a model from Maastricht Medical School (Source Cleland and Rethans [43])
>
> **Priority** – start feedback by answering the student's (learner's) questions about the achievement of his or her individual learning goals. After this, the SP can broaden feedback to matters that felt significant and relevant to the SP or in response to inquiry from the learner or peer group.
>
> **Domain** – only give feedback with regard to his or her own experiences as a patient during the encounter with the student (i.e. no feedback on medical content).
>
> **Perspective** – SPs should give feedback from their own point of view, using 'I statements', for example, 'I didn't feel comfortable during the conversation since I didn't understand your questions' instead of 'You should be more clear because people don't understand your questions and then feel uncomfortable'.
>
> **Neutrality** – SP should not give judgments about the student's performance, positive nor negative, and focus this feedback to the individual student whilst refraining from making comparisons with fellow students, for example 'You listened to me very well' instead of 'You listened better than the other student I have spoken with'.

may come with a great depth of abilities, experiences and expectations about how they might contribute to the learning experience. If the faculty member/educator is not familiar with the use of SPs, they may well underutilize the skills available or inadvertently redirect the focus of the session. In this respect the situation is similar to that in any form of SBE. Much will depend on the educator's skills and familiarity with the educational resources available in order to achieve the learning objectives intended.

Assessment of SP preparation

Having clear objectives and competences for SP training enables assessment criteria to be developed, described by Adamo [41] as training and post-training characteristics (Box 6.6).

Ideally these should be tailored to the educational context for which the SP is being prepared, and hence will underpin 'fitness for purpose' for the SP in relation to this work. The rigour of this assessment will be determined by available resources and informed by the level of complexity and consequences of the SP role, especially if they are to have a role in providing feedback or summative assessment. The consequences of unsatisfactory performance by an SP may affect the learners behaviours and practice for some time, and in turn could influence patient care.

Assessment methods to provide assurance that an SP is prepared sufficiently include self and peer evaluation and portraying their case to the teaching faculty before being used to teach and/or assess students. Assessment should include:

• Accuracy – how clearly does the SP replicate the picture?
• Consistency – how reproducible is the representation by the SP?
• Replicability – does the portrayal of the same patient on different occasions or by different SPs achieve the same interaction?
• Portability – can the simulation be produced at different sites?

Wind *et al.* [42] developed a written checklist (the Maastricht Assessment of Simulated Patients, MaSP) which addresses authenticity of portrayal and feedback following consultation and was based on interviews with students, teachers and experts involved with SPs. The psychometric properties of this tool were shown to be satisfactory when SP encounters take place for educational purposes, emphasizing the value of authenticity of role play and the quality of feedback in these circumstances. The authors emphasized that consistency and uniformity of role play becomes increasingly relevant when the SP participates in high-stakes assessment exercises.

Box 6.6   Training and post-training characteristics used to assess SP preparation (Source Adamo [41])

Training characteristics
The SP should be able to demonstrate:
• Promptness and preparedness.
• Ability to adapt to varying interviewing styles.
• Ability to sustain affective portrayal per case requirement.
• Ability to adapt behaviour as a result of coaching /feedback
• Active listening skills.
• Ability to extrapolate from training experiences to varied stimuli in application.

Post-training characteristics
In order to be deemed suitable as an SP at the end of a training process the SP will:
• Be able to demonstrate stable findings on repeated physical examination.
• Provide evidence of consistent recording accuracy to enable accurate feedback by the faculty educator or the SP
• Be able to deliver constructive feedback from the patient perspective in role or out of role, referenced to specific episodes during the learner interaction, and under supervision or unsupervised according to requirements

---

Professional and personal development

The recruitment and preparatory processes for new and existing SPs is an investment made by the institution responsible for the SP service and a fundamental component of the quality assurance framework. There is little published about standards of practice (i.e. selection, training, assessment, ongoing development) but the subject is currently being debated within learned organizations in medical and healthcare education in various countries and statements are anticipated shortly. These will identify features of good practice agreed at a personal or organizational level, and will enable commissioners and regulatory bodies for healthcare education to consider how they are referenced and monitored in quality assurance processes.

For those managing SP services, key areas that need to be addressed include:

• Evidence of maintaining key skills and development of new capabilities, through keeping a personal portfolio which is shared with the service managing the SPs for monitoring and appraisal purposes.

• Reviewing personal attitudes and beliefs, which might form part of an annual appraisal process.

• Reviewing personal physical and mental health, mediated via GPs or occupational health services in order to maintain confidentiality.

• Developing an appraisal tool kit and passport that details relevant qualifications and professional development activities.

SUMMARY

The benefits of developing high-quality SB educators as faculty (whether they be clinicians, academics, simulated patients, technical or administrative staff) needs to be recognized at several levels within healthcare: the individual educator, the team(s) or service in which they practice or support health care delivery, and the organization itself that has responsibility for overall quality and safety of care to individual patients and communities.

The SB educator can have an important contribution individually in the clinical environment through personal supervision, instruction, facilitation or assessment of performance of learners. This may include integrating the use of simulation alongside practice to enhance learning opportunities, or by helping translate and embed learning from a separate simulated experience into the clinical context.

The translation of learning between different contexts and levels of complexity is a critical insight to develop in learners, especially if attempting to support the trajectory of learning from achieving competency to that of proficiency, mastery and even expert performance. The educator plays a critical role in sharing this mental model, and in reinforcing the need for learners to reflect 'in practice', 'on practice' and 'for practice' in order to improve individual performance.

As simulated patients also become more professionalized, the need for accrediting individual SPs (or agencies) and quality assuring training and assessment of SP capabilities is emerging. This is particularly pertinent in relation to the role of SPs in high-stakes assessments, professional development and revalidation and aligns with the implementation of standards for clinical educators/supervisors (e.g. from regulatory bodies such as the UK General Medical Council). The US ASPE and the UK Association for Simulated Practice in Healthcare (ASPiH) are currently discussing the place of accreditation and certification of SP educators (i.e. those who recruit and train the SPs) and SPs.

Advantages for the professionalization of SPs relate to improving employability and pay conditions and the portability of qualifications within healthcare education systems. An 'SP passport' will provide evidence of training, qualifications, accredited professional development activity, appraisals by approved managers, and perhaps some form of individual certification (especially if wishing to participate in high-stakes assessment). The extent to which SPs will replace clinical educators in teaching and assessment also remains to be seen, but there are strong arguments to suggest this is a possibility.

Future developments will focus on developing the opportunities and establishing motivation to support collaboration amongst the different stakeholders and interested parties on national and international scales. This will enable a consensus on relevant standards of SP practice which recognize and support the professional and valuable contribution SPs make towards workforce development and health improvements.

✓ **Key points**

- The ethical and professional values of SB educators and simulated patients are the same as for all educators.
- The contextual roles and approaches an effective SB educator has to adopt are wide and varied.
- SB educators can and should be educational leaders.
- SPs provide a valuable service in offering learners the patient's perspective.
- Developing and supporting SB educators and SPs requires institutional support and continuing professional development in alignment with national and international trends towards professionalization.
- The attributes required to support effective feedback and debriefing are a fundamental influence on effective learning.

REFERENCES

1. Higher Education Academy (HEA) (2011). *The UK Professional Standards Framework*. York: HEA. Available from http://www.heacademy.ac.uk/ukpsf (accessed 6 Match 2013).

2. Academy of Medical Educators (2012). *Professional Standards*. London: AoME http://www.medicaleducators.org/index.cfm/profession/profstandards/ (accessed 6 March 2013).

3. General Medical Council (2012). *Recognising and Approving Trainers: the Implementation Plan*. London: GMC. Available from http://www.gmc-uk.org/education/10264.asp (accessed 6 March 2013).

4. Gaba D (2004) The future vision of simulation in health care. *Quality & Safety in Health Care* **13:** i2–i10.

5. Schön D (1987). Teaching artistry through reflection-in-action. In: *Educating the Reflective Practitioner*. San Francisco: Jossey-Bass: 22–40.

6. Harden R, Crosby J (2000) AMEE Educational Guide No 20. The good teacher is more than a lecturer – the twelve roles of the teacher. *Medical Teacher* **22:** 334–347.

7. Issenberg *et al* (2005) Features and uses of high-fidelity medical simulations that lead to effective learning: a BEME systematic review *Medical Teacher* **27:** 10–28.

8. McGaghie WC, Issenberg SB, Petrusa ER, Scalese RJ (2010) A critical review of simulation-based medical education research: 2003–2009. *Medical Education* **44:** 50–63.

9. Hesketh E, Bagnall G, Buckley EG, *et al.* (2001) A framework for developing excellence as a clinical educator *Medical Education* **35:** 555–564.

10. Barrows H (1993). An overview of the uses of standardized patients for teaching and evaluating clinical skill. *Academic Medicine* **68:** 443–453.

11. Association for Standardized Patient Educators (2011) http://www.aspeducators.org/terminology-standards (accessed 6 March 2013).

12. Collins JP, Harden RM (1998) AMEE Medical Education Guide No. 13: Real patients, simulated patients and simulators in clinical examinations. *Medical Teacher* **20:** 6; 508–521.

13. Barrows H, Abrahamson S (1964). The programmed patient: a technique for appraising student performance in clinical neurology. *Journal of Medical Education* **39:** 802–805.

14. Harden R, Stevenson M, Downie WW, Wilson GM (1975) Assessment of clinical competence in using objective structured examination. *British Medical Journal* **1:** 447–445.

15. Van der Vleuten C, Swanson D (1990) Assessment of clinical skills with standardised patients: state of the art. *Teaching and Learning in Medicine* **2:** 58–76.

16. Miller G (1990). The assessment of clinical skills/competence/performance. *Academic Medicine* **65:** S63–67.

17. Hargie O, Dickson D, Boohan M, Hughes K (1998) A survey of communication skills training in UK Schools of Medicine: present practices and prospective proposals. *Medical Education* **32:** 25–34.

18. Kneebone R, Kidd J, Nestel D, *et al.* (2002) An innovative model for teaching and learning clinical procedures. *Medical Education* **36:** 628–634.

19. Ker S (2003) Developing professional skills for practice – the results of a feasibility study using a reflective approach to intimate examination. *Medical Education* **37** (Suppl 1)**:** 34–41.

20. Grant C, Nicholas R, Moore L, Salisbury C (2002) An observational study comparing quality of care in walk-in-centres with general practice and NHS Direct using standardised patients *British Medical Journal* **324:** 1556.

21. Rethans J, Sturmans F, Drop R, van der Vleuten C (1991) Assessment of the performance of general practitioners by the use of standardised (simulated) patients. *British Journal of General Practice* **41:** 97–99.

22. Hazelkorn H, Robins L (1996). Actors play patients. Using surrogate patients to look into private practice. *Public Health Reports* **111:** 129–132.

23. Pickard S, Baraitser P, Rymer J, Piper J (2003). Can gynaecology teaching

associates produce high quality effective training for medical students in the United Kingdom? *British Medical Journal* **327:** 1389–1392.

24. Nestel D, Muir E, Plant M, *et al.* (2002) Modelling the lay expert for the first-year medical students: the actor-patient as teacher. *Medical Teacher* **24:** 562–564.

25. Stillman P, Ruggill JS, Rutala PJ, Sabers DL (1980) Patient instructors as teachers and evaluators. *Journal of Medical Education* **55:** 186–193.

26. Stillman PL, Regan MB, Philbin M, Haley HL (1990) Results of a survey on the use of standardised patients to teach and evaluate clinical skills. *Academic Medicine* **65:** 288–292.

27. Vu N, Marcy MM, Colliver JA, *et al* (1992) Standardized (simulated) patients' accuracy in recording clinical performance check-list items. *Medical Education* **26:** 99–104.

28. Fraser RC, McKinley RK, Mulholland H (1994) Consultation competence in general practice: testing the reliability of the Leicester assessment package. *British Journal of General Practice* **44:** 293–296.

29. Allen J, Rashid A (1998) What determines competence within a general practice consultation? Assessment of consultation skills in simulated surgeries. *British Journal of General Practice* **48:** 1259–1262.

30. Rethans J, van Boven C (1987) Simulated patients in general practice: a different look at the consultation. *British Medical Journal (Clinical Research Education)* **294:** 809–812.

31. Elman D, Hooks R, Tabak D, *et al.* (2004) The effectiveness of unannounced standardised patients in the clinical setting as a teaching intervention. *Medical Education* **38:** 969–973.

32. Tamblyn R (1998) Use of standardised patients in the assessment of medical

practice. *Canadian Medical Association Journal* **158**: 205–207.

33. Kinnersley P, Pill R (1993) Potential of using simulated patients to study the performance of general practitioners. *British Journal of General Practice* **43**: 297–300.

34. O'Connell CA, Thayer-Doyle C (1993) Examining whether certain Myer-Briggs 'personality preferences' can be used to select standardized patients. *Academic Medicine* **68** 931.

35. Naftulin D, Andrew B (1975) The effects of patient simulations on actors. *Journal of Medical Education* **50**: 87–89.

36. Bokken L, van Dalen J, Rethans JJ (2004) Performance–related stress symptoms in simulated patients. *Medical Education* **38**: 1089–1094.

37. Woodward C, Gliva-McConvey G (1995) The effect of simulating on Standardised Patients. *Academic Medicine* **70**: 418–420.

38. McAvoy B (1998) Teaching clinical skills to medical students: the use of simulated patients and videotaping in general practice. *Medical Education* **22**: 193–199.

39. McDowell B, Nardini DL, Negley SA, White JE (1999) Evaluating clinical performance using simulated patients. *Journal of Nursing Education* **23**: 37–39.

40. Bokken L, Linssen T, Scherpbier A, *et al.* (2009) Feedback by simulated patients in undergraduate medical education: a systematic review of the literature. *Medical Education* **43**: 202–210.

41. Adamo G (2003) Simulated and standardised patients in OSCEs: achievements and challenges 1992–2003. *Medical Teacher* **25**: 262–270.

42. Wind L, Van Dalen J, Muijtjens AM, Rethans JJ (2004) Assessing simulated patients in an educational setting: the MaSP (Maastricht Assessment of Simulated Patients). *Medical Education* **1**: 39–44.

43. Cleland, AK, Rethans JJ (2009) The use of simulated patients in medical education. AMEE Guide No. 12. *Medical Teacher* **31**: 477–486.

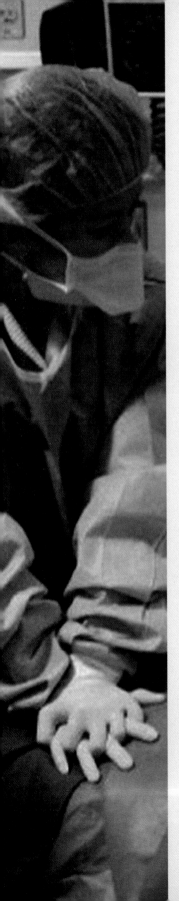

CHAPTER 7

Surgical technical skills

Rajesh Aggarwal and Amit Mishra   Imperial College London, London, UK

Overview

Delivery of high-quality and safe clinical care is the aggregate of a host of factors. Sound organizational structures, adequate resources for service and education provision and a comprehensive health policy provide a conducive framework in which health professionals can use their skills to deliver the best-quality care. The acquisition of appropriate clinical skills over time, allows medical professionals to effectively assess and recognize problems and to formulate management plans. For effective patient management, specialized medical professionals are required who have good technical skills and the non-technical skills of leadership, communication and appropriate decision-making strategies to deliver this care.

Technical skills have traditionally been held as the most important quality for a surgeon and as the specialty has expanded to incorporate innovations such as laparoscopic surgery, single incision laparoscopic surgery (SILS) and natural orifice transluminal surgery (NOTES) into standard practice, the training challenges have grown. Towards the end of the twentieth century, an exponential increase in computing power, technological advances in imaging and fibreoptics have prompted the development of many new interventional techniques in non-surgical specialties such as endoscopic procedures in gastroenterology and interventional cardiology. Additionally, the advent of interventional radiology in the latter half of twentieth century has created a new branch of clinical medicine.

For such training situations, simulation can be a very effective technical skills training tool offering a

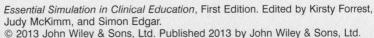

Essential Simulation in Clinical Education, First Edition. Edited by Kirsty Forrest, Judy McKimm, and Simon Edgar.
© 2013 John Wiley & Sons, Ltd. Published 2013 by John Wiley & Sons, Ltd.

Overview (ctd)

controlled and risk-free environment where trainees can be taught, trained and objectively assessed in simple technical skills such as suturing through to full surgical or anaesthetic procedures. There can be no substitute for real clinical and operative experience, which is how surgical skills were traditionally taught via an apprenticeship model, neatly summarized by the mantra of 'see one, do one, teach one'. The increasing range of skills surgeons need to acquire means that this model cannot accommodate modern training needs, especially not without compromising patient safety. Simulators allow the inevitable errors that occur during the early stages of skills acquisition to occur in a safe environment without any adverse events involving real patients. Patient safety and quality of care have become central considerations in healthcare worldwide. Simulation has had great success in other fields at improving safety, as training errors and learning curves are removed from real life consequences and it is in this critical role that they play in patient safety that is proving to be the real driver in their development.

This chapter will consider the use of simulation in surgical technical skills training for teaching, assessment, continuing professional development and revalidation, and the training infrastructure that needs to be developed for effective delivery.

Technical skills

Technical skills are of fundamental importance in surgical practice and are at the heart of achieving good surgical outcomes. Technical skills have traditionally been taught in an apprenticeship model where the trainee learns their operative experience under the supervision and guidance of an experienced trainer.

However, in the last two decades, advances in fibreoptics have allowed endoscopic surgical techniques to develop and flourish, often as a first-line choice [1]. The advent of endoscopic surgery has revolutionized surgical practice across specialties, with thoracoscopic, laparoscopic and arthroscopic surgical skills becoming part of the required repertoire of surgeons in those fields. These surgical modalities present a completely different set of psychomotor requirements from those of open techniques. The challenges include operating ambidextrously using rigid instruments through small incisions which causes a fulcrum effect, all in a confined three-dimensional (3D) surgical field while simultaneously observing the field on a separate two-dimensional (2D) screen. These skills need

to be learned in addition to open surgical skills in often a reduced training period [2].

Laparoscopic abdominal surgery was one of the earliest forms to be incorporated into standard practice. Within 5 years of the first reported video-assisted laparoscopic cholecystectomy, performed by Philip Mouret in France in 1987 [3], the procedure had become established, not only as a credible alternative to open cholecystectomy [4] but was indeed being considered as the gold standard for the treatment of symptomatic cholelithiasis [5,6,7,8,9]. It was during these early years when the pace of surgical developments was so rapid that doubts regarding the safety and technical skills ability of established expert surgeons performing these new procedures surfaced. Particularly evident were the increased risk of errors and complications during the initial learning stages. It was initially thought that previous surgical experience would allow for rapid uptake of the new skills, but it was found that previous experience was not a factor, and across all levels of experience errors were increased during the learning curve stage of new skills acquisition [10,11,12].

As new technical skills requirements have mushroomed, there has been a growing realization by surgeons that they must adopt a different operational model. The 2008 UK Healthcare Commission found that breaches in patient safety had a major impact on clinical outcomes and patients' experiences; 3–16% of inpatient surgical procedures being associated with major complications, resulting in permanent disability or death in 0.4–0.8% [13]. In addition to the human cost of patient adverse events, the ensuing financial and reputational cost to the clinician and organization is often irreparable. This places increasing pressure on organizations to address deficiencies in the factors that affect patient safety. While non-technical skills play a large role in patient safety, the role of technical skills errors still remains significant. Lessons from other high-reliability organizations, particularly civil and military aviation have therefore been adapted to great effect in technical skills training.

Table 7.1 Validity in surgical simulation	
Validity in surgical simulators	
Contruct validity	Ability of simulator to discriminate between different levels of expertise
Content validity	Does simulator test technical skills specifically *(rather than anatomical knowledge for example)*
Face validity	Extent to which the simulated tasks resembles real operative tasks
Predictive validity	Ability of performance on simulator to predict operative performance

Adapted from Reznick *et al.* 1993. Teaching and testing technical skills. American journal of surgery [16].

Simulation in technical skills training

Throughout human history the link between excellence in organizational performance and simulated practice has been well known. Josephus, a contemporary historian, observed of the ancient Roman Army 'They do not begin to use their weapons first in time of war as they have never any truce from warlike exercises.' [14]. By the 1990s, the use of simulators in technical skills training was already established as an integral part of training in other high-reliability organizations such as aviation and nuclear energy, yet their use in medical training lagged behind, perhaps partly due to much greater visibility and publicity of adverse events in the other industries.

Within technical skills training, a range of simulation modalities have evolved as technology has allowed, but for practical use in training programmes, simulators must demonstrate their effectiveness both for skills acquisition and as assessment tools. Evaluation of effectiveness should be based on sound evidence to justify the high levels of investment: financial, space and human resources required to establish and maintain good-quality training infrastructure. Simulation training systems must demonstrate validity, reliability and feasibility in both teaching and assessment [15,16] (Table 7.1).

Box trainers simulation (endotrainers)

Box trainers or endotrainers were used early on for laparoscopic skills training, offering a simple, versatile and relatively inexpensive training tool [17]. These consisted of a box approximating the size of a human abdomen covered with an opaque membrane to represent the outer abdominal wall. Through this wall, real instrument ports can be inserted either using trochars or through prefabricated slits in the membrane, following which laparoscopes and real laparoscopic instruments are inserted and used to manipulate the contents of the trainer (Figure 7.1). These can vary from simple objects used to teach basic psychomotor skills such as transferring rings across different pegs using a grasper, through to animal tissue, including porcine gallbladders, used to simulate handling of real organic tissue. The trainee can thus familiarize themselves with the look, tactile experience and motor properties of the real instruments they would use intraoperatively and, especially when combined

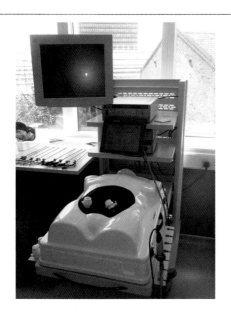

Figure 7.1 Box trainer.

with the use of animal tissue, the trainer provides a similar haptic experience to real surgery. Such tasks provide the backbone of the training and evaluation systems which utilize the box trainers. As box trainers and associated training programmes have developed contemporaneously with the development of laparoscopy, this has allowed the development and testing of structured training systems.

Of the existing training systems, one of the most extensively researched is MISTELS (McGill Inanimate System for Training and Evaluation of Laparoscopic Skills), which was developed at McGill University in Montreal in the late 1990s. Using a panel of experienced laparoscopic surgeons, the main challenges of laparoscopic surgery compared with open surgery were identified from a series of videos of different laparoscopic procedures. From these, specific domains were selected for focused training and evaluation and standardized tasks devised to teach them [18]. This ultimately led to MISTELS. MISTELS consists of a standardized set of five tasks performed on an endotrainer. The trainee first watches a video demonstrating proper performance of these tasks and then carries out these tasks and is scored for time (classed as effi-

ciency) with a penalty score applied for errors being deducted from efficiency to give a final score for each task.

The validity of the MISTEL score was assessed in a multicentre study involving 250 subjects from across five countries and demonstrated a significant difference in scores between junior, intermediate and senior level surgeons, with scores increasing with level of training, furthermore this result was independent of the testing site and shown to correlate highly with intraoperative technical skills measurements [19]. MISTELS provides a robust example of a structured technical skills training programme, which has identified key technical skills; developed objective and valid metrics to assess these skills, shown an acquisition and improvement of these skills with practice on the system and demonstrated translation of this into the operating theatre with improved operative performance. MISTELS provided the technical skills component of a more comprehensive laparoscopic training skills program developed by the Society of American Gastrointestinal Endoscopic Surgery (SAGES) known as Fundamentals of Laparoscopic Surgery (FLS). FLS also includes digital written chapters on the theory and principles of laparoscopic surgery and written assessments, combining teaching and assessment of both the principles and theoretical knowledge underpinning laparoscopy with the technical skills training. Extensive testing of validity and reliability has solidified the effectiveness of FLS as a global laparoscopic skills training programme [19,20,21,22,23,24]. Now recommended by SAGES for all senior residents wishing to demonstrate laparoscopic competency, FLS represents a comprehensive program with simulation at the heart of technical skills acquisition.

Combined with the relative maturity of endotrainer-based programs, relatively low acquisition and maintenance costs have allowed them to become the most widespread training modality available [2]. As minimally invasive techniques have spread, these trainers prove especially valuable providing a relatively cheap and proven education tool in healthcare systems which have significantly less financial resources and lack the IT support and infrastructure required to field more complex computer simulation systems.

Animal training models

At first glance this method might offer a solution for simulation training. Practising procedures on live anaesthetized animals, usually porcine or canine models to approximate human sizes and anatomy, offers the most realistic comparison to the real operative environment. Trainees are able to practice full procedural technical skills on live tissue, with face validity, haptic (tactile) and visual feedback closely resembling real human procedures. Additionally, faculty can integrate non-technical skills training such as team communication into the simulation to provide a truly comprehensive experience.

However, significant issues prevent the large-scale use of animals. Providing full operating theatre facilities, the use of actual operative equipment and the provision of proper animal welfare make this a very costly endeavour compared to other simulators which limits the frequency of their use. It is also difficult to objectively measure psychomotor parameters of performance without the increased expense of developing technologies such as eye and hand motion tracking to accurately assess progress. Perhaps more relevantly in Europe, huge ethical issues are involved in breeding and keeping live animals for operating practice. While there are surgical skills training centres that use animal models in Europe, their use in the United Kingdom is currently illegal. Ultimately these factors rule out animal models as a viable model for large-scale technical skills training.

Virtual reality simulators

Used to great effect in aviation where it is now an indispensable part of training, virtual reality (VR) simulation has seen a slow and at times stagnant role in surgical skills training. Insufficient computing power to accurately simulate the complex environment and tasks involved, combined with a lack of funding comparison with that which military and corporate aviation receives, led to educators not truly utilizing the enormous potential offered by VR until relatively recently. The exponential increase in computing power throughout the 1990s combined with a concurrent fall in cost and a strong emphasis on safety now provide the ideal environment for full use of this modality in technical skills training. The nature of modern minimally invasive interventions, such as endoscopic surgery and interventional radiology, as procedures are visualized on a 2D screen, lend themselves easily to VR simulation. VR simulators offer a versatility and adaptability not seen in other modalities. Computer systems can be constantly upgraded, new programs can be added with relative ease, and VR offers a natural education medium for the current generation of trainees. However, before their integration into formal programmes, VR simulations must face the same scrutiny and demonstrate all the required criteria of any other system, with the added dimension that while there are only a few kinds of box trainer, there are many different companies producing hugely different VR simulators with different capabilities and tasks. The added corporate pressure on generating sales to cover the development costs, which can be many times that of a box training system, and ultimately a profit, can further complicate the issue as companies must compete to gain academic validation and institutional sales.

At the most basic level, VR simulators comprise a computer core, visual display and psychomotor input devices, usually in the case of laparoscopic simulators a pair of instrument handles. Beyond this, they vary greatly in terms of tasks, graphics and fidelity of simulation. The earlier systems offered an array of abstract tasks such as grasping and manipulation of simple virtual objects and, as graphical power grew, they allowed the representation of simulated tissue with increasing fidelity and visual face validity. Minimally invasive surgery (MIS) uses mainly visual and tactile, sensory modalities. Realistic tactile feedback has been more difficult to incorporate into VR than other simulation methods, but limited haptic feedback (discussed later in the chapter) has been incorporated into newer systems.

Minimally invasive surgery trainer–virtual reality

As with all technology ventures, there can be a high attrition rate, with many products being shelved in the early development stages. One system that has proven itself repeatedly is the minimally invasive surgery trainer–virtual reality (MIST-VR).

Developed in the mid-1990s in the UK, the MIST-VR has evolved into one of the most extensively tested systems available and is now available commercially via Mentice, a Swedish company based in Gothenburg [25]. MIST-VR consists of a PC linked to an apparatus containing two laparoscopic instruments held in position-sensing gimbals, the movements of which are translated into a real-time graphical display of the instruments interacting with virtual objects within an operative field represented by a virtual cube. Whereas prior systems had attempted to provide an accurate visual representation of tissues, the designers of MIST-VR had a more novel approach. They first tried to define the specific technical skills required in minimally invasive surgery and how these skills (rather than the procedure itself) could be taught. Initially, an ergonomic analysis of the psychomotor skills involved in performing a laparoscopic cholecystectomy was performed, through this a series of simplified part tasks were identified which would represent the basic skills needed for ambidextrously holding and manipulating tissue and application of electrocautery [26]. These were then represented by a series of real-time abstract tasks, which would show movement and errors in real time, culminating in the development of core skills modules.

Technical skills training content, assessment and validity

The core skills modules form the foundation of the system: beginning with the simple manipulation and passing of a virtual sphere from one instrument to the other, with tasks increasing in complexity and difficulty, to maintaining the virtual sphere's position in a confined space with one instrument and applying diathermy to randomly appearing objects on the sphere's surface (Figure 7.2) [27]. Precise measurement of motion of the instruments in 3D space and their interaction with virtual objects allowed performance to be broken down into specific parameters. While it was known that experienced surgeons performed tasks more quickly, MIST-VR provided an ideal test bed to elucidate what other parameters are experience dependent

and allowed for a more detailed analysis of technical skills. Taffinder *et al.* [28] demonstrated construct validity of the error, economy of motion and time parameters providing the opportunity for an objective target level of skill to be set. Pooled data from expert performance were used to provide a benchmark which trainees can aim for, with competition being a strong motivating factor.

Curriculum development

Once simulators had evolved to the degree where they could effectively teach technical skills and practice would improve these skills, the problem of structure remained. VR simulation again offered a solution; first by giving instant objective feedback to trainees set against objective data on expert performance, which provided a well-defined set of targets. Second, VR simulators provided incremental levels of difficulty to stretch the trainee's skills set. Practising increasingly technically challenging tasks would theoretically increase trainees' skills until they reached these objective targets, enabling a proficiency-based model of education as opposed to one based on time spent in training or numbers of procedures performed. A structured curriculum in VR skills training needed to be developed, and a team from Imperial College London and Toronto jointly developed the MIST-VR curriculum. While the skills acquisition properties of the MIST-VR had been well demonstrated [28,29,30], subjects had been trained using a random series of tasks or an arbitrary number of repetitions without any evidence to demonstrate how many repetitions, and at what level, of a task were required to reach proficiency.

A study was conducted where subjects were familiarized with the core skills modules by performing all 12 tasks, then randomized into two groups, one continuing to train on all the tasks and the other continuing only with the two most complex. Those in the latter group reached proficiency (in the two most complex tasks) in a shorter time than in the former. This allowed the development of an evidence-based VR training curriculum for the MIST-VR with proficiency as defined by expert level objective performance as the goal. This provided a prescriptive training programme that

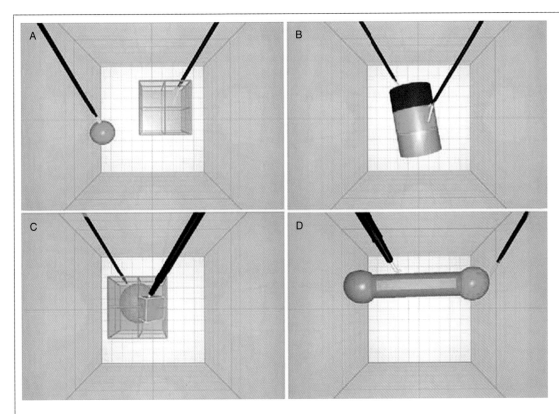

Figure 7.2 MIST-VR core skills tasks. Tasks on the MIST-VR laparoscopic simulator: A. Acquire Place. B. Traversal. C. Task 6, Core Skills 1, Manipulate Diathermy. D. Task 6 Core Skills 2, Stretch Diathermy.

gave novices the technical skills required to be safe participants and assistants in real laparoscopic procedures [31]. The concept of proficiency-based graded training curricula, developed and validated initially on MIST-VR, provided a general framework for the development of similar curricula on future simulators (Table 7.2) [32].

Translation into the operating room

Translation of simulation training into improved patient outcomes remains the ultimate vindication of VR simulation training programmes; however, given the multitude of other factors that have to be controlled for and the resulting size and complexity of any studies, demonstrating this remains difficult. Despite this, solid evidence for VR training improving operative performance and technical skills justify its formal inclusion in curricula [33,34,35,36] (Figure 7.3). Conclusive validation of a proficiency-based curriculum and demonstrated operative benefits lend great credence to the incorporation of a MIST-VR-based training programme into formal education. As a mature and relatively inexpensive VR system, MIST-VR provides for large-scale surgical education, combined with video tutorials and theoretical manuals, and is an integral part of junior surgical training in many places. Although newer simulators might be eclipsing MIST-VR in technological terms, its proven effectiveness in technical skills acquisition warrants its inclusion into basic skills courses, at least while other systems are still in the testing stages. It certainly fills a niche in the training market for a basic laparoscopic skills trainer that is simple, inexpensive and uses simple abstract tasks to teach basic laparoscopic skills. In this sense

Table 7.2 Translation of MIST-VR training to operative performance, whats the evidence?

Study	Methodology	Training model	Assessment task	Assessment method	Result
Hamilton *et al.* (2001)	Randomized trial	Time-based training	Laparoscopic cholecystecomy (human)	Blinded rater: Global Rating Scale	Operative performance improved with training
Ahlberg *et al.* (2002)	Randomized trial	Time-based training	Laparoscopic appendicectomy (porcine)	Blinded rater: video analysis	Operative performance no better with training (VR performance correlated with OR performance)
Seymour *et al.* (2002)	Randomized trial	Proficiency-based training	Laparoscopic cholecystecomy (human)	Blinded rater: video analysis	Operative performance improved with training
Grantcharove *et al.* (2003)	Randomized trial	Fixed repetitions	Laparoscopic cholecystecomy (human)	Blinded rater: video analysis	Operative performance improved with training

Adapted from Seymour (2008) [36] VR to OR: a review of the evidence that virtual reality simulation improves operating room performance.

it is relatively future-proof as its utility as a trainer does not depend on high-fidelity graphics or haptics.

High-fidelity simulators: LapSim

Expanding computer graphics capabilities have allowed for increasingly realistic representations, and a great deal of research interest has now shifted to more high-fidelity simulators. LapSim, developed by Surgical Science AB, Sweden, demonstrates the natural evolution of MIS simulators. The basic skills modules consist of simulated tasks which trainees could expect to perform in theatre, including camera and instrument navigation, tissue grasping and clip application in a reasonably high-fidelity visual environment. In addition to these basic tasks, trainees must complete a procedural module, which includes dissection of Calot's triangle, clipping and cutting the cystic ducts and avoiding damage to the adjacent structures (Figure 7.4). LapSim was devel-

oped at a time when the zeitgeist had firmly shifted towards VR simulation in training, as older trainees became new consultants, attitudes towards VR became much more accepting and brought with it more widespread interest and funding.

With an established development pathway from validation, to curriculum implementation to operative transference devised with earlier simulators, progress with LapSim was even more rapid. Protocols and experiments already devised to test and develop the MIST-VR programme were replicated and reused and introduced in 2001, it was extensively validated a few years later [37,38,39]. Similarly an experimentally validated proficiency-based curriculum was devised, utilizing a similar protocol to the MIST-VR proficiency-based curriculum. Again, pooled expert performance was used to establish proficiency criteria. Trainees completed basic tasks at increasing difficulty levels and practised on more technically complex tasks at the

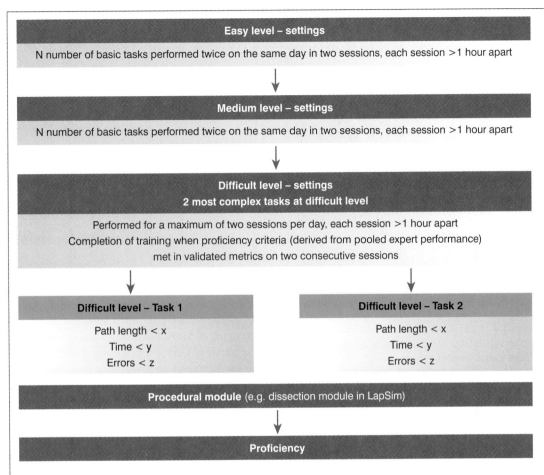

Figure 7.3 Virtual reality training curriculum for technical skills training. A general example of a proficiency based VR training curriculum for the acquisition of technical skills. Adapted from Aggarwal *et al.* 2006. A competency-based virtual reality training curriculum for the acquisition of laparoscopic psychomotor skill [31] and Aggarwal *et al.* 2006. An evidence based virtual reality training program for laparoscopic surgery [32].

higher difficulty setting. The addition of a simulated gallbladder dissection task allowed trainees to practice at least part of a real surgical procedure. This was incorporated into the curricula as the final task, and it was expert performance on this task that was used to determine proficiency. The candidate would work through the curriculum, which demonstrated a defined learning curve with improvements in time, economy of movement and errors, until achieving the pre-set criteria for the simulated procedural task, at which point they would be deemed proficient [32].

When the LapSim curriculum was used in a randomized trial to train novice laparoscopic surgeons using already established principles for VR simulator validation and curricula, both the tool and the course could be tested. Those who had structured VR training performed significantly better on cadaveric porcine models than those who didn't. This difference eventually disappeared as more porcine operations were performed but this demonstrates exquisitely one of the original aims of simulation in training: to reduce the learning curve on real operative procedures, while minimizing risk to the patient (Figure 7.5). The incorporation of the transfer effectiveness ratio (TER) from the airline industry also demonstrated that one minute on the simulator was roughly equivalent to two and a half minutes on the porcine cholecystectomy. The TER provides an objective measure of the time and cost-effectiveness of this particular simulator and gives an effective comparison of different systems, which in the future can be used to decide which systems receive educational funding [40].

Haptic feedback

Visual fidelity continues to increase in all computing mediums; it remains however only one sensory modality in MIS, for true fidelity the tactile experience must also be simulated. Simulators must therefore provide haptic feedback via a series of motors incorporated into the simulated instruments. Currently haptic simulation is in its infancy. Like the rudimentary graphics of early simulators, the haptic experience often remains crude and unrealistic. The motors are currently unable to match the subtleties of differing human tissues, compounded by the fact that inherently there is greater variation in human perception of haptics. Whereas a trainee can easily see a photo of Calot's triangle and therefore recognize the structures on a screen or intra-operatively

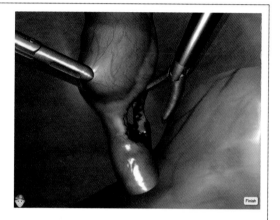

Figure 7.4 Example of procedural task, dissection module on LapSim. Reproduced with permission from Wolters Kluwer Health.

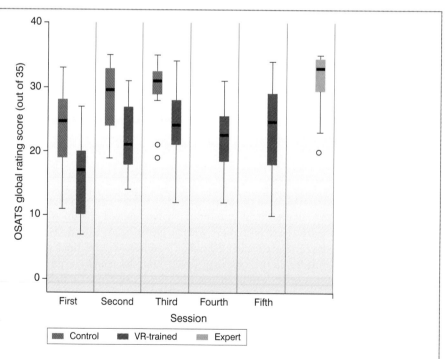

Figure 7.5 Reduced learning curve after training on virtual reality simulator (Aggarwal *et al.* 2007).

they must grasp a real gallbladder to first 'feel' the haptic experience. The Simbionix LAP Mentor is at the forefront of haptic technology in MIS simulation. One of the first procedural simulators, it can simulate the intra-abdominal parts of performing a laparoscopic cholecystectomy in high graphic fidelity. In addition to instant measurement of psychomotor parameters, the LAP Mentor also offers full video recording of virtual procedures enabling the assessment of procedural skills via objective rating scales such as Objective Structured Assessment of Technical Skill (OSATS). LAP Mentor's use as a procedural training tool has been validated [41] and these skills have been shown to be transferrable between procedures, with use improving performance extending to unrelated laparoscopic procedures. Lucas *et al.* found that medical students who trained on the VR LC module performed better procedurally on live porcine laparoscopic nephrectomy as measured by the OSATS rating tool [42].

Tactile feedback can be disengaged allowing the device to be its own control and accurately assess the effect of haptics on training. At present this has been somewhat anticlimactic with studies showing limited impact on training, and it remains to be seen whether haptic simulators' utility as psychomotor and procedural skills trainers are significantly enhanced by the haptic feedback which adds greatly to costs [43,44]. Despite disappointing results so far, it would be presumptuous to discount the effects of incorporating tactile responses. Like all nascent technologies, the underlying factors that comprise effective simulated haptic feedback remain to be fully explored. These include questions about how best to model the tissues and the physical response they give which could be simulated by having deformable materials within the simulator or by subtle motors [45].

Future potential of procedural simulators

The full potential of procedural simulators remains untapped; they can offer an unprecedented level of preparation, 3D imaging modalities such as CT or MRI can be used to generate VR models and construct a library of varying anatomies and challenging scenarios [45]. A significant percentage of surgical resources in the developed world are devoted to the multidisciplinary management of cancer with patient pathways ensuring that expert surgeons prior to any operation review detailed imaging with consultant radiologists. Surgical oncology provides a uniquely varied and challenging experience and one could foresee the incorporation of imaging in constructing anatomically accurate procedural simulations allowing senior surgeons to practise the more challenging cases. Developing this potential of VR simulation becomes even more imperative when we consider that the consultant surgeons of the future will have spent a fraction of the hours training compared to the cohort now approaching retirement. A catalogue of difficult cases with unexpected challenges could be included in expert certification assessments, ensuring lead surgeons are familiar with scenarios they may never have seen in the real operating environment.

Ultimately close collaboration is required between clinicians, materials scientists and IT specialists to provide a detailed multidisciplinary perspective in accurate and effective simulation training and indeed in determining what level of accuracy is most appropriate given the financial constraints on health systems worldwide.

Widespread dissemination of the principles and development pathways of VR simulator training (Figure 7.6) has allowed for its organic proliferation across interventional specialities; arthroscopic, thoracoscopic and endovascular simulators are being developed and researched internationally in what promises to be an exciting future [46,47,48]. In particular the adoption of endovascular techniques potentially offers an even larger technical skills jump from traditional open surgery especially in the visual component. Abdominal and thoracic surgeons can still visualize the operative field in full colour video through endoscopes but vascular trainees must acquire visual recognition skills more akin to interventional radiology with the extensive use of intraoperative fluoroscopy. In this too VR training has proved effective [49].

Simulation in Interventional Specialities

Once the dividing line was clear between craft and non-craft specialities, basically surgeons cut,

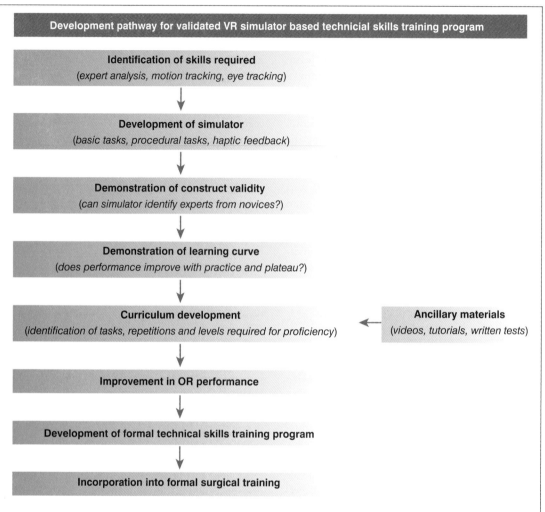

Figure 7.6 Development pathway for validated virtual reality simulator-based technical skills training programme.

physicians did not. This has been the case for the better part of half a century. While the endoscopic camera was the key to minimally invasive surgery, it also heralded a shift in other fields with specialties such as gastroenterology and respiratory medicine incorporating minimally invasive interventional procedures into their service provision. The most radical shift has been the advent of interventional radiology (IR), which has displaced surgery as the first line treatment for some patient groups. Percutaneous coronary artery stenting, endovascular aortic aneurysm repair (EVAR) and radiological guided embolization of bleeding vessels all represent procedures available to patients which would have previously required a surgeon to treat the underlying pathology. These other craft specialities face the same challenges as surgery, namely an ever increasing technical skills set requirement coupled with an decrease in training time and opportunities;.

VR simulators for training seem the ideal choice in such a procedure intensive specialty in which the operator must combine viewing radiological imaging both static and dynamic with fine motor skills. Similar to surgical VR simulators, IR and endoscopic simulation systems require a similar process to develop as fully fledged training tools requiring multidisciplinary involvement during the development stages, validation as training and assessment tools and development of structured curricula. Aside from these general principles however, IR technical skills vary greatly from MIS. Instead of rigid instruments visualized continuously through a full colour camera, IR operators must often navigate endoluminal channels of differing anatomy with flexible guide wires, catheters and stents while visualizing position and orientation through a sequence of static radiological images.

While the principles behind simulation training are well-known, they remain to be widely applied to the field of IR with a relative scarcity of research compared to MIS trainers.

In terms of the specific systems developed, the Procedicus Vascular Interventional System Trainer (VIST) is among the most studied. This consists of a mechanical system housed within a plastic manikin, which is connected to a PC with a dual screen display. Modified instruments can be inserted through an access port, inside which a series of motorized carts lock onto it allowing the subject to manipulate the instrument in real-time and providing simulated haptic feedback [50]. As with other systems, objective performance criteria both generic and unique to the specialty must be identified and validated. In terms of generic measures, time has been identified as being dependent on expertise, with experienced operators requiring less total fluoroscopy time, thereby limiting radiation exposure to patients and staff. Specialty specific metrics can also be accurately measured and recorded including contrast use and accuracy of stent placement, both of which are of importance in patient outcomes. Face and construct validity have been demonstrated in a number of trials already and the system has progressed to commercialization with modules available for training in atherosclerotic disease (carotid, renal and iliofemoral regions) and interventional cardiology procedures [50]. The Procedicus VIST also remains the only major system to have demonstrated transfer of skill to actual in vivo procedures. Specifically trainees who completed the ilio-femoral modules have demonstrated improved objective performance in both porcine models and real

patients [49,50,51]. In such a rapidly developing specialty, the ability of VR trainers to adapt and incorporate new techniques and procedures will ensure their development and use will continue to expand and evolve.

Integration of simulation into formal technical skills training

Surgical training pathways vary globally and technical skills training is just one of many components. In general, training can be divided into undergraduate training, general junior grades with both medical and surgical rotations and specialty training. At the undergraduate level, many schools do not offer a formal technical skills course, the merits of programmes at this level can be debated. When considering that most interns/foundation trainees will have some exposure to the operating theatre it may be wise to include basics such as knot tying and suturing as a mandatory part of training. In North America and increasingly in the United Kingdom, trainees are specializing earlier and joining formal structured training programmes. Formal technical skills training should be a required part of this early on and many programmes already include simulation on models and endotrainers, for example the Basic Surgical Skills course run by the UK Royal Colleges provides simulated practice on porcine cadaveric tissue and laparoscopic box trainers. Beyond this however, there is no one standard simulation course. It is at this stage where VR simulation could feasibly be incorporated.

A proposed model for surgical simulation training

Taking general surgery training, the MIST-VR trainer provides a good basis for a basic laparoscopic skills course. Such a course would include lectures and videos on the principles and practice of endoscopic surgery including camera and instrument handling; training would follow on the simulator using a validated curriculum with proficiency-based assessment at the end. Once this has been completed trainees would receive formal certification allowing them to progress up the training ladder.

The next step would be training on procedural simulators such as the LAP Mentor, again using a formal curriculum and proficiency-based assessment, which could include a global rating of a simulated procedure. At the end of this a trainee would have a portfolio of certification at each level, complete with trainee specific objective data such as learning curves, performance on specific parameters and a full global rating scale assessment of procedural skills. Armed with such preparation the trainee would enter theatre with a detailed knowledge of the underpinning theory and principles and an extensive simulated experience of the technical skills. Continued intra-operative assessment from supervisors could highlight areas of weakness, which need to be addressed. The trainee would then return to the simulation lab and practice these without having to wait for further cases. While clinical experience will remain the main determining factor in technical skills, VR simulation especially would provide a key component of training, reducing learning curve errors on real patients and ensuring trainees are adequately prepared before real operative experience (Case study 7.1).

Case study 7.1 Laparoscopic cholecystectomy

Laparoscopic cholecystectomy (LC) remains the gold standard treatment of symptomatic gallstone disease and will represent one of the most common procedures a junior surgical trainee will perform. Hence technical skills training in this procedure is of great importance.

A hypothetical training ladder, which would impart these skills, would involve the following steps.

1. Theoretical and anatomical teaching of principles underlying procedure and technical skills required.
2. Basic training using a box trainer/endotrainer using the FLS course
3. Completion of MIST-VR structured curriculum (conferring basic psychomotor skills such as instrument handling and localization)
4. Completion of LapSim structured curriculum (conferring part task skills such as clip applying and cutting).
5. Completion of LAP Mentor structured curriculum (conferring full procedural skills with haptic feedback)
6. Training on porcine models (allowing trainee to gain high fidelity visual and haptic experience)
7. Assistance on full patient LC with supervisor feedback.
8. Further training if required on simulators, addressing issues highlighted
9. Completion of full patient LC under supervision
10. Continued assessment, feedback and further training
11. Attainment of expertise with further operative and simulated experience.

Beyond technical skills training: selection, stressors and revalidation

As valid assessors of technical skills, the integration of these tools in surgical practice can be expanded beyond the training ladder itself, feasibly being used to decide who gets onto the ladder and who exits at the top. With other high reliability organizations, candidate selection is a critical step in producing high quality, highly skilled human resources, without this step thousands of hours of training and money can be wasted on candidates ultimately unsuitable for the role.

While an extensive set of criteria are used in candidate selection, technical skills (specifically the potential to rapidly and effectively acquire them) should be an integral part of the selection process. Simulators have demonstrated discriminative validity, some have specifically recognized a subset of trainees who have particular difficulty in skills acquisition [52] and while it may seem callous to exclude these potential surgeons from training, if we are to improve patient safety, more stringent selection criteria must be applied. Other high reliability organizations have stringent exclusion criteria, for example candidates who are unable to cope with the complex spatial perception requirements of air traffic control are excluded early on. Similarly, within the UK ballistic missile submarine fleet, officer selection pushes candidates to their psychological limit in terms of stress, with significant communication and information overload, those who meet the requirements are further tested to determine their own personal failure points. Selection and training has led to both organizations having improved safety records with the majority of workers being able to perform their duties under considerable pressures at a high level of performance [53].

While surgeons are not entrusted with such large scale and potentially globally devastating responsibilities, a surgeon who has difficulties acquiring new technical skills can have distressing consequences on individual patients and their families. Notwithstanding the increased length of time needed to train and remediate such individuals on training programmes, further research is required across the board to demonstrate if VR simulators can identify those with difficulty in skills acquisition and exclude those who would present the greatest patient risk. As with all performance, technical skills vary within individuals from day to day in response to external stressors. Surgeons must cope with the challenges of mental and physical stress and fatigue, all of which have an effect on technical performance but have not been fully been explored. VR Trainers offer a safe and ethical way in which to assess the effects of these stressors in a scientific manner, identify which individuals are most at risk and determine which countermeasures are most effective. Stress, sleep deprivation and alcohol are all examples of factors which have been demonstrated to adversely affect psychomotor performance on VR simulators, ethically providing evidence to incorporate strategies which reduce their effects on surgical practice [54,55,56,57,58]. This evidence vastly strengthens the case for limiting these effects and

selecting candidates most resilient to these stressors in a profession, which has been known for an element of cultural bravado. Trainees may dismiss these effects but there can be no arguing with an objectively measured drop in performance.

As surgical procedures evolve, patient outcomes and consumer pressure increases demand for newer techniques. It was patient demand as well as reduced complications that ultimately led to the widespread uptake of MIS. If these same principles carry forward to other techniques like single incision laparoscopic surgery (SILS) it will again redefine the skill set required of expert surgeons. In such a rapidly changing environment the expert can again become a novice in the space of a few years. VR simulator development has been increasingly streamlined and future proofed, meaning that as new procedures and techniques are developed, the relevant training simulator modules and programs can be developed and incorporated into existing systems at an equal pace. Experts will require reaccreditation or revalidation as techniques and surgery evolve, VR simulation with its proven efficacy and adaptability provides the best tool to ensure that experts remain just that.

Infrastructure

Apple Computers began life in a garage and, as the company's products metamorphosed into the ubiquity we see today, extensive infrastructure capabilities were required to rapidly design, test, produce and maintain its products and customer base. VR Simulation can be viewed in a similar way, a relatively obscure and novel technology now maturing into an effective tool. As such, manufacturing companies require streamlined development and production capabilities to deliver quality products at reasonable cost and the support services to maintain them. Apart from the commercial dimension, education and professional certification organizations require a whole different set of infrastructure requirements. Investment in a simulation based training program requires careful consideration of the needs of learners, the financial and space resources of the organization and the availability of good trainers.

A future 'virtual' reality

Major cities such as London represent one example; a global city with numerous medical institutes of academic renown, with high population density, a large number of surgical trainees on centralized training programs and the resources to provide the highest quality tools. These factors would justify the investment in developing a centralized simulation centre, providing simulation in minimally invasive surgery, endoscopy and radiology. This could incorporate lecture theatres, VR simulation suites adopting developed training curricula with a full time complement of educational and support staff. Once developed it could provide high volume, high-quality skills education, combining a variety of aspects of performance including non-technical skills, to trainees with the potential to produce highly skilled, motivated professionals delivering a world class level of quality.

Conversely smaller centres could incorporate skills laboratories into hospital education centres perhaps with smaller regional hubs. As technology grows, obsolete tools could be recycled or donated and utilized in low resource settings, providing valuable skills training in health systems, which cannot field such costs on their own.

SUMMARY

From a novelty in its early days, simulation has developed into a complete pedagogy. Evolving from simple box trainers to rudimentary VR simulators in the nascent days of personal computing, well-validated simulation systems now employ proven and structured curricula to teach technical skills in a safe and reliable way. These skills can then be transferred into real operations improving patient outcomes and safety.

What is required is a full commitment by the profession and the incorporation of a long-term strategic view of this medium. Health authorities and governments must then provide the resources to deliver this high quality training on a large scale ultimately delivering high quality care to patients.

✓ Key points

- Simulation is an adjunct to clinical and operative experience NOT a replacement.
- The primary driving force of simulation in technical skills education is patient safety by reducing errors.
- Simulation systems must be validated and feasible as training tools.
- Training should be structured into validated curricula with objective proficiency based assessment.
- Simulation based training should demonstrate improved operative outcomes, most importantly in the learning curve stage, for it to improve patient safety.

REFERENCES

1. Harrell AG, Heniford BT (2005) Minimally invasive abdominal surgery: lux et veritas past, present, and future. *American Journal of Surgery* [Comparative Study Review] **190:** 239–243.

2. Roberts KE, Bell RL, Duffy AJ (2006) Evolution of surgical skills training. *World Journal of Gastroenterology* [Review] **12:** 3219–3224.

3. Litynski GS (1999) Profiles in laparoscopy: Mouret, Dubois, and Perissat: the

laparoscopic breakthrough in Europe (1987–1988). *Journal of the Society of Laparoscopic Surgeons* [Biography Historical Article Portraits] **3**: 163–167.

4. Olsen DO (1991) Laparoscopic cholecystectomy. *American Journal of Surgery* **161**: 339–344.

5. Trade M, Troidl H, Herfarth C, *et al.* (1992) [Should laparoscopic cholecystectomy be already regarded as the gold standard in bland cholecystolithiasis?]. *Langenbecks Archiv fur Chirurgie* **377**: 190–194.

6. Sain AH (1996) Laparoscopic cholecystectomy is the current 'gold standard' for the treatment of gallstone disease. *Annals of Surgery* [Comment Letter] **224**: 689–690.

7. Begos DG, Modlin IM (1994) Laparoscopic cholecystectomy: from gimmick to gold standard. *Journal of Clinical Gastroenterology* [Review] **19**: 325–330.

8. Moss G (1995) Laparoscopic cholecystectomy and the gold standard. *Journal of Laparoendoscopic Surgery* [Editorial] **5**: 63–64.

9. Ido K, Kimura K (1996) [Endoscopic treatment of digestive system diseases. 5. Laparoscopic cholecystectomy has become the gold standard of cholecystectomy]. *Nihon Naika Gakkai Zasshi* **85**: 1450–1453.

10. Hawasli A, Lloyd LR (1991) Laparoscopic cholecystectomy. The learning curve: report of 50 patients. *The American Surgeon* **57**: 542–544; discussion 5.

11. Cagir B, Rangraj M, Maffuci L, Herz BL (1994) The learning curve for laparoscopic cholecystectomy. *Journal of Laparoendoscopic Surgery* **4**: 419–427.

12. Moore MJ, Bennett CL (1995) The learning curve for laparoscopic cholecystectomy. The Southern Surgeons Club. *American Journal of Surgery* [Research Support, U.S. Gov't, Non-P.H.S.] **170**: 55–59.

13. Vincent C, Neale G, Woloshynowych M (2001) Adverse events in British hospitals: preliminary retrospective record review. *British Medical Journal* [Research Support, Non-U.S. Gov't] **322**: 517–519.

14. Josephus F, Thompson E, Price WC, Rouben Mamoulian Collection (Library of Congress). *The Works of Flavius Josephus.* London: Printed for Field and Walker 1777.

15. Reznick RK (1993) Teaching and testing technical skills. *American Journal of Surgery* **165**: 358–361.

16. Moorthy K, Munz Y, Sarker SK, Darzi A (2003) Objective assessment of technical skills in surgery. *British Medical Journal* [Research Support, Non-U.S. Gov't Review] **327**: 1032–1037.

17. Sackier JM, Berci G, Paz-Partlow M (1991) A new training device for laparoscopic cholecystectomy. *Surgical Endoscopy* **5**: 158–159.

18. Derossis AM, Fried GM, Abrahamowicz M, *et al.* (1998) Development of a model for training and evaluation of laparoscopic skills. *American Journal of Surgery* [Research Support, Non-U.S. Gov't] **175**: 482–487.

19. Fried GM, Feldman LS, Vassiliou MC, *et al.* (2004) Proving the value of simulation in laparoscopic surgery. *Annals of Surgery* [Clinical Trial, Randomized Controlled Trial, Research Support, Non-U.S. Gov't Validation Studies] **240**: 518–525; discussion 25–28.

20. Peters JH, Fried GM, Swanstrom LL, *et al.* (2004) Development and validation of a comprehensive program of education and assessment of the basic fundamentals of laparoscopic surgery. *Surgery* [Validation Studies] **135**: 21–27.

21. Vassiliou MC, Ghitulescu GA, Feldman LS, *et al.* (2006) The MISTELS program to measure technical skill in laparoscopic

surgery: evidence for reliability. *Surgical Endoscopy* [Evaluation Studies, Research Support, Non-U.S. Gov't] **20**: 744–747.

22. Swanstrom LL, Fried GM, Hoffman KI, Soper NJ (2006) Beta test results of a new system assessing competence in laparoscopic surgery. *Journal of the American College of Surgeons* [Evaluation Studies Research Support, Non-U.S. Gov't] **202**: 62–69.

23. Vassiliou MC, Feldman LS, Andrew CG, *et al.* (2005) A global assessment tool for evaluation of intraoperative laparoscopic skills. *American Journal of Surgery* [Evaluation Studies, Research Support, Non-U.S. Gov't] **190**: 107–113.

24. McCluney AL, Vassiliou MC, Kaneva PA, *et al.* (2007) FLS simulator performance predicts intraoperative laparoscopic skill. *Surgical Endoscopy* [Validation Studies] **21**: 1991–1995.

25. Wilson MS, Middlebrook A, Sutton C, *et al.* (1997) MIST VR: a virtual reality trainer for laparoscopic surgery assesses performance. *Annals of the Royal College of Surgeons England* [Research Support, Non-U.S. Gov't] **79**: 403–404.

26. McCloy R, Stone R (2001) Science, medicine, and the future. Virtual reality in surgery. *British Medical Journal* [Review] **323**: 912–915.

27. Gallagher AG, Boyle E, Toner P, *et al.* (2011) Persistent next-day effects of excessive alcohol consumption on laparoscopic surgical performance. *Archives of Surgery* [Comparative Study, Randomized Controlled Trial] **146**: 419–426.

28. Taffinder N, Sutton C, Fishwick RJ, *et al.* (1998) Validation of virtual reality to teach and assess psychomotor skills in laparoscopic surgery: results from randomised controlled studies using the MIST VR laparoscopic simulator. *Studies in Health Technology and Informatics* [Comparative Study] **50**: 124–130.

29. Gallagher AG, Satava RM (2002) Virtual reality as a metric for the assessment of laparoscopic psychomotor skills. Learning curves and reliability measures. *Surgical Endoscopy* **16**: 1746–1752.

30. Chaudhry A, Sutton C, Wood J, *et al.* (1999) Learning rate for laparoscopic surgical skills on MIST VR, a virtual reality simulator: quality of human-computer interface. *Annals of the Royal College of Surgeons England* [Research Support, Non-U.S. Gov't] **81**: 281–286.

31. Aggarwal R, Grantcharov T, Moorthy K, *et al.* (2006) A competency-based virtual reality training curriculum for the acquisition of laparoscopic psychomotor skill. *American Journal of Surgery* **191**: 128–133.

32. Aggarwal R, Grantcharov TP, Eriksen JR, *et al.* (2006) An evidence-based virtual reality training program for novice laparoscopic surgeons. *Annals of Surgery* **244**: 310–314.

33. Hamilton EC, Scott DJ, Fleming JB, *et al.* (2002) Comparison of video trainer and virtual reality training systems on acquisition of laparoscopic skills. *Surgical Endoscopy* [Comparative Study Research Support, Non-U.S. Gov't] **16**: 406–411.

34. Seymour NE, Gallagher AG, Roman SA, *et al.* (2002) Virtual reality training improves operating room performance: results of a randomized, double-blinded study. *Annals of Surgery* [Clinical Trial, Randomized Controlled Trial, Research Support, Non-U.S. Gov't] **236**: 458–463; discussion 63–64.

35. Grantcharov TP, Kristiansen VB, Bendix J, *et al.* (2004) Randomized clinical trial of virtual reality simulation for laparoscopic skills training. *British Journal of Surgery* [Clinical Trial, Randomized Controlled Trial, Research Support, Non-U.S. Gov't] **91**: 146–150.

36. Seymour NE (2008) VR to OR: A review of the evidence that virtual reality

simulation improves operating room performance. *World Journal of Surgery* **32**: 182–188.

37. Duffy AJ, Hogle NJ, McCarthy H, *et al.* (2005) Construct validity for the LAPSIM laparoscopic surgical simulator. *Surgical Endoscopy and Other Interventional Techniques* **19**: 401–405.

38. Woodrum DT, Andreatta PB, Yellamanchilli RK, *et al.* (2006) Construct validity of the LapSim laparoscopic surgical simulator. *American Journal of Surgery* **191**: 28–32.

39. van Dongen KW, Tournoij E, van der Zee DC, *et al.* (2007) Construct validity of the LapSim: Can the LapSim virtual reality simulator distinguish between novices and experts? *Surgical Endoscopy and Other Interventional Techniques* **21**: 1413–1417.

40. Aggarwal R, Ward J, Balasundaram I, *et al.* (2007) Proving the effectiveness of virtual reality simulation for training in laparoscopic surgery. *Annals of Surgery* **246**: 771–779.

41. Aggarwal R, Crochet P, Dias A, *et al.* (2009) Development of a virtual reality training curriculum for laparoscopic cholecystectomy. *British Journal of Surgery* **96**: 1086–1093.

42. Lucas SM, Zeltser IS, Bensalah K, *et al.* (2008) Training on a virtual reality laparoscopic simulator improves performance of an unfamiliar live laparoscopic procedure. *Journal of Urology* **180**: 2588–2591.

43. Salkini MW, Doarn CR, Kiehl N, *et al.* (2010) The role of haptic feedback in laparoscopic training using the LapMentor II. *Journal of Endourology* **24**: 99–102.

44. Thompson JR, Leonard AC, Doarn CR, *et al.* (2011) Limited value of haptics in virtual reality laparoscopic cholecystectomy training. *Surgical Endoscopy and Other Interventional Techniques* **25**: 1107–1114.

45. Basdogan C, Sedef M, Harders M, Wesarg S (2007) VR-based simulators for training in minimally invasive surgery. *IEEE Computer Graphics* **27**: 54–66.

46. Gomoll AH, O'Toole RV, Czarnecki J, Warner JJ (2007) Surgical experience correlates with performance on a virtual reality simulator for shoulder arthroscopy. *American Journal of Sports Medicine* **35**: 883–888.

47. Solomon B, Bizekis C, Dellis SL, *et al.* (2011) Simulating video-assisted thoracoscopic lobectomy: a virtual reality cognitive task simulation. *Journal of Thoracic and Cardiovascular Surgery* [Research Support, Non-U.S. Gov't] **141**: 249–255.

48. Tedesco MM, Pak JJ, Harris EJ, Jr., *et al.* (2008) Simulation-based endovascular skills assessment: the future of credentialing? *Journal of Vascular Surgery* **47**: 1008–1001; discussion 14.

49. Chaer RA, Derubertis BG, Lin SC, *et al.* (2006) Simulation improves resident performance in catheter-based intervention: results of a randomized, controlled study. *Annals of Surgery* [Randomized Controlled Trial] **244**: 343–352.

50. Neequaye SK, Aggarwal R, Van Herzeele I, *et al.* (2007) Endovascular skills training and assessment. *Journal of Vascular Surgery* [Review] **46**: 1055–1064.

51. Berry M, Lystig T, Beard J, *et al.* (2007) Porcine transfer study: virtual reality simulator training compared with porcine training in endovascular novices. *Cardiovascular and Interventional Radiology* [Comparative Study Randomized Controlled Trial] **30**: 455–461.

52. Gallagher AG, Lederman AB, McGlade K, *et al.* (2004) Discriminative validity of the Minimally Invasive Surgical Trainer in Virtual Reality (MIST-VR) using criteria levels based on expert performance. *Surgical Endoscopy and Other Interventional Techniques* **18**: 660–665.

53. Rogers PN (2010) Safety in surgery: is selection the missing link? *World Journal of Surgery* **34:** 2001–2002.

54. Moorthy K, Munz Y, Dosis A, *et al.* (2003) The effect of stress-inducing conditions on the performance of a laparoscopic task. *Surgical Endoscopy and Other Interventional Techniques* **17:** 1481–1484.

55. Rotas M, Minkoff H, Min D, Feldman J (2007) The effect of acute sleep deprivation and alcohol consumption on simulated laparoscopic surgery. *Obstetrics and Gynecology* **109:** 9s-s.

56. Taffinder NJ, McManus IC, Gul Y, *et al.* (1998) Objective assessment of the effect of sleep deprivation on surgical psychomotor skill. *British Journal of Surgery* **85:** 1578–1579.

57. Dorafshar AH, O'Boyle DJ, McCloy RF (2002) Effects of a moderate dose of alcohol on simulated laparoscopic surgical performance. *Surgical Endoscopy and Other Interventional Techniques* **16:** 1753–1758.

58. Crochet P, Aggarwal R, Mishra A, *et al.* (2009) Caffeine and taurine reverse the deterioration in laparoscopic and cognitive skill following sleep deprivation. *Journal of the American College of Surgeons* **209:** S111–S.

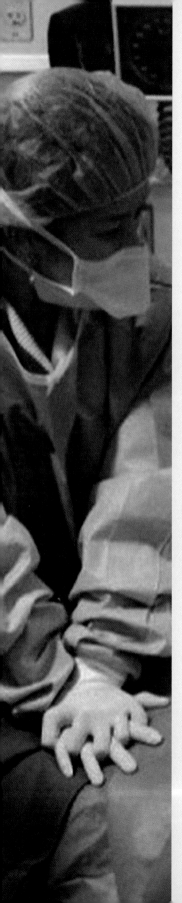

CHAPTER 8
The non-technical skills

Nikki Maran[1], Simon Edgar[2] and Alistair May[1]   [1]Scottish Clinical Simulation Centre, Larbert, UK, [2]NHS Lothian, Edinburgh, UK

Overview

There is increasing awareness of the existence and importance of non-technical skills (NTS) in clinical practice including the introduction of classification frameworks relating to clinical care. Simulated practise can raise awareness of the importance of NTS for learners to enhance more than just psychomotor skills. This chapter provides an introduction to NTS and ideas and techniques for incorporating NTS learning outcomes into simulation based education.

We discuss how teachers can incorporate NTS based learning outcomes into simulation scenarios and explain the different meanings of terms such as non-technical skills (NTS), Cockpit/Crew/Crisis Resource Management (CRM) and Human Factors. This chapter also highlights the key aspects of non-technical clinical performance and the benefits and challenges inherent in incorporating non-technical learning outcomes into scenario design.

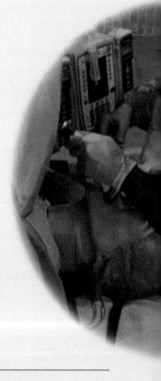

Essential Simulation in Clinical Education, First Edition. Edited by Kirsty Forrest, Judy McKimm, and Simon Edgar.
© 2013 John Wiley & Sons, Ltd. Published 2013 by John Wiley & Sons, Ltd.

Human factors and non-technical skills in safety

Research in a number of high-reliability domains such as aviation, oil production and nuclear power generation has demonstrated that, despite high levels of technical skills training, the majority of incidents and accidents are caused by human error. The term 'human factors' refers to the 'environmental, organisational and job factors, and human and individual characteristics which influence behaviour at work in a way which can affect health and safety' [1]. By studying the science of human factors, psychologists use theory, principles, data and methods to design systems in order to optimize human well-being and overall system performance. This includes a range of approaches, including studying tasks and technologies (ergonomics), the skills of individuals (NTS) and organizational culture.

NTS are the cognitive and social skills used by experienced professionals. They underpin and enhance technical skills, improving safety by helping people to anticipate, identify and mitigate against errors. We know from accident analyses and psychological research in other high-reliability domains that failures of NTS such as poor teamwork, communication and leadership and flawed decision making contribute to many adverse incidents and accidents.

Much of the early work in this area was carried out in the airline industry, which quickly realized that these issues were not being addressed by the very comprehensive but highly technically focused training which was delivered at the time. The response to this was to develop training to help staff understand the problems of human error and human performance limitation and to develop the NTS required to avoid, mitigate and manage emergency situations. This training, known as cockpit resource management **(CRM)** was initially developed for pilots but was rapidly extended to include all staff (crew resource management). The 'CRM' skills highlighted on these courses were not new – they had always been accepted as part of 'good airmanship' – but in identifying and making the particular skills more explicit, it allowed more effective training to be developed. In order to allow NTS to be assessed more accurately, **behavioural marker**

systems such as NOTECHS (NOn-TECHnical Skills) [2] were developed. By providing objective examples of specific observable behaviours these frameworks can be used to give focused formative feedback during simulator and line-of-flight training and assessment. For example, in the category of **cooperation**, the sub-element of **supporting others** has a behavioural (observable) example of 'Giving help to other crew members in cases where they need assistance.' In recent years, summative assessment of NTS has been incorporated into both initial assessment and ongoing relicensing procedures.

CRM training in healthcare

Growing concerns about safety in healthcare in the mid-1990s led to specific studies looking at the causes of adverse events. In the USA, David Gaba and colleagues were among the first to recognize that many of the principles of CRM training could be applied to healthcare, particularly in the management of anaesthetic critical incidents. Their early simulator studies [3] demonstrated that anaesthetists were often slow to recognize critical incidents, and even when they did so they often failed to work effectively with others to manage the problem effectively. Gaba *et al.* [4] identified principles from CRM which could be applied in the operating room to improve early identification and management of crises. These CRM key principles (Box 8.1) became the focus of the development of their simulator based Anaesthesia Crisis Resource Management (ACRM) courses [5].

As we discuss later, these CRM key points make an excellent platform for scenario design and focus of debriefing on non-technical aspects of performance.

Non-technical skills in healthcare

There is growing evidence that NTS are important in supporting safety in various medical disciplines including surgery [7,8,9,10,11,12,13] and that poor non-technical skills contribute to technical failures and play an important part in adverse events [14,15]. However, until relatively recently, non-technical skills (other than communication skills)

Box 8.1 CRM key points [6]

1. Know the environment
2. Anticipate and plan
3. Call for help early
4. Exercise leadership and followership with assertiveness
5. Distribute the workload (10-for-10 concept)
6. Mobilize all available resources
7. communicate effectively – speak up
8. Use all available information
9. Prevent and manage fixation errors
10. Cross- and double-check (never assume anything)
11. Use cognitive aids
12. re-evaluate repeatedly (apply the 10-for-10 concept)
13. Use good teamwork – coordinate with and support others
14. Allocate attention wisely
15. Set priorities dynamically

have not appeared explicitly in any medical speciality curricula as expected statements of competence for doctors in training in the UK.

To train and assess non-technical skills in any given domain, the skills specific to that area must first be identified. This may be done using accident and incident analyses, cognitive interviews (an advanced interview technique where cognitive prompts and cues are used to help the interviewee recall and outline a process or timeline), questionnaires and observations in the workplace. The identified skills are then organized and refined into a framework or taxonomy, which classifies items arranged in a hierarchical structure that encompasses identification, description, and agreed nomenclature.

A combination of these methods has been used to develop non-technical skills frameworks for anaesthetists (Anaesthetists' Non Technical Skills, ANTS) [16], surgeons (Non-technical Skills for Surgeons: NOTSS) [17] and theatre scrub practitioners (Scrub Practitioners' List of Intraoperative Non-Technical Skills: SPLINTS) [18]. Each taxonomy has a hierarchical structure. At the highest

level the skills can be divided into cognitive (thinking) and social (interpersonal) categories. Each category is then subdivided into a number of elements, each of which comprises a set of descriptor behaviours with examples of good and poor practice. These observable behavioural descriptors are not designed to be exhaustive.

An example of the hierarchical nature of the ANTS taxonomy [16] is shown in Figure 8.1. To raise awareness of, and train individuals in the aspects of the category of 'good teamwork', five sub-elements each have their own set of behavioural descriptors for good and poor practice that can be used to focus a debriefing conversation during simulated or 'real life' clinical performance.

Comparison of current behavioural marker systems (ANTS, NOTSS, etc.) highlights that some of the skills are generic to all taxonomies (for example situation awareness), although the behaviours indicative of good and poor practice vary between different specialty groups. These marker systems can be used to raise awareness of and develop skills through observation and feedback and can be used to design training interventions and objectives [19].

ANTS, NOTSS and SPLINTS have been designed to focus on an individual's non-technical skills as the 'building blocks' on which teams are built. This also allows them to fit within individual competency frameworks and assessment tools; both ANTS and NOTSS elements have now begun to appear in the most recent anaesthetic and surgical specialty curricula and assessment tools. Other non-technical skills systems such as surgical NOTECHS and OTAS (Observational Teamwork Assessment for Surgery) [20]) are designed to support observation of entire theatre teams and therefore may be more appropriate tools to use for feedback during whole team training.

Use of behavioural marker systems for feedback

In the context of NTS frameworks, simulation (or observed practice in the clinical setting) provides the opportunity for formative assessment of performance in 'real' life contextually relevant scenarios. The comparison of observed performance

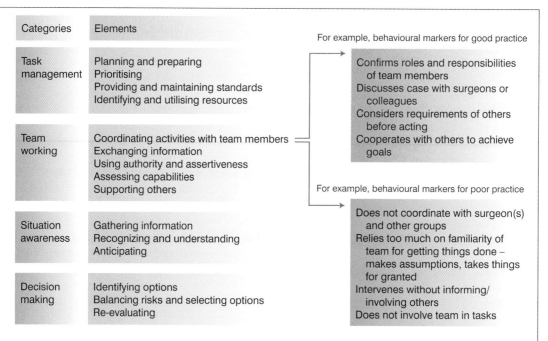

Figure 8.1 ANTS taxonomy [16]. Reproduced with permission of University of Aberdeen and Scottish Clinical Simulation Centre.

to the generic or specialty framework (e.g. ANTS) enables the facilitator to structure a conversation that focuses on performance, raises awareness at an individual or team level of current ability and identifies potential areas for improvement in the domains of knowledge , skills and non-technical aspects of performance (Figure 8.2).

The benefit to an educator of using skills frameworks is that they possess the extra sophistication of behaviours closely linked (anchored) to the domain descriptors. This can aid debrief by identifying specific behavioural examples during performances with illustration of the positive and negative impacts of these actions thus allowing learners to focus on developing specific aspects of practice (Box 8.2).

First, acquire the technical skill – then make the context real

It is clear that realistic high-fidelity scenario simulation creates an ideal environment in which to observe behavioural aspects of practice. Commenting on those behaviours through associated debrief-

ing is an ideal environment to highlight and develop NTS as the primary focus of learning. However, even the most simple simulator-based learning focusing on what appears to be predominantly 'technical' skills (such as carrying out a lumbar puncture or intubating the trachea using a part task trainer), when embedded in a realistic environment can help to highlight the requisite NTS required for expert performance.

It is very difficult for a novice clinician who is focusing attention on development of new practical skills to think beyond this psychomotor sequence until initial competence is achieved. This is one of the obvious reasons that it is so important for trainees to develop initial psychomotor skills in the controlled environment of the clinical skills training facility. However, in order to put basic skills into practice in a clinical environment, that skill needs to be underpinned with the appropriate NTS to support safe practice.

In the following sections we present a stepwise approach to using simulation-based learning to **surface**, **highlight** and **develop** NTS.

Figure 8.2 A cycle of observation and feedback.

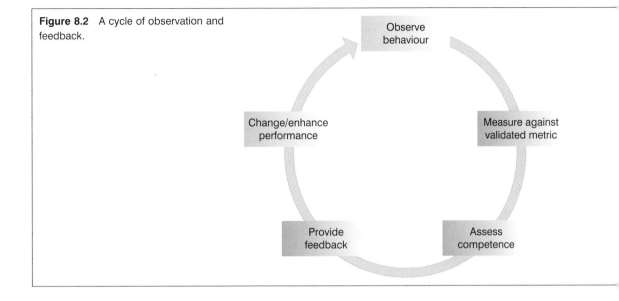

Box 8.2 Example

When observing a trainee doctor who is not communicating well with assistant staff during a procedure, the feedback can either be:

'You need to work on communicating better.'

Or

'During the procedure I noticed that your assistant was unsure as to the next item of equipment to hand to you next. How could you have helped your assistant understand what you were planning to do next in this situation?'

Surfacing non-technical skills associated with practical procedures

To aid this discussion, we can think about insertion of central venous catheter (CVC) as an example of a practical procedure taught to many postgraduate doctors in training grades. The technical skills associated with CVC insertion include advancing the needle, inserting the guide wire and railroading the CVC followed by suturing. This is traditionally taught as a defined sequence of psychomotor skills.

These skills should be safely learned and rehearsed in a simulated environment using part task training in order to focus on development of the necessary technical skills without the distractions of 'real' clinical life such as patient discomfort or time pressure. However, there is clearly more to safe, successful and skilful performance of this task than mere technical ability. It is the awareness and demonstration of the key aspects of related NTS that adds value, enhances performance and promotes safe practice.

In order to surface the NTS through simulation, the basic psychomotor skills need to be set in a more realistic environment. This may at first be as simple as 'blending' a part task trainer into a more realistic setting such as pairing a CVC insertion model with a rhythm generator to allow the ECG to be 'connected' to the patient or with a simulated patient to encourage explanation of the task and appropriate patient reassurance and interaction during the procedure. You may also provide appropriate sterile equipment to encourage performance of the complete task and the presence of an assistant with whom the learner should also interact. This allows the learner to carry out something more akin to the 'entire' procedure and allows surfacing of the various non-technical skills associated with putting the technical task into practice.

The following are examples of observable NTS which would support the 'technical' task of CVC insertion.

- **Task management** associated behaviours would include:
  - setting out equipment in the order it is to be used (planning & preparing)
  - ensuring that ECG monitoring is attached to the patient prior to starting (maintaining standards)
- **Situation awareness** would be demonstrated by
  - identifying surface landmarks for insertion and then obtaining clear ultrasound views of the area (information gathering)
  - correctly identifying structures from the ultrasound views (recognizing and understanding information)
  - looking at ECG monitoring when inserting guide wire, anticipating arrhythmias associated with guide wire proximity to the heart (anticipating)
- **Team working** may be demonstrated by
  - communicating management plan to assistant prior to commencing procedure (establishing a shared understanding)
  - allocation of patient monitoring and documentation to able assistant during line insertion (appropriate delegation of tasks)

Using scenarios to highlight non-technical skills

Simulation-based training is often used to allow learners to demonstrate their ability to recognize signs of acute illness and apply appropriate treatments. Modern simulators can provide appropriate visual cues such as chest excursion and palpable pulses, physiological cues using monitor emulators such as pulse oximetry and non-invasive blood pressure and patient 'interaction' through voice control from a distant operator. This allows observation of behaviours that are more realistic than is possible when cues such as statement of blood pressure or changes in colour are fed by an instructor within the room. These behaviours include not only technical skills but also NTS such as establishing and maintaining situation awareness by using patient and monitor cues, making decisions in real time

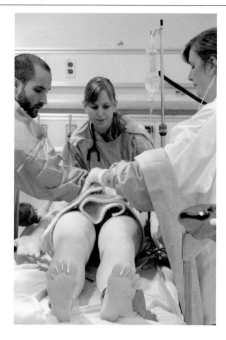

Figure 8.3 Simulation training allows non-technical skills, such as maintaining situation awareness and making decisions in real time, to be observed. Photo by Laura Seul, copyright Northwestern Simulation.

and sharing this within a team (Figure 8.3). By increasing the reality of interventions such as real administration of oxygen, intravenous fluids and drugs which have appropriate effects in real time, we can also begin to look at the ability of learners to delegate tasks to ensure all jobs are completed and to recognize the effects of their decisions or actions in real time and to recognize when treatments are inappropriate or ineffective. These NTS are indeed key to successful management of the patient and should be identified as explicit learning objectives within the scenario.

The following is an example from one of our patient safety courses run for medical and nursing undergraduates at the Scottish Clinical Simulation Centre. It illustrates the process of identifying NTS within an acute care scenario which can then be highlighted during debriefing and become key themes of patient safety to be reiterated during the day.

The design process

Stage 1: scenario learning objectives

Learning objectives (Box 8.3) within the scenarios are mapped to the competences within the Scottish Doctor curriculum [21] with the core learning being focused on surfacing generic NTS around the identification and management of the acutely unwell patient.

As the highlighted text in Boxes 8.4, 8.5 and 8.6 indicates, the overall list of scenario experiences (Box 8.3) has at its core, learning objectives describ-ing behaviours in all three domains: knowledge, technical skill and non-technical aspects of performance. Furthermore, some of the objectives are in the knowledge domain but describe knowledge pertaining to NTS.

Not every one of these learning objectives could or should be addressed within the debrief so as not to overwhelm the students. However, clearly defining key learning objectives for the suite of scenarios within a programme of learning allows the facilitator to ensure that by the end of the programme, all objectives have been met.

Box 8.3   Learning objectives.

Reproduced with permission of University of Aberdeen and Scottish Clinical Simulation Centre
Scenario Title: Hypoglycaemia
Target learners: Final Year medical students
Learning Objectives
At the end of this scenario and debriefing, the learners will be able to:
- Demonstrate a systematic approach to assessment of the critically unwell patient
- Recognise airway obstruction and use simple airway maneuvers for the obstructed airway
- Discuss important aspects of effective clinical leadership and team working
- Discuss the importance of prioritisation of clinical tasks in the emergency situation
- Demonstrate strategies for appropriate allocation of tasks
- Recognise hypoglycaemia and institute appropriate treatment
- Utilise resources to ensure rapid treament
- Indentify personal limitations and call for help
- Demonstrate a structured help request (SBAR)

Box 8.4   Learning objectives.

Reproduced with permission of University of Aberdeen and Scottish Clinical Simulation Centre
Scenario Title: Hypoglycaemia
Target learners: Final Year medical students
Learning Objectives
At the end of this scenario and debriefing, the learners will be able to:
- **Demonstrate a systematic approach** to assessment of the critically unwell patient
- Recognise airway obstruction and use simple airway maneuvers for the obstructed airway
- **Discuss** important aspects of effective clinical **leadership and team working**
- **Discuss** the importance of **prioritisation** of clinical tasks in the emergency situation
- Demonstrate strategies for appropriate allocation of tasks
- **Recognise hypoglycaemia** and institute appropriate treatment
- Utilise resources to ensure rapid treament
- Indentify personal limitations and call for help
- Demonstrate a structured help request (SBAR)

Box 8.5   Learning objectives.

Reproduced with permission of University of Aberdeen and Scottish Clinical Simulation Centre
Scenario Title: Hypoglycaemia
Target learners: Final Year medical students
Learning Objectives
At the end of this scenario and debriefing, the learners will be able to:
• Demonstrate a systematic approach to assessment of the critically unwell patient
• Recognise airway obstruction and **use simple airway maneuvers for the obstructed airway**
• Discuss important aspects of effective clinical leadership and team working
• Discuss the importance of prioritisation of clinical tasks in the emergency situation
• Demonstrate strategies for appropriate allocation of tasks
• Recognise hypoglycaemia and **institute appropriate treatment**
• Utilise resources to ensure rapid treament
• Indentify personal limitations and call for help
• **Demonstrate a structured help request (SBAR)**

Box 8.6   Learning objectives.

Reproduced with permission of University of Aberdeen and Scottish Clinical Simulation Centre
Scenario Title: Hypoglycaemia
Target learners: Final Year medical students
Learning Objectives
At the end of this scenario and debriefing, the learners will be able to:
• Demonstrate a systematic approach to assessment of the critically unwell patient
• **Recognise airway obstruction** and use simple airway maneuvers for the obstructed airway
• Discuss important aspects of effective clinical leadership and team working
• Discuss the importance of prioritisation of clinical tasks in the emergency situation
• **Demonstrate** strategies for **appropriate allocation of tasks**
• Recognise hypoglycaemia and institute appropriate treatment
• **Utilise resources** to ensure rapid treament
• **Indentify personal limitations** and call for help
• Demonstrate a structured help request (SBAR)

Stage 2: storyboard: technical aspects of performance

Using the Scottish Clinical Simulation Centre storyboard template, realistic clinical scenarios are created to provide clinical experiences which will facilitate the participant achieving the intended learning objectives.

From the example in Table 8.1, the **baseline** state of the patient at the start of the scenario will facilitate the learner engaging with both knowledge-based objectives relating to assessment and recognition of airway obstruction and technical aspects of performance in the use of simple airway manoeu-

vres to facilitate airway patency. At undergraduate level, *demonstrating* effective leadership would be exemplary but the scenario is designed to be able to use debriefing to *discuss* important aspects of effective clinical leadership and team working as the learning objective states.

This illustration of the baseline state should be considered in the context of general issues relating to scenario design. It can be seen that the 'story' and clinical setting incorporating the patient physiology and appearance are all designed around enabling the learners to achieve the learning objectives thus meeting their educational requirements.

Table 8.1 Example using the Storyboard template

Scenario Storyboard				
STATE NAME	STATE	DESIRED LEARNER BEHAVIOURS & TRIGGERS TO MOVE ON		
1. Baseline	**Patient** Snoring **Physiology** SpO$_2$ 91% RR 14 HR 105 BP 120/70 **Events**	**Learner Actions:** Begin to assess patient Recognise airway problem Use simple airway maneuvers	**Transition Trigger:** (Actions OR Time) O$_2$ on, Air way open	**Teaching Points:** Systematic approach K Airway management S Leadership role NTS allocation

K, knowledge; S, skill; NTS, non-technical skill.
Reproduced with permission of University of Aberdeen and Scottish Clinical Simulation Centre.

Stage 3: storyboard: non-technical integration

Consider now the completed storyboard (Table 8.2) alongside the generic CRM components from Gaba set out in Box 8.1.

As well as enabling the demonstration of technical competences, the **baseline** state can enable the participant to engage with aspects of leadership, teamwork and task allocation, but to do this the scenario participant cannot be performing alone. Thought therefore must be given to scenario design with respect to numbers and ratio of participants and faculty (confederates). Scenarios involving multiple personnel will, by definition, allow exploration of the interpersonal skills required for effective teamwork but are more complex and expensive to organize.

The second state (**'airway open'**), relates to a number of the learning objectives targeting non-technical aspects of performance such as prioritization, and task allocation. The scenario design needs to balance the number of participants within the scenario to the expected number of tasks to be undertaken. For example, four participants in this scenario plus the faculty plant or confederate (see Chapter 11 for definition and role of the confederate) making a team of five may be able to achieve

all necessary tasks with ease and minimal thought to planning. Decrease the number of participants by 50% and suddenly the team 'leader' requires to not only prioritize the required tasks but allocate them to a smaller number of willing volunteers. In fact, reducing the number of participants will necessitate the 'leader' undertaking tasks themselves, adding a potential new dimension to the performance of 'attention allocation' as the leader becomes distracted by tasks.

State 3 **'improves'** relates to recognition of the need for help. As indicated in the storyboard, this learning objective is translated through the scenario to a number of learning and teaching points relating to the recognition of the need for help, the route to appropriate help and also using a structure for communication with a senior colleague either face-to-face or via telephone (for example SBAR, Situation, Background, Assessment, Recommendation). This is much more comprehensive and involved than merely 'call for help early' or 'communicate effectively' and ultimately more useful to the learners. If the specific observed positive, and less positive behaviours exhibited when dealing with the communication challenge within the scenario are used to describe the performance, the participant has tangible aspects (or anchors) to concentrate on maintaining or developing when back in the clinical domain.

Table 8.2 Storyboard: non-technical integration

Scenario Storyboard

State Name	State	Desired Learner Behaviours & Triggers to Move On		
1. Baseline	**Patient** Snoring **Physiology** SpO$_2$ 91% RR 14 HR 105 BP 120/70 **Events**	**Learner Actions:** Begin to assess patient Recognise airway problem Use simple airway maneuvers	**Transition Trigger:** (Actions OR Time) O$_2$ on, Air way open	**Teaching Points:** Systematic approach K Airway management S Leadership role NTS allocation
2. Airway open	**Patient** Stop Snoring **Physiology** SpO$_2$ 97% RR 14 HR 100 BP 120/70 **Events** Nurse gets dextrose	**Learner Actions:** Continue to assess patient Detect hypoglycaemia Delegate tasks and treat -IV Access -Dextrose / Glucagon -Protocol	**Transition Trigger:** (Actions OR Time) Treatment given	**Teaching Points:** Information NTS gathering Priorities NTS Task allocation NTS Resource utilization NTS Microteaching medical K management
3. Improves	**Patient** Wakes up, initially confused. **Physiology** SpO$_2$ 97% RR 14 HR 10 BP 120/70 **Events**	**Learner Actions:** Plan for subsequent monitoring Phone senior	**Transition Trigger:** (Actions OR Time) Decides on increased BM vigilance	**Teaching Points:** Next step Senikor input NTS SBAR S

K, knowledge; S, skill; NTS, non-technical skill.
Reproduce with permission of University of Aberdeen and Scottish Clinical Simulation Centre.

⊙ Top tip

Clearly defining the appropriate behaviours expected in any one scenario and its stages will enhance the running of the scenario and greatly improve the focus of debrief.

Designing scenarios to develop non-technical skills

The key first step in designing scenarios to develop NTS in participants, is the appropriate selection and statement of learning objectives for the intended scenario participants.

In some circumstances, the *primary* aim of the scenario may be to highlight and develop NTS. In this case, the NTS become the key objectives and the technical or clinical skills have less importance. This is likely when training is for more senior staff when knowledge and technical skills are more likely to be already established. By designing scenarios to address a certain aspect of NTS (such as situation awareness), participants can focus on developing behaviours which are most effective in these situations.

For those who are as yet unfamiliar with using the NTS behavioural marker systems such as ANTS or NOTSS, or for those who are inexperienced at designing scenarios specifically to NTS objectives, it is perhaps easier to start by using the Gaba CRM principles in Box 8.1. Choosing a combination of key points such as 'use cognitive aids', 'distribute the workload' and 'exercise leadership and followership' allows learners to focus on development of appropriate skills to improve performance in these areas. The scenario should therefore involve the use of a protocol, the physical presence of the protocol, enough personnel so that it is possible to have a leader and followers and enough personnel to whom tasks can be distributed. Management of diabetic hyperglycaemia is just one example of a clinical scenario which would allow many of these key behaviours to be surfaced, observed or addressed in the debriefing conversation, but there are many other realistic clinical scenarios that can be used. To add more dimensions, the scenario may be designed specifically to start with inadequate personnel to manage such a situation with the objective being that extra help must be sought early (mobilize all available resources) in order to minimize task overload.

For the novice simulation educator, the Gaba CRM points provide some broad NTS to consider. However, to make the debriefing diagnostic and developmental, attention must be paid to the specific behaviours you would expect to see within those broad CRM points. Taking 'prevent and manage fixation errors' as an example, you may ask 'What did you do to try and manage those fixation errors? What kind of things could you have done to have prevented that fixation error?' The debriefing conversation must be directed towards the specifics that underlie broad CRM points and the educator must spend time thinking about this in advance. The speciality domain specific NTS frameworks such as ANTS and NOTSS are almost ready-made for diagnostic conversations but are not generally applicable to other professional domains.

Designing and running your own scenarios with embedded non-technical skills

A scenario that runs as intended, moving smoothly through scenario stages which relate to the states of the patient and providing opportunities to engage with all intended learning outcomes, is the goal of all educators using scenario-based simulation methodology. As mentioned, it is generally easier to start creating scenario states based on **technical** learning objectives and then overlay the **non-technical objectives** with slight changes as described earlier. With a focus on NTS and to ensure the maximum educational benefit through an appropriate and intended experience, the simulation educator should consider **four** key areas when designing and running NTS-based scenarios.

1. Learning objectives: 'where's the challenge?'

The key to educationally excellent non-technical scenarios is not complexity but appropriate and unambiguous learning objectives. Being explicit about adapting basic scenario design for different levels of experience through focusing on diverse areas of performance (as in the undergraduate example mentioned earlier) will smooth the progress from basic knowledge and psychomotor skills development to expert performance encompassing essential non-technical aspects.

As with all outcomes based education, educators must ensure that learning objectives are appropriate and staged to the level of training of the participants.

2. Fidelity and engagement

Consider the difference between a scenario designed to enhance the NTS of surgeons in an operative environment for a laparoscopic procedure, compared with a scenario designed to enhance NTS within the hypoglycaemia patient example discussed earlier. Attention to key aspects of fidelity in both of these scenarios is extremely important but subtly different.

The **technical** fidelity required to challenge and engage the surgeon with the psychomotor aspect of the laparoscopy is paramount. An 'unbelievable' aspect to the craft piece will promote disbelief and disengagement resulting in inappropriate or unrealistic behaviours, making it difficult for the non-technical behaviours to be assessed.

When focusing on behavioural markers, especially the CRM aspects, the **environmental** and **psychological** fidelity is paramount. Only when the scenario 'feels real' to the participant, can their behaviour and performance be meaningfully used for observation, discussion and comment.

In contrast, it is not meaningful to debrief around NTS if the learner did not get relevant and realistic cues during the scenario. In this situation, the behaviour in the scenario might be compromised by inappropriate or inadequate fidelity and therefore not be a true reflection of clinical performance. Consequently, the facilitator may lose some or all of the material on which to base a formative developmental conversation.

Therefore it is key that the scenario design is realistic *enough* and runs to an anticipated plan to ensure a performance that allows a debriefing conversation between faculty and participants to comment on behaviour and interactions.

3. Analysis and take home messages – understanding the message

In the facilitated discussion after the simulated episode, it is important that the conversation is explicit about the behaviours and examples that made the non-technical aspects of performance 'good', and the areas on which to improve, including specific clarification. Avoid ending up with vague take home messages like 'do teamwork better' as this is unhelpful for your learners. The analysis of the learning event and summation of the discussion into key learning points or 'take home messages' (THMs) must be specific enough to allow post-event reflection on behaviours to focus on and develop.

For example, consider the 'Identify personal limitations and call for help' learning outcome example from state 3 (Box 8.3 and Table 8.3). It is important that the THMs are more explicit than 'call for help' or 'call for help earlier'. The debriefing conversation should have allowed discussion around

why help was (or was not) called and what it was that triggered the call when it eventually came. What were the participants thinking at the time? What was the final trigger that initiated the call for 'help'– was it a physiological parameter, or merely a realization of being out of ones depth?

Having directed the debriefing conversation to deliberately address the intended learning outcomes, the resulting THMs will be much richer and more explicit, thereby allowing participants to better understand and implement them in their clinical practice.

4. Safe learning environment

Most medical students and doctors in training have had some experience of simulation-based clinical education (SBCE). SBCE focusing on non-technical aspects of behaviour is of educational benefit to all in the clinical environment. However, many established clinicians who have been practising for some time have not had the opportunity to learn using simulation as a methodology. For many of these clinicians, the prospect of performing in an unknown clinical situation, while being videoed in front of a group of peers and then critiqued, is somewhat alien and incredibly challenging. Being critiqued around non-technical aspects of performance (such as leadership and team working) can feel even more personal and threatening.

Although creating a safe environment for learning is a consistent message in SBCE, it should be specifically identified and promoted as a key component of any courses focusing on non-technical aspects of performance. The debriefs associated with behaviours in stressful clinical situations can be some of the most challenging to engage with both from facilitator and participant perspective.

> ⓘ **Top tip**
>
> Simulation and debriefing focused on non-technical aspects of performance is more 'real'. The conversations will lead into personal territory. This can be extremely threatening to more experienced clinicians. Do it sensitively and well!

Using simulation-based education to raise awareness of key aspects of NTS is one of the real benefits of this methodology. It should however not be seen as a complex added extra, but designed in the same way as all other scenarios i.e. with NTS as the main or one of the key learning objectives for the scenario.

One of the main challenges of beginning to use the NTS frameworks, is that often trainees and their supervisors are novices in the vocabulary used to describe the categories, elements and behavioural markers. Terms such as 'situation awareness' although increasingly used in medical parlance, are very often perceived and understood differently by healthcare professionals. However, as these descriptors are embedded in clinical speciality training, the frameworks will become more widely recognized, used and understood. The benefits of using a shared common language to describe performance enhancing behaviours, is that in the initial phase of learning, novices can become aware of key aspects of development needed, over and above that of pure knowledge and technical skill.

Authors have indicated that achieving consistency across the behavioural marker systems between assessors is generally challenging [22]. The skill of using non-technical aspects of performance as the basis for debrief should not therefore be underestimated in its complexity and challenge. It should be seen as a specific skill set that novice clinical educators need to be trained for and learn as part of their own educator development.

Effective debriefing focussing on non-technical aspects of performance is more complex and challenging than simple knowledge and technical skills enhancement. The novice clinical educator approaching this type of debriefing must have a working knowledge base of NTS frameworks and understand that NTS debriefing is a specific and learned skill, very much improved with deliberate practice.

✓ Key points

- Non-technical skills are the cognitive and social skills used by experienced professionals to deliver a high-quality and safe clinical performance.
- Scenario-based simulation training provides the optimal environment in which to explore and highlight NTS.
- When using simulation for teaching NTS, scenarios must include learning objectives in the NTS domain and be designed accordingly.
- Embedding NTS into scenario design will enhance the learning and development gained by healthcare professionals from engagement with simulated practice.
- CRM key points provide an excellent platform to begin focussing on generic non-technical aspects of performance in scenario design.

REFERENCES

1. Health and Safety Executive (1999) *Reducing Error and Influencing Behaviour.* HSG48. London: HSE Books, 5.

2. Avermaete van J, Kruijsen E (1998) (eds). *NOTECHS. The Evaluation of Non-Technical Skills of Multi-Pilot Aircrew in Relation to the JAR-FCL Requirements.* Final Report NLR-CR-98443. Amsterdam: National Aerospace Laboratory (NLR).

3. DeAnda A, Gaba D (1991) The role of experience in the response to simulated critical incidents. *Anesthesia and Analgesia* **72:** 308–315.

4. Gaba D, Fish K, Howard S (1994) *Crisis Management in Anesthesiology.* New York: Churchill Livingston.

5. Gaba DM, Howard SK, Fish KJ, *et al.* (2001) Simulation-based training in anesthesia crisis resource management (ACRM): a decade of experience. *Simulation & Gaming* **32:** 175–193.

6. Gaba D, Rall M (2010) Impact of human performance on patient safety. In: *Miller's Anaesthesia* (R Miller, *et al.* eds), 7th edn, London: Churchill Livingstone, 93–109.

7. Carthey J, de Leval MR, Wright DJ, *et al.* (2003) and all UK paediatric cardiac centres. Behavioural markers of surgical excellence. *Safety Science* **41:** 409–425.

8. Catchpole K, Giddings A, Wilkinson M, Hirst G, *et al.* (2007) Improving patient safety by identifying latent failures in successful operations. *Surgery* **142:** 102–110.

9. McCulloch P, Mishra A, Handa A, *et al.* 2009. The effects of aviation-style non-technical skills training on technical performance and outcome in the operating theatre *Quality & Safety in Health Care* **18:** 109–115.

10. Mishra A, Catchpole K, Dale T, McCulloch P (2008) The influence of non-technical performance on technical outcome in laparoscopic cholecystectomy. *Surgical Endoscopy* **22:** 68–73.

11. Moorthy K, Munz Y, Adams S, *et al.* (2005) A human factors analysis of technical and team skills among surgical trainees during procedural simulations in a simulated operating theatre. *Annals of Surgery* **242:** 631–639.

12. Fletcher G, McGeorge P, Flin R, *et al.* (2002) The role of non-technical skills in anaesthesia: a review of current literature. *British Journal of Anaesthesia* **88:** 418–429.

13. Flin R, Maran N (2004) Identifying and training non-technical skills for teams in acute medicine. *Quality & Safety in Health Care* **13**(Suppl 1)**:** i80.

14. Bromiley M (2008) Have you ever made a mistake? *Bulletin of The Royal College of Anaesthetists* **48:** 2442–2445.

15. Hull L, Arora S, Aggarwal R, *et al.* (2011) The impact of nontechnical skills on technical performance in surgery: systematic review. *Journal of the American College of Surgeons* **214:** 214–230.

16. University of Aberdeen and Scottish Clinical Simulation Centre (2001) Anaesthetists' non-technical skills system handbook v1.0. Available from http://www.abdn.ac.uk/iprc/documents/ants/ants_handbook_v1.0_electronic_access_version.pdf (accessed April 2012).

17. University of Aberdeen (2006) The non-technical skills for surgeons system handbook v1.2. Available from http://www.abdn.ac.uk/iprc/notss (accessed April 2012).

18. University of Aberdeen (2009) Scrub Practitioners List of Intraoperative Non-Technical Skills Handbook v1.0. Available at http://www.abdn.ac.uk/iprc/splints/ (accessed April 2012).

19. Flin R, O'Connor P, Crichton M (2008). Training methods for non-technical skills.

In: *Safety at the Sharp End: a Guide to Non-technical Skills*. Farnham: Ashgate, 243–267.

20. Imperial College London (2011) Observational teamwork assessment for surgery, user training manual. Available from http://www1.imperial.ac.uk/resources/018F4A1D-5129-444E-96CF-04C524C2EA99/otas_manual.pdf (accessed April 2012).

21. University of Edinburgh, Learning Technology Section (2011) The Scottish doctor. Available from http://www.scottishdoctor.org/index.asp (accessed April 2012).

22. Flin R, Patey R, Glavin R, Maran N (2010) Anaesthetists' non-technical skills. *British Journal of Anaesthesia* **105:** 38–44.

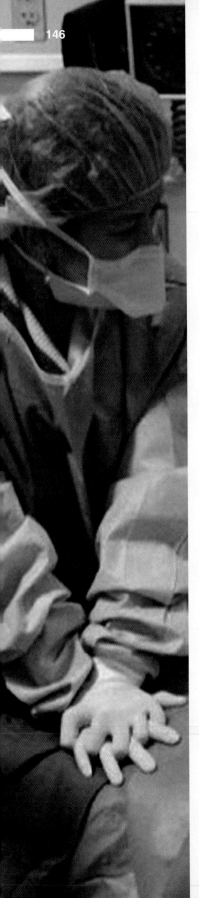

CHAPTER 9
Teamwork

Jennifer M. Weller   University of Auckland, Auckland, New Zealand

A team is called a team for a very good reason; there is an expectation that there will be sufficient co-operation and communication amongst its members to minimise the risk of harm to the patient. For a team to function as such there must be a sense of collective responsibility for ensuring patient safety [1].

Overview

This chapter explores a number of different aspects relating to how teams function and can be developed to improve teamwork in healthcare. It considers the political, social and organizational drivers and barriers to improving teamwork, offering different definitions of what a 'team' is and providing evidence from the literature and perspectives on team training. It goes on to evaluate how simulation can contribute to team training in terms of what to teach, the teaching environment, designing effective interventions and implementing them, concluding in considering assessment: what to assess and measurement tools.

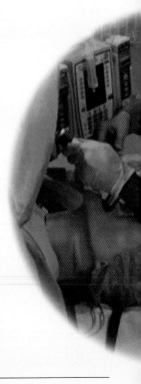

Essential Simulation in Clinical Education, First Edition. Edited by Kirsty Forrest, Judy McKimm, and Simon Edgar.
© 2013 John Wiley & Sons, Ltd. Published 2013 by John Wiley & Sons, Ltd.

Introduction

Teamwork failures have been identified as a major contributor to adverse patient outcomes. With increased complexity of healthcare delivery, there is an ever-increasing need for health professionals to work effectively as a team to best serve the interests of the patient. However, until recently, changing models of healthcare delivery have not been accompanied by systematic organizational or educational changes to support the development of new teamwork competencies. While some disciplines, particularly chronic care disciplines such as palliative care, have formally established multidisciplinary healthcare teams, this is not generally the case in more acute settings.

Simulation-based team training (SBTT) is increasingly used by a range of disciplines to improve teamwork and communication. However, its availability is patchy, depends on local champions and is not widely adopted at an institutional level. SBTT is resource intensive and implementation is often hampered by lack of evidence about the critical components that improve the performance of healthcare teams; validity of SBTT; reliability and validity of the measurement tools and the transfer of learning from simulation to clinical practice.

A call for improved teamwork in healthcare: drivers and barriers

Drivers for team training

The training of healthcare professionals has traditionally focused on developing the knowledge and skills of individual clinical practitioners. However modern healthcare is increasingly being delivered by teams of health professionals with the expectation that this will lead to improved healthcare delivery processes, better outcomes for patients and lower costs than non-team approaches [2].

Adverse events are common in hospitals worldwide, with studies reporting that between 6% and 16% of all hospital admissions are associated with an adverse event, resulting in disability or longer hospital stay [3,4,5]. Failures in teamwork and communication make a substantial contribution to adverse events and suboptimal care [6,7,8,9,10,11,12]. Lingard *et al.* [13], observing communication between members of operating room teams, found that over a quarter of all communications failed due to poor timing, inaccurate or missing content or failure to resolve issues. Many of these failures had observable deleterious effects, including inefficiency, tension between team members, wasted resources, delays or procedural errors.

A study of recently graduated doctors and nurses revealed fundamental problems with team formation, sharing of information and common understanding of the goals of patient care. Institutional structures, organization of work, lack of leadership in team development and maintenance, and limited understanding of the requirements for effective team collaboration were all considered contributing factors [14].

National policy documents continue to reinforce the importance of team work in the delivery of healthcare [2]. The Institute of Medicine in the USA recommended interdisciplinary medical team training as a key strategy to reduce patient harm due to medical errors [15]. Furthermore, educational providers now include team collaboration and communication as core competencies in the training of physicians. For example, the US Accreditation Council for Graduate Medical Education [16] includes aspects of communication and collaboration in the competencies required of graduating doctors, as does the Canadian CanMEDS curriculum framework for basic medical education [17]. There have been similar calls from national patient safety organizations [18] such as the Agency for Healthcare Research and Quality which launched a project in 2007 to establish national training and support network for the US TeamSTEPPS programme [19]. TeamSTEPPS was developed to improve communication and teamwork skills among healthcare professionals and increasing numbers of reports of team training initiatives are appearing in the healthcare literature.

Barriers to team training

However, evidence of change and success tends to be at local level and a review of teamwork interventions in healthcare concluded that the critical components of teamwork in healthcare are still not well understood [2]. Progress towards a culture of teamwork and interdependence between the professions at an institutional level is hampered by the complexity of interprofessional relationships, compounded by established professional silos, entrenched individualism, lack of application of the safety lessons from other complex disciplines, hierarchical structures and diffuse accountability [20]. The development of effective clinical teams requires more than simply an isolated training intervention or the grouping or clustering of health professionals in a clinical area with the expectation that they will work effectively as a team.

Fluid teams

Teams can be conceived of as 'fluid', moving and changing across the contexts of setting, disease or patient. While much of the literature on teamwork focuses on stable teams, this is not helpful in healthcare, where a fundamental requirement is adaptability and the ability for healthcare practitioners to function effectively in new and fluid teams.

Attitudes, traditions and hierarchies

Different professional groups have different approaches and attitudes towards teamwork [21] which may impede the development of a well-functioning team. Horsburgh *et al.* [22] found medical, nursing and pharmacy students differed in how they believed clinical work should be organized even before they started their training. Medical students believed that clinical work should be the responsibility of individuals. In contrast, nursing students had a collective view and believed that work should be systemized, whereas pharmacy students were at a mid-point in this continuum.

The attitude of the 'heroic doctor' relying on his or her individual talents to save the patient is not relevant in today's complex healthcare environment [23]. In the interests of patient safety, input from more than one team member into problem-solving and decision-making is desirable. Bleakley [23] talks of the need for 'democracy' in healthcare, as a prerequisite for shared input into decision-making.

The traditional communication style of medical leadership in healthcare team can be considered as monological (i.e. a monologue; statements and closed questions), rather than dialogical (i.e. a dialogue; inviting input and stimulating exchange). In displaying a deeply monological communication style, a surgeon, for example, may display an authoritarian attitude that discourages or denies input or democratic decision-making from other members of the operating room team. This creates a poor climate for patient safety, where team members are inhibited from contributing information or ideas, raising concerns or challenging decisions.

Cultural differences

Internationalization of the health workforce may also create additional challenges for effective team functioning. For example, attitudes of doctors towards the roles of nurses, and nurses towards doctors, and attitudes to speaking up and challenging authority varies across cultural groups [24].

Organizational structure

The organizational structures within healthcare institutions may also inhibit the development of effective healthcare teams. Teams are often formed *ad hoc*, with constantly changing membership. Patients may be cared for by multiple teams based on healthcare disciplines rather than centred on the patient. Changes in how work is organized and how healthcare is delivered, increasing sub-specialization and changes in junior doctor working hours (reducing continuity of care) have all impacted on the development of stable, patient-centred healthcare teams [25,26,27].

Educational system

The educational system can further entrench professional isolation. Traditionally, different health professional groups learn in isolation, from undergraduate education through postgraduate training and ongoing professional development. While much is published on interprofessional education as a means to increase interprofessional collaboration, embedded, effective interprofessional learning at undergraduate level is still aspirational rather than the norm, and certainly, at postgraduate level, there is little evidence of widespread interdisciplinary approaches to mainstream continuing professional development.

On teams, teamwork and training: definitions, evidence and perspectives

A team refers to two or more individuals each with specific roles, working toward a common goal, and with concrete boundaries. Teams work on complex tasks requiring dynamic exchange of resources (e.g. information), coordination of effort and adaptation to changing situational factors. Teamwork is the vehicle through which such coordination occurs. It is defined in terms of the behaviours (e.g. closed loop communication) cognitions (e.g. shared mental models) and attitudes (e.g. collective efficacy, trust) that combine to make adaptive interdependent performance possible [28].

Despite a large body of literature on group dynamics in healthcare, medical education is only now seriously asking 'what do we mean by a *team*?' [23]. While many different definitions of teams have been proposed, basically a team comprises two or more individuals who have specific roles, perform interdependent tasks, and share a common goal [29].

The clinical setting may dictate the appropriate structure for the team and health professionals may identify with a number of different teams. For example a junior doctor may identify primarily with his or her medical team, but also with the team of health professionals looking after a patient, or even at an institutional level [30]. The operating room 'team' is sometimes described as three parallel teams (surgical, anaesthetic, nursing) with their own priorities, tasks and goals. Where a patient has complex and diverse needs however, a multidisciplinary approach to patient care, with specialized input from a range of health professionals is required [31].

Evidence on team training

A meta-analysis of studies of 2650 non-clinical teams found that nearly 20% of variance in team processes and outcomes could be accounted for by team members' participation in team training, underscoring the potential of team training to change team behaviour [32]. These outcomes applied equally to teams who did or did not regularly work together. While unique factors affect healthcare teams (dynamic team membership, different patient populations, disease types and care delivery settings), there is some evidence that team training initiatives targeting medical teams exhibit similar effects to those observed in aviation and *ad hoc* laboratory teams, although these studies are restricted to quantitative indicators [33]. While individual studies on teamwork interventions may show positive results in particular dimensions [34], the ability to generalize these positive results to other contexts is limited. The diverse nature of the studies makes it difficult to attempt to pool evidence on such a complex intervention as team training in healthcare. Comparisons are problematic because of the multiple contexts of team training, the range of approaches, the lack of consistency and validation of measurement tools, and the different outcome measures [34].

Kirkpatrick [35] provides us with a useful hierarchical framework against which to evaluate the strength of the evidence on the effectiveness of educational interventions (Box 9.1).

Box 9.1   Kirkpatrick's levels of evidence for educational interventions [35]

Level1	Participation in educational experiences
Level2a	Change of attitudes
Level2b	Change of knowledge and/or skills
Level3	Behavioural change
Level4a	Change in professional practice
Level4b	Benefits to patients/society

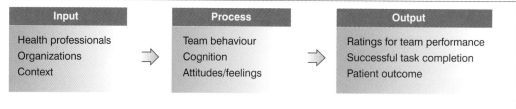

Figure 9.1   A framework for studying team function (Source: Rousseau [40]).

Although observational studies of long-term change in professional practice, or objective evidence of benefits to patients through team training initiatives are lacking, some qualitative data from participant interviews provides evidence at level 4, where participants in team training interventions report subsequent changes they have made to their practice, and cite specific clinical events where the new teamwork skills have, in their opinion, improved the outcome for a particular patient [36,37].

To measure patient outcomes in terms of morbidity and mortality, the traditional end points of quantitative research methodologies, would require a very large sample size, beyond the capacity of current SBTT initiatives. The contribution of qualitative approaches to supporting the evidence of team interventions is therefore valuable. The concept of evidence-based medicine requires the assessment of all available evidence and not just that available from quantitative studies [38]. Quantitative studies are appropriate when seeking predefined, measurable outcomes; they represent a positivist view on evidence, often coming more naturally to clinicians accustomed to the medical science tradition, searching for 'the truth'. A more constructivist perspective, applying qualitative research methods, while bounded by context and limited in terms of generalizability, provides useful insight into team working and the effect of educational interventions.

Numerous models have been proposed to study teamwork and its components. Common ground in these models is the input–process–output (I-P-O) framework, taking into account also the dynamic nature of teams, and the social, cultural, hierarchical, environmental and organizational factors influencing each step [39].

Based on the I–P–O framework, Rousseau *et al.* [40] consider team function in terms of input (individuals, organization and context), team processes (teamwork behaviours, cognition, feelings) and team outputs (patient and team) (Figure 9.1).

'Teamwork behaviours' can be broken down into components: behaviours required for maintaining a team, behaviours required to accomplish a task and behaviours required to ensure collaboration between team members (Figure 9.2). The requirement and importance of each of these components varies with the nature of the task the team is undertaking. Task complexity, routine or novel tasks, uncertain goals and the interdependence of tasks, all affect the demands on the team in terms of these behaviours. A complex task may demand more collaborative behaviours in order to coordinate different but interdependent tasks. An unstructured task with ambiguous outputs requires high levels of preparation in order to accomplish the task (i.e. working out what needs to be done) and assessing progress towards achieving the goals (i.e. monitoring how the situation is progressing in response to actions).

To illustrate the components outlined in Figure 9.2, consider a patient presenting to the emergency department with acute respiratory distress, cause unknown. To manage this uncertain situation, a large component of teamwork behaviours in the 'Preparing for the task' component will be required. With complex, high workload events, some team members may become overloaded, requiring more 'Adjusting behaviours to achieve the task'. In highly structured tasks where each team member knows exactly what is to be done there is less need for these behaviours. This model provides a theoretical framework on which to build simulated scenarios for training and assessing teams.

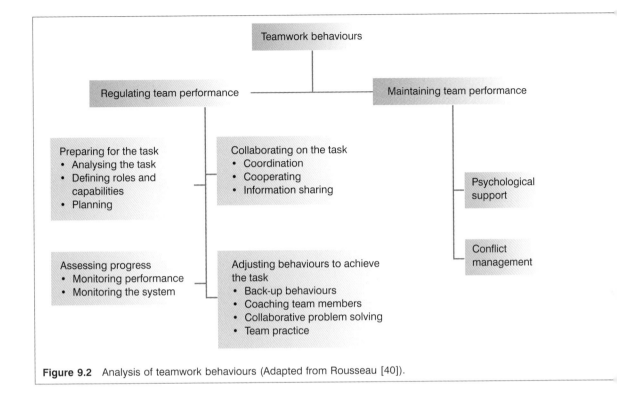

Figure 9.2 Analysis of teamwork behaviours (Adapted from Rousseau [40]).

Many other models have been proposed. Salas *et al.* [41] proposed that the important dimensions of team behaviour are team leadership, mutual performance monitoring, back-up behaviour, adaptability and team orientation. Three coordinating, or enabling, mechanisms facilitate these dimensions: mutual trust; shared mental models; and closed loop communication (Figure 9.3). These reflect the elements of the Rousseau model, and can be seen echoed in the major categories of other team measurement scales, though perhaps with a different emphasis on leadership. The application of these models to SBTT is further discussed in the next section.

Team training: content, environment, design and implementation

The majority of reported team training initiatives involve simulation [28]. Unlike other educational modalities, simulated training environments can recreate the tasks and complexity of the clinical working environment in a controlled manner, thus allowing manipulation and enhancement of the clinical experience to address the domains and competencies of interest. SBTT allows learners to engage in the dynamic processes of teamwork enhanced by structured, facilitated reflection on the experience. It provides an opportunity for multidisciplinary teams to work together on relevant clinical tasks to develop and practise a range of teamwork behaviours including communication, task coordination, sharing information and collaborative problem solving. It also provides the opportunity to explore cognitive processes underlying observed actions, and assumptions, attitudes and other influences on team performance including environmental factors such as organizational structures, resources, equipment and workspace design [36,39,42,43,44].

What to teach: teamwork behaviours

The 'teamwork behaviours', described in detail earlier are often the focus of simulation-based team

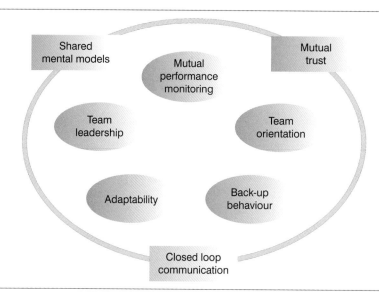

Figure 9.3 The five dimensions of teamwork and the enabling mechanisms (Adapted from Salas [41]).

training, and the crew resource management (CRM) [45] model, taken originally from aviation and translated to acute care medicine, is widespread in SBTT, with much of the literature coming from the disciplines of Surgery, Emergency Medicine, Anaesthetics, Obstetrics and Gynaecology and Paediatrics. The task characteristics of these medical disciplines – multiple and concurrent tasks, uncertainty, changing plans and high workload [46] – make CRM training in these contexts highly relevant. These have been usefully translated into key learning points for healthcare teams [47] (Box 9.2). Other approaches based on task analysis in clinical fields identify broadly similar theoretical frameworks around which to structure team training, based on discipline-specific work around non-technical skills in anaesthesia, surgery and other acute specialties [48,49,50] (Table 9.1).

Teamwork behaviours lend themselves to the development of measurement tools based on objectively identifiable 'observable markers'. A structured framework against which instructors observe a simulation and provide feedback to participants is an essential element of effective SBTT [51]. A formal extension of this is a recently validated behaviourally anchored rating scale for structuring observation of teamwork [52] (Table 9.2). Behavioural anchors for each item assist observers (and partici-

> **Box 9.2   Key points of crisis management (adapted from Gaba *et al.* [44])**
>
> 1. Know, modify and optimize your environment
> 2. Anticipate and plan
> 3. Take a leadership role
> 4. Communicate effectively
> 5. Call for help (or a second opinion) early enough
> 6. Allocate attention wisely and use all available information – avoid fixation errors
> 7. Distribute the workload and use all available resources

pants) in identifying good and suboptimal performance. Furthermore, this instrument appropriately incorporates the behaviours of the entire team, not just the leader.

In addition to these overall teamwork assessment instruments, an increasing and valuable number of specific tools illustrated here are being used to address components of team behaviour:
• ISBAR (Identify self, Situation, Background, Assessment, Recommendations) [54] is a tool to

Table 9.1 Anaesthesia Non Technical Skills (source Flin *et al*. [53])

The ANTS system

Team working	Task management
• Coordinating activities with team • Exchanging information • Using authority and assertiveness • Assessing capabilities • Supporting others	• Planning and preparing • Prioritizing • Providing and maintaining standards • Identifying and utilizing resources
Situation awareness	**Decision-making**
• Gathering information • Recognizing and understanding • Anticipating	• Identifying options • Balancing risks and selecting options • Re-evaluating

Table 9.2 Team Behavioural Rater (Adapted from Weller *et al*. [51])

Team Behavioural Rating Tool

ITEM	Descriptors
1. A leader was clearly established	**Excellent**: One person centralized information and decision-making and coordinated the actions of the team. **Poor**: Unclear who was taking the lead, information not centralized, action of individuals not coordinated.
2. The leader maintained an overview of the situation	**Excellent**: Kept on top of all the information available, and how tasks were being implemented. Avoided taking on tasks that could be delegated. **Poor**: Leader slow to notice new information, failed to notice that some tasks weren't being done.
3. Each team member had a clear role	**Excellent** The leader explicitly designated roles to team members by name. All required roles were taken on. No duplication or confusion over roles was evident. **Poor**: No designation of roles occurred. Some roles were unassigned. It was unclear what team members should be doing.
4. The leader's instructions were explicit	**Excellent**: Instructions were clearly audible, easy to understand, with sufficient detail to avoid any potential confusion. **Poor**: Unclear, inaudible, or imprecise instructions. etc., e.g. 'give some adrenaline'.
5. The leader's verbal instructions and verbal communications were directed.	**Excellent**: Used person's name when giving instruction. **Poor**: Use of 'someone', no indication of who the communication was meant for.
6. When team members received instructions they closed the communication loop	**Excellent**: For critical instructions, team members repeated it back for confirmation. **Poor**: No acknowledgement that the instruction had been heard or would be acted upon.

(Continued)

Table 9.2 *(Continued)*	
Team Behavioural Rating Tool	
ITEM	Descriptors
7. The leader's plan for treatment was communicated to the team	**Excellent**: Relevant team members informed of the plan in sufficient detail for them to understand what was required of them. **Poor**: No treatment plan was shared by the leader to the team.
8. Priorities and orders of actions were communicated to the team	**Excellent**: When more than one task/action was needed at any time, the leader clarified what was most important. **Poor**: the leader issued multiple requests without prioritizing.
9. The leader verbalized to the team possible future developments or requirements.	**Excellent**: Leader anticipated and verbalized potential future development and what might be required. **Poor**: The leader failed to inform team members of possible developments that they would have to prepare for.
10. The team leader responded appropriately to questions or requests for clarification from team members.	**Excellent**: Input invited. Answered questions, acknowledged concerns, gave explanation or clarification in response to questioning from team members. **Poor**: Input not invited and actively discouraged. Ignored or dismissed questions or concerns from team members.
11. When expressions of concern to the leader did not elicit an appropriate response, team members persisted in seeking a response, or took action	**Did this occur? Yes/No. If yes,** **Excellent**: The team member, after having their initial concern ignored, raised the issue again until it was resolved. **Poor**: The team member didn't pursue their concern, or persisted with low level probing and the issue remained unresolved.
12. The leader verbalized important clinical interventions to the team.	**Excellent**: The leader always/almost always told the team s/he was doing and what was happening, **Poor**: The leader rarely or never told the team what s/he was doing, or what was happening.
13. Team members verbalized their clinical actions to the leader	**Excellent**: Team members consistently told the leader what they were doing, when undertaking critical tasks, and when these have been completed. **Poor**: The team members rarely or never told the team leader what they were doing.
14. Team members verbalized situational information to the leader	**Excellent:** *All* team members consistently told the leader important situational information. (patient information, vital signs, monitor data, etc.). **Poor**: Team members didn't inform leader of new information or change in patient status that the leader may not have noticed.

Table 9.2 (*Continued*)	
Team Behavioural Rating Tool	
ITEM	**Descriptors**
15. **Team members sought assistance from each other**	**Excellent**: Explicitly asked each other for help with tasks. **Poor**: Team members never asked for help when it was clear they had too much to do.
16. **Team members offered assistance to one other**	**Excellent**: Explicitly offered to help with tasks, with the purpose of making sure everything got done in a timely fashion. **Poor**: Team members never asked for help when it was clear they had too much to do.
17. **The team leader invited suggestions from the team members when problem-solving.**	**Excellent**: Asks for suggestions about possible other causes or strategies to manage a problem. E.g. I think this is due to blood loss does anybody have any other ideas? **Poor**: leader never asked for anyone's opinion, suggestion or idea, even when this would have potentially helped the situation.
18. **When faced with a problem, the team leader sourced external assistance**	**Did a situation arise where outside help could have improved management? Yes/No.** If yes **Excellent:** The team leader sourced external advice/help in a timely way. e.g. anticipates difficulties and calls a colleague or senior. **Poor:** External help was never called even though this could have helped resolve the situation.
19. **The team leader gave a situation update to the team when the situation changed.**	**Excellent**: Described patient status, their assessment of the situation and proposed plan (e.g. SNAPPI, etc.). **Poor**: Leader did not inform the team members of any relevant changes or new information in patient status.
20. **Task implementation was well coordinated**	**Excellent**: All tasks were managed efficiently, all components done, and done in the correct order. **Poor**: Tasks were only ever partially completed, generally muddled, interruptions and distractions impeded smooth and efficient completion of tasks.
21. **Global behavioural performance**	Overall impression of the team performance.

improve information sharing in patient handover between team members, or when referring a patient to another health profession for their input (Box 9.3).

• PACER (Probe, Alert, Challenge, Emergency, Response) [55], and the Two Challenge Rule [56] are tools to assist team members to speak up or challenge decisions by the team leader (Boxes 9.4 and 9.5).

• SNAPPI (Stand back and get attention, Notify team of the situation, Assessment of situation, Plan and Priorities, Invite ideas) [57] is a tool to structure a team call out, where the team is brought together to ensure shared situational assessment, shared goals and inviting team input into the problem (Box 9.6). These tools can be used in team training either in the debriefing of scenarios where good examples of these have been seen or where they could have

---

Box 9.3 ISBAR (Source: Marshall *et al.* [54])

ISBAR – handover tool
Identify who you are
Situation – describe the problem
Background – clinical context
Assessment – what you think is going on
Recommendation/**R**equirement – what you
  think needs to be done, what you need the
  other person to do
Example: Junior house officer to consultant.
I: *I'm the medical house officer from ward 41*
  looking after Mrs Smith.
S: *She is a 75-year-old woman who has*
  become acutely short of breath overnight
  raised respiratory rate, and low oxygen
  saturation. Her chest sounds clear.
B: *She had a total knee joint replacement 3*
  days ago but was previously well on no
  medication.
A: *I think she may have a pulmonary*
  embolus, but other options to consider
  would be chest infection or pulmonary
  oedema.
R: *I think we should get a chest X-ray, blood*
  gas and chest CT. Would you please come
  and see her to confirm my assessment of
  the situation?

Box 9.4 PACER (Source: Patient Safety Centre [55])

Pacer
Probe
Alert
Challenge
Emergency
Response
Example: Anaesthetic technician to
anaesthetic registrar
P: *Do you think the patient is adequately*
  fasted for anaesthesia.
A: *The patient may vomit during the induction*
  of anaesthesia.
C: *I don't think you should proceed with the*
  induction.
E: *The patient's life will be in danger if you*
  proceed.
R: *I'm calling the supervisor.*

Box 9.5 Two challenge rule

'If a pilot is clearly challenged twice about an
unsafe situation during a flight without a
satisfactory reply, the junior is empowered to
take over the controls.'
  Juniors are expected to express their
concerns.
  Seniors are expected to listen and reply.
Example: Anaphylaxis in theatre.
Junior: I'm concerned about the low blood
  pressure and that new rash. Could this be
  anaphylaxis?
Senior: No, everything's fine. Just histamine
  release.
Junior: The blood pressure is falling further,
  the rash is getting worse.
Senior: No answer.
Junior: I'm calling the anaesthetic
  co-ordinator, and drawing up adrenaline.

---

been useful, or modelled in video simulations depicting team behaviours.

Referring back to Rousseau's model of team function (Figure 9.1), the factors influencing team processes are teamwork behaviours, cognition, and attitudes. A number of instruments have been developed to observe and measure teamwork behaviours (Box 9.2, Tables 9.1 and 9.2) and these are commonly used to frame debriefing and reflection after a simulation. But from Rousseau's model, it can clearly be seen as only one of a number of conditions affecting team function that could be amenable to SBTT. More difficult to observe are the attitudes of team members to each other and their role in the team, and their cognitive processes – how do they engage in individual or team problem solving?

> ## Box 9.6   SNAPPI call out
>
> **S**tand back and get the attention of the team
> **N**otify the team of patient status (vital signs etc.)
> **A**ssessment of the situation (what you think is going on)
> **P**roposed plan for treatment
> **P**riorities (what needs to be done first, etc.)
> **I**nvite ideas and suggestions
>
> Example: *'Hold on everyone, let's take stock for a moment. The patient is hypoxic, and has reduced air entry on the right but the airway is clear. It could be consolidation or collapse, or maybe pneumothorax. We need to provide immediate treatment and at the same time work out what's going on. We should give oxygen and then do a chest X-ray and then do a blood gas. Any other ideas?*

What to teach: cognition

This section focuses on team cognition, or the sharing of information between team members, identified in Salas *et al.*'s [41] model as one of the fundamental enablers of effective teamwork. These relate to 'cognition', a factor influencing team processes, in Rousseau's framework for team performance (Figure 9.2). The team cognition process is often referred to as developing 'shared mental models' and affects team performance in several ways: problem solving, task management and supporting other team members.

Shared cognition is fundamental to teams adapting their performance processes under varying task conditions, interpreting environmental cues in a similar or complementary way and making compatible decisions. SBTT can provide an opportunity to explore, through facilitated debrief, how information is filtered and distributed among the team. There is evidence in other fields that information sharing, or lack thereof, is causally connected to team effectiveness [39]. Lack of shared cognition can derail the process of building shared understanding of the situation and thus impair perform-

ance and cause errors [39,58]. There are numerous examples in healthcare where failures to work within shared mental models have led to poor outcomes for patients [14].

The team can be the 'unit of cognition' [39], where problem solving is a shared activity. In this sense the team shares the collective responsibility for collecting, managing and retrieving information. Think of the situation between a group of old friends trying to remember an event in the past. One starts with a piece of information, that sparks a memory in another and so on, until the entire event is pieced together, in a way that no single member of the group could have achieved. Think also of a novel problem, where different members of the group have different experiences and abilities to call on, contribute new ideas, or see something others have missed or a situation where a nurse knows about how a patient copes on the ward, a doctor knows what the treatment is and the social worker has explored the home situation. Sharing these separate pieces of information provides a better solution and care pathway for the patient. In terms of the components in the Rousseau teamwork model (Figure 9.2) this is mission task analysis, planning and collaborative problem solving.

An example of the team as a superior unit of cognition can be demonstrated in the NASA Moon Game, an entertaining exercise which can be usefully included in team training programmes. First, participants individually rank the items they would include in their kit if their spacecraft crashed on the moon. Next the team works together to rank the items, resulting in the team coming up with a better answer. A full description can be found at http://starchild.gsfc.nasa.gov/docs/StarChild/space_level2/activity/problems_space.html.

Where tasks are interdependent (i.e. all tasks are required to achieve the goal), coordinated task management is facilitated by shared mental models, by ensuring a common understanding of who is responsible for the different tasks and identifying what information people need to know to complete that task. This allows them to coordinate their tasks. This relates to 'group specification' in the Rousseau teamwork model (Figure 9.2).

Finally, a shared mental model allows team members to anticipate one another's needs, for example to prepare equipment, alert other hospital departments or services, request additional resources, or offload some of their team member's tasks. This relates to 'back up behaviours' in Rousseau's model.

While the concept of a shared mental model may seem theoretical and 'difficult', approaches to achieving this are in fact practical, and may not be too difficult to implement. For example the success of the WHO surgical safety checklist may in part be due to the team briefing at the beginning of the case [59] where for just a moment, the team comes together to make sure they all agree on the operation they are about to embark on together, and identify any issues that may be a concern for them. Methods to approach team training for shared mental models can include 'pause and discuss',

where a scenario is stopped, and at that point each team member is asked to describe their understanding of the situation, or during a debrief, where the team can be asked to share their understanding of what went on or what they were thinking at a certain point of time shown on video replay. The former allows the team to actually share the mental model and then proceed. The latter may demonstrate the consequences of a lack of a shared mental model. Both approaches can be effective in learning what and when to communicate information. When individuals in a team become aware, through debriefing of the extent to which others in the team had very different understanding of the simulated case or plan or potential problems, learning can be profound.

🔍 Example 1   What were you thinking?

During an in situ simulation of malignant hyperthermia(MH), the anaesthetist asked the circulating nurse to get ice. The nurse phoned the orderly who noted the request down on her list of tasks. The ice didn't come for 25 minutes.

During the debrief, the nurse and anaesthetist were asked what they were thinking at the time of the request for ice. The anaesthetist wanted ice urgently to cool the patient with life threatening MH and a temperature of 42°C. The nurse didn't know what MH was or the urgency of the request for ice, but was focussed on the need to manage the patient's cardiovascular instability. Participants considered how the management of the case would have been improved if the whole team had a clear understanding of what the problem was and a shared understanding of the goals of treatment. They further discussed how this could have been implemented realistically, what were the barriers (an opportunity to explore attitudes, roles) and how these barriers could be overcome.

What to teach: attitudes

Returning to 'The two challenge rule' in SBTT (Box 9.5), while this behaviour can be learned, a number of other factors will affect its actual use in clinical practice. These include lack of confidence in one's own opinion; expectation that the other person knows what they're doing; expectation of hostile response (conflict avoidance); not your responsibility (professional silos, lack of focus on patient); workplace culture (don't challenge seniors); or team climate that doesn't invite input from members (the 'monologic' leader).

SBTT creates a situation that triggers a response from the team. The situation can be manipulated

to replicate or amplify these responses in order to explore their effect on team effectiveness and their consequences on patient care. Examples can be reviewed through videotape replay, and with skilled facilitation, assumptions can be exposed, challenged and, potentially, attitudes changed.

Teaching environment: where, when, what and who

Where

Options include a purpose-built simulation facility; *in situ* simulations where scenarios are conducted within the clinical environment, for example in an

Example 2 Why didn't you say something?

A senior male doctor was working with a junior female nurse in a simulation of a case of a cardiac arrest. During the arrest the doctor was performing cardiac compressions at 60 per minute. In the subsequent debrief we asked the nurse what she was thinking at the time. She admitted to thinking this was too slow but didn't like to say anything. When asked why she didn't speak up, she said she was only junior, didn't think it was her place to speak up, and wasn't entirely confident that she was right. The doctor was amazed that the nurse felt unable to speak up, and realized he may need to explicitly voice his own uncertainties and invite suggestions from team members to get their input. The nurse was pleased to know that her ideas or suggestions would have been welcome and valued, and realized that her failure to speak up could have compromised patient outcome.

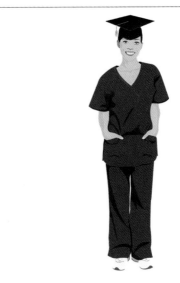

Figure 9.4 Avatar example. Courtesy of Henry Fuller. http://secondlife6750.wordpress.com.

unused operating theatre or empty room on a ward or clinic or in a virtual world, with the team at a distance, communicating through avatars (Figure 9.4). The purpose-built simulation facility reduces the chance of work interfering with training, and increases control and potentially quality of the simulation, but is expensive and resource intensive. *In situ* simulations can engage an entire department, potentially leading to mutual reinforcement of lessons learned, can test the interaction with the environment and might be considered more authentic. Disadvantages may include managing the clinical environment safely (e.g. patients, other staff informed, simulated drugs or equipment not mixed with real drugs, interference with work). Online (avatar based) team training has the advantages of flexibility and easier access but many people may need training or persuasion to engage in what they might see as a game.

When

The main options are a one-off workshop or an ongoing programme. The former may be more feasible, but the latter will potentially have a greater impact. For development of new skills, regular, spaced sessions are more effective than a single exposure, especially where there are opportunities to apply and effective teamwork skills in increasingly challenging situations [60].

What

Most SBTT interventions described in the literature have been confined to a single context. The patient moves between different environments, and in fact the transitions between these environments and between teams may be the periods of high risk. Consider the options for linking the SBTT to the other components of the patient journey through the system, for example a trauma patient transferred from the emergency department to the intensive care unit via radiology.

Who

A major challenge in healthcare team collaboration is interprofessional communication. However, most reports of SBTT interventions focus on a single professional group. While this may be a useful and non-threatening beginning, in reality health professionals work in multidisciplinary teams. Different professions have different ways of coding, retrieving, prioritizing and communicating information; therefore, some of the bigger challenges in teamwork are likely to come from interactions across professional groups. Understanding the capabilities of other professional groups, and the information they need to know to do their job, may be limited. During the process of professional socialization, typically attributes of the group a professional belongs to are seen as positive, and of other groups as less desirable. Stereotypical representation of other groups may be inaccurate or even derogatory and can potentially be reinforced during uniprofessional team training, for example through consistently simulating negative aspects of other professions, or through language permitted in uniprofessional discussions (e.g. unhelpful, obstructive, idle). Learning how to negotiate these differences would seem to be a fundamental requirement for SBTT and the requirement for a multidisciplinary faculty to facilitate multidisciplinary team training would appear to be equally fundamental.

Designing and implementing SBTT

The fundamental goal of SBTT is to improve patient outcomes. SBTT has the potential to change processes, perceptions or cultures in the workplace at individual, team and organization level. When designing an SBTT intervention, the first step is to decide which aspect of teamwork, out of all the possibilities outlined, is the target: what are the desired outcomes of the intervention, what needs to happen to reach those outcomes, how can these changes be achieved, where does simulation fit in this, and how will goals be evaluated? For SBTT, have the lessons learned in the simulation been transferred to clinical practice [28]? Clear objectives are required, with appropriate construction of the learning environment, incorporating feedback, and an opportunity to practice (Box 9.7) [61].

Furthermore, we can draw on change management strategies in the development of the SBTT, for example involving the learners. There is value in

role modelling desired behaviours, being explicit about the expected standard of performance and allowing participants to practise these behaviours and observe each other. Structured teamwork assessment tools can improve the ability of instructors to give specific and accurate teamwork and enable participants to reflect on their own performance: reflection through, on and for action. Training the instructors in both the theory and practice of teamwork and in the art of feedback is of critical importance [28]. Current understanding of memory decay and retention of new learning supports the suggestion to evaluate some time out from the intervention.

Salas *et al.* [39] further emphasizes the value of exploring beyond observed behaviours to understand what underlies them, or what impact they had on other team members. The ability to dig deeper in SBTT beyond the observed behaviours depends on the facilitation skills of the instructors and their understanding of teamwork, and on the ability to design scenarios to elicit the desired behaviours. While some teamwork skills can be learned and practised as in the Advanced Cardiac Life Support (ACLS) algorithm (or ISBAR) and readily applied to practice, others can be learnt in a simulation suite, but may be more difficult to actually implement in the workplace (or even a realistic, immersive simulated workplace). Consider, for example, trying to teach the skill of 'Speaking up'. Exploring the factors that inhibit or facilitate team members speaking up in a team, perhaps showing video of the type of language used that invited or repressed other team members from contributing, may be a way of getting to the underlying causes of what stops team members from speaking up thus inhibiting the development of optimal shared mental models.

Assessing teams: what to assess, measurement tools and common outcomes

If you can't measure it you can't improve it. (Attributed to Lord Kelvin)

A key component of SBTT is providing feedback on observed behaviours, exploring the cognitive and

---

Box 9.7 Strategies for design and implementation of SBTT.
Source: Issenberg [61]

Course design
- Involve participants in development of training.
- Base learning objectives on theoretical models of teamwork and team training.
- Clearly define the learning outcomes for and benchmarks for performance.
- Take learner level into account and increase task difficulty with progress.

Learning methods
- Model the desired behaviours.
- Adapt the simulation to complement multiple learning approaches.
- Provide for individualized as well as team learning from the simulations.

Simulations
- Aim for cognitive fidelity – i.e. trigger the cognitive processes involved in effective teamwork in the clinical environment.
- Control the environment for learners (e.g. rules of engagement).
- Ensure the simulation is valid for the learning task.

- Address complexity – e.g. changing environment, clinical variation, ad hoc teams.

Feedback/debriefing
- Use a structured assessment tool to improve feedback.
- Explore the outcomes of team behaviours (e.g. impact of behaviour on other team members), not just identify the behaviours.
- Explore team cognition

Ongoing learning
- Integrate simulation into the overall curriculum
- Provide opportunities to practice.

Instructor training
- Train the trainers.

Programme evaluation
- Evaluate at delayed time to evaluate retention of learning.
- Look for transfer of learning to clinical practice.

---

attitudinal basis of these behaviours, and facilitating new learning from the experiences. Feedback is more constructive if it is structured, specific and accurate.

The range of published instruments developed to assess teamwork behaviours was reviewed by Shapiro *et al.* [62] and has been further extended. Many focus on an individual in a team, often the leader, for example Anaesthesia Non-Technical Skills (ANTS) [48]. Some consider whole team performance such as NOTECHS (Non-TECHnical Skills) and the Team Behavioural Rater [52,63]. Other tools are available to measure attitudes [64] and team climate [65].

While devising a single, robust measure of a healthcare team's performance would be desirable, there are a number of difficulties in developing

effective team performance measures. These include complexity of healthcare teams stemming from different contexts, often changing personnel, and dynamic interactions between multiple, different people; multiple perspectives on the outcome measure of interest, which could include team processes (e.g. communication, problem solving, team climate), or patient outcomes; teams and team performance changes over time; the effect of the observer on performance; and in simulation-based education, the effect of the synthetic environment.

That being said [18], Salas *et al.* [18] have proposed a best-practice guide to developing or choosing team performance measurement scales on the assumption that these will be helpful on every occasion where an observer (instructor) watches participants in a simulation (or indeed in real life) with the purpose of providing accurate, specific and constructive feedback on performance. While the focus of these is on observable behaviours and not directly measuring participant cognition, attitudes or feelings, this approach more accurately identifies what happened, enabling, for example, a discussion of cognitive processes, assumptions, influence of actions on others. Key items to consider when developing assessment tools for teams include the following (adapted from Salas *et al.* [18]).

Develop measures from a theoretical framework

In previous sections, some theoretical frameworks for considering the components of teamwork have been explored (Figures 9.2 and 9.3) which can be identified in other team measurement scales. If these are taken as the key components to be measured, then measures should be developed to capture each of these. Other models may have different priorities and may need to be adapted to specific contexts as the nature of the task may vary, e.g. differences in leadership structure, interdependencies.

Define the purpose of the assessment, and design the measure to meet this purpose

An assessment can be for diagnostic purposes, e.g. to discover the factors impeding team performance, for formative assessment to facilitate learning or for summative purposes. For team performance measures, the aims are likely to be diagnostic and to facilitate learning, to provide accurate feedback to improve performance.

Design the measure based on the competencies required in the particular context

Specific teamwork competencies may vary between different professional groups and published lists of general teamwork competencies may not be relevant. A task analysis of the context under study may therefore be required.

Measure different components of performance

Teams may perform poorly for a number of different reasons. Team members may have inadequate knowledge or procedural skills to perform the task. Alternatively, individually they may have the knowledge and skills, but lack the ability to put this into practice due to poor teamwork skills.

Furthermore, the problem may be at an individual or whole team level. A leader with limited communication skills will deprive the team of the knowledge they need to do the required tasks. Alternatively, the team may fail to identify a leader, and subsequently fail to decide what needs to be done.

Link measures to scenario events

SBTT allows performance to be observed in situations that faithfully replicate important features of the real world and incorporate specific events requiring critical competencies. A checklist can then be constructed to target the competencies that the event is designed to elicit which could have high diagnostic value [18]. Scenario-specific checklists can be used in conjunction with a more global teamwork measurement tools. The latter can provide reliable assessments of teamwork performance over time, but their diagnostic accuracy may not be as high as a purpose-designed checklist for specific competencies. For example, if a training objective is to develop strategies to resolve conflict, include in the scenario an event where conflict will arise, and create a checklist of the desirable behaviours that one hopes to elicit in the team members.

Focus on observable markers

Global ratings of team performance can provide a reliable overall measure, but to get the level of detail required for specific and constructive feedback it is necessary to include the different components of teamwork that can be observed and addressed, for example, 'Each team member had a clear role' rather than 'workload management'.

Train the instructors

Training instructors to assess team performance is crucial. Instructors should be trained in the use of a structured teamwork observation chart. This is generally achieved by watching tightly scripted and structured training scenarios, scoring the team performance and then reconciling scores with other instructors to ensure common interpretation of items and agreement on required standard. Regular calibration may be required to ensure adequate inter-rater reliability and limit drift in scoring.

This chapter has considered the imperatives for effective multidisciplinary approaches to teamwork training and some theoretical models which help us to better understand the dimension of teamwork. The chapter has also considered what simulation has to offer and presented some different approaches to team training interventions and discussed the need for measurement tools to enable structured and accurate feedback and to know if interventions are effective.

Future developments should consider utilizing theoretical models and empirical evidence from other organizations and disciplines to develop a better understanding of teamwork in healthcare, refining measurement tools and incorporating measurement of transfer to the clinical environment. The future should see much more emphasis on training together those who work together, i.e. authentic, interprofessional and often *ad hoc* teams.

SUMMARY

 Key points

- Effective teamwork and communication between team members is crucial to patient safety.
- Simulation-based environments offer enormous potential for team training.
- Development and implementation of simulation-based team training (SBTT) courses should be based on theoretical understanding of teamwork, and sound educational approaches.
- SBTT can incorporate specific behavioural strategies to improve team performance, address team cognition and problem solving, and challenge attitudes and perceptions of other professional groups.
- Team training in healthcare should be multidisciplinary, to overcome communication barriers between different health professional groups.
- Observation, assessment and feedback on team performance can be improved using structured observation charts.
- Training of instructors is vital.

REFERENCES

1. Health and Disability Commissioner (2002) A Report by the Health and Disability Commissioner. (Case 00/06857). Health and Disability Commission. Available from http://www.hdc.org.nz/media/2695/00HDC06857%20surgeon.pdf (accessed 6 March 2013).

2. Bosch M, Faber MJ, Cruijsberg J, *et al.* (2009) Effectiveness of patient care teams and the role of clinical expertise and coordination: A literature review. *Medical Care Research & Review* **66**(Suppl): 5S–35S.

3. Davis P, Lay-Yee R, Schug S, *et al.* (2001) Adverse events in New Zealand public

hospitals – principal findings from a national survey. Wellington. Available from http://www.health.govt.nz/publication/adverse-events-new-zealand-public-hospitals-principal-findings-national-survey (accessed 6 March 2013).

4. Wilson R, Runciman W, Gibberd R, *et al.* (1995) The Quality in Australian Health Care Study. *Medical Journal of Australia* **163:** 458–471.

5. Leape L, Brennan T, Laird N, *et al.* (1991) The nature of adverse events in hospitalized patients: The results of the Harvard Medical Practice Study II. *New England Journal of Medicine* **324:** 377–384.

6. Alvarez G, Coiera E (2006) Interdisciplinary communication: An uncharted source of medical error? *Journal of Critical Care* **21:** 236–242.

7. Manser T (2009) Teamwork and patient safety in dynamic domains of healthcare: a review of the literature. *Acta Anaesthesiology Scandinavica* **53:** 143–151.

8. Webb RK, Currie M, Morgan CA, *et al.* (1993) The Australian incident monitoring study: an analysis of 2000 incident reports. *Anaesthesia & Intensive Care* **21:** 520–528.

9. Bognor M (1994) *Human Error In Medicine*, 1st edn. New Jersey: Lawrence Erlbaum Association Inc.

10. Helmreich R (ed.) (2000) *Threat and Error in Aviation and Medicine: Similar and Different. Special Medical Seminar, Lessons For Health Care: Applied Human Factors Research.* Australian Council of Safety and Quality in Health Care & NSW Ministerial Council for Quality in Health Care.

11. Reader TW, Flin R, Cuthbertson BH (2007) Communication skills and error in the intensive care unit. *Current Opinion in Critical Care* **13:** 732–736.

12. Reason J (1990) *Human Error*, 1st edn. Cambridge: Cambridge University Press.

13. Lingard L, Espin S, Whyte S, *et al.* (2004) Communication failures in the operating room: an observational classification of recurrent types and effects. *Quality & Safety in Health Care* **13:** 330–334.

14. Weller J, Barrow M, Gasquoine S (2011) Interprofessional collaboration among junior doctors and nurses in the hospital setting. *Medical Education* **45:** 478–487.

15. Institute of Medicine (2000) *To Err Is Human: Building a Safer Health System.* Washington DC: National Academy Press.

16. US Accreditation Council for Medical Graduates (2001) *ACGME Core Competencies.* Chicago: ACGME.

17. Frank J (ed.) (2005) *The CanMEDS 2005 Physician Competency Framework: Better Standards. Better Physicians. Better Care.* Ottawa: The Royal College of Physicians and Surgeons of Canada.

18. Salas E, Almeida SA, Salisbury M, *et al.* (2009) What are the critical success factors for team training in health care? *Joint Commission Journal on Quality & Patient Safety* **35:** 398–405.

19. US Agency for Healthcare Research and Quality. TeamSTEPPS: National Implementation. US Department of Health and Human Services. Available from http://teamstepps.ahrq.gov/abouttoolsmaterials.htm (accessed 26 October 2012).

20. Leape L, Berwick D (2005) Five years after to err is human: what have we learned? *Journal of the American Medical Association* **293:** 2384–2390.

21. Hall P (2005) Interprofessional teamwork: professional cultures as barriers. *Journal of Interprofessional Care* **19:** 188–196.

22. Horsburgh M, Perkins R, Coyle B, Degeling P (2006) The professional subcultures of students entering medicine, nursing and pharmacy programmes. *Journal of Interprofessional Care* **20:** 425–431.

23. Bleakley A (2010) Social comparison, peer learning and democracy in medical education. *Medical Teacher* **32**: 878–879.

24. Kobayashi H, Pian-Smith M, Sato M, *et al.* (2006) A cross-cultural survey of residents' perceived barriers in questioning/challenging authority. *Quality & Safety in Health Care* **15**: 277–283.

25. Morris-Stiff GJ, Sarasin S, Edwards P, *et al.* (2005) The European Working Time Directive: One for all and all for one? *Surgery* **137**: 293–297.

26. Ramsey RA, Anand R, Harmer SG, *et al.* (2007) Continuity of care and the European working time directive: a maxillofacial perspective. *British Journal of Oral & Maxillofacial Surgery* **45**: 221–222.

27. Tsouroufli M, Payne H (2008) Consultant medical trainers, modernising medical careers (MMC) and the European time directive (EWTD): tensions and challenges in a changing medical education context. *BMC Medical Education* **8**: 31.

28. Weaver SJ, Lyons R, DiazGranados D, *et al.* (2010) The anatomy of health care team training and the state of practice: a critical review. *Academic Medicine* **85**: 1746–1760.

29. Baker DP, Day R, Salas E (2006) Teamwork as an essential component of high-reliability organizations. *Health Services Research* **41**: 1576–1598.

30. Weller J (2010) Interdisciplinary simulations to reduce communication failures and improve outcomes. CMHSE Research Seminar; 2010. University of Auckland.

31. Jaarsma T (2005) Inter-professional team approach to patients with heart failure. *Heart* **91**: 832–838.

32. Salas E, DiazGranados D, Klein C, *et al.* (2008) Does Team training improve team performance? A meta-analysis human factors. *Journal of the Human Factors and Ergonomics Society* **50**: 903–933.

33. Salas E, DiazGranados D, Weaver S, King H (2008) Does team training work? Principles for health care. *Academic Emergency Medicine* **11**: 1002–1009.

34. McCulloch P, Rathbone J, Catchpole K (2011) Interventions to improve teamwork and communications among healthcare staff. *British Journal of Surgery* **98**: 469–479.

35. Kirkpatrick DL (1994) *Evaluating Training Programmes: the Four Levels.* San Francisco: Berrett-Koehler.

36. Weller J, Janssen A, Merry A, Robinson B (2008) Interdisciplinary team training: a qualitative analysis of team interactions in anaesthesia. *Medical Education* **42**: 382–388.

37. Weller J, Wilson L, Robinson B (2003) Survey of change in practice following simulation-based training in crisis management. *Anaesthesia* **58**: 471–473.

38. Jensen L, Merry A, Webster C, *et al.* (2004) Evidence-based strategies for preventing drug administration errors during anaesthesia. *Anaesthesia* **59**: 493–504.

39. Salas E, Cooke NJ, Rosen MA (2008) On teams, teamwork, and team performance: discoveries and developments. *Human Factors* **50**: 540–547.

40. Rousseau V, Aube C, Savoie A (2006) Teamwork behaviors: a review and an integration of frameworks. *Small Group Research* **37**: 540–570.

41. Salas E, Sims D, Burke C (2005) Is there a 'big five' in teamwork? *Small Group Research* **36**: 555.

42. Hunt EA, Shilkofski NA, Stavroudis TA, Nelson KL (2007) Simulation: translation to improved team performance. *Anesthesiology Clinics* **25**: 301–319.

43. Paige JT, Kozmenko V, Yang T, *et al.* (2009) High-fidelity, simulation-based, interdisciplinary operating room team

training at the point of care. *Surgery* **145:** 138–146.

44. Shapiro MJ, Morey JC, Small SD, *et al.* (2004) Simulation based teamwork training for emergency department staff: does it improve clinical team performance when added to an existing didactic teamwork curriculum? *Quality & Safety in Health Care* **13:** 417–421.

45. Helmreich RL, Merritt AC, Wilhelm JA (1999) The evolution of crew resource management training in commercial aviation. *International Journal of Aviation Psychology* **9:** 19–32.

46. Xiao Y, Moss J (2001) Practices of High Reliability Teams: Observations in Trauma Resuscitation. *Proceedings of the Human Factors and Ergonomics Society Annual Meeting* **45:** 395–359.

47. Gaba D, Fish K, Howard S (1994) *Crisis Management in Anesthesiology*, 1st edn. Edinburgh: Churchill Livingston.

48. Fletcher G, Flin R, McGeorge P, *et al.* (2003) Anaesthetists' Non-Technical Skills (ANTS): evaluation of a behavioural marker system. *British Journal of Anaesthesia* **90:** 580–588.

49. Flin R, Maran N (2004) Identifying and training non-technical skills for teams in acute medicine. *Quality and Safety in Health Care* **13** (Suppl 1)**:** i80–i84.

50. Yule S, Flin R, Paterson-Brown S, Maran N (2006) Development of a rating system for surgeons' non-technical skills. *Medical Education* **40:** 1098–1104.

51. Rosen MA, Salas E, Wilson KA, *et al.* (2008) Measuring team performance in simulation-based training: adopting best practices for healthcare. *Simulation in Healthcare* **3:** 33–41.

52. Weller J, Frengley R, Torrie J, *et al.* (2011) Evaluation of an instrument to measure teamwork in multidisciplinary critical care teams. *BMJ Quality & Safety* **20:** 216–222.

53. Flin R, Glavin R, Patey R (2003) Framework for observing and rating anaesthetists' non-technical skills. University of Aberdeen. Available from http://www.abdn.ac.uk/iprc/documents/ants/ants_handbook_v1.0_electronic_access_version.pdf (accessed 6 March 2013).

54. Marshall S, Harrison J, Flanagan B (2009) The teaching of a structured tool improves the clarity and content of interprofessional clinical communication. *Quality & Safety in Health Care* **18:** 137–140.

55. Patient Safety Centre (2009) *Recognition and management of the deteriorating patient.* Brisbane: Queensland Government. Available from http://www.health.qld.gov.au/patientsafety/documents/deter_paper.pdf (accessed 14 October 2011).

56. Pian-Smith MCM, Simon R, Minehart RD, *et al.* (2009) Teaching Residents the two-challenge rule: a simulation-based approach to improve education and patient safety *Simulation in Healthcare* **4:** 84–91.

57. Weller J, Torrie J, Hendersdon K, Frengley R (2010) The Anaesthetist as a Team Player: Speed Dating and Other Useful Skills. In: Australian and New Zealand College of Anaesthetists Annual Scientific Meeting Christchurch 2010.

58. Stout RJ, Cannon-Bower JA, Salas E, Milanovich DM (1999) Planning, shared mental models, and coordinated performance: an empirical link is established. *Human Factors* **41:** 61.

59. Haynes A, Weiser T, Berry W, *et al.* (2009) A surgical safety checklist to reduce morbidity and mortality in a global population. *New England Journal of Medicine* **360:** 491–499.

60. Ericsson KA (2004) Deliberate practice and the acquisition and maintenance of expert performance in medicine and related domains. *Academic Medicine* **79**(Suppl)**:** S70–81.

61. Issenberg S, McGaghie W, Petrusa E (2005) Features and uses of high fidelity medical simulations that lead to effective learning: a BEME systematic review. *Medical Teacher* **27:** 10–28.

62. Shapiro M, Gardner R, Godwin S, *et al.* (2008) Defining team performance for simulation-based training: methodology, metrics, and opportunities for Emergency Medicine. *Academic Emergency Medicine* **15:** 1088–1097.

63. Mishra A, Catchpole K, McCulloch P (2009) The Oxford NOTECHS system: reliability and validity of a tool for measuring teamwork behaviour in the operating theatre. *Quality & Safety in Healthcare* **18:** 104–108.

64. Helmreich R, Sexton JB, Merritt AC (1997) *The Operating Room Management Attitudes Questionnaire (ORMAQ)*. Austin: University of Texas.

65. Anderson NR, West MA (1998) Measuring climate for work group innovation: development and validation of the team climate inventory. *Journal of Organizational Behaviour* **19:** 235–58.

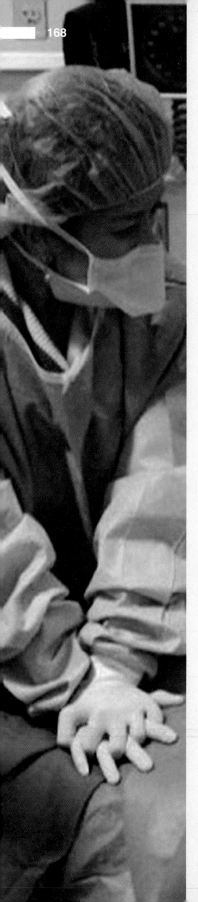

CHAPTER 10

Designing effective simulation activities

Joanne Barrott[1], Ann B. Sunderland[1], Jane P. Micklin[1] and Michelle McKenzie Smith[2]   [1]Leeds Metropolitan University, Leeds, UK; [2]Montagu Hospital, Mexborough, UK

Overview

Designing and establishing a simulation facility, whether large, small or even a single educational intervention, begins with a thorough assessment, from evidencing the need to early engagement with key internal and external stakeholders. Throughout the chapter, we discuss lessons learned from the experiences of large, small and independent facilities providing courses, with hints and tips of what has worked well in actual cases, the challenges they faced and how these were overcome. The chapter provides practical steps and guidance through the processes of planning, identifying and management of resources, identification of roles and responsibilities, running a facility or course and planning for the future through sustainability and/or income generation.

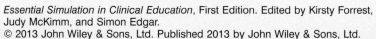

Essential Simulation in Clinical Education, First Edition. Edited by Kirsty Forrest, Judy McKimm, and Simon Edgar.

Introduction

Good organization and forward planning are key to starting, running and sustaining effective healthcare simulation activities. Indeed, prior to accepting the challenge of planning, designing, resourcing and running any simulated activity, the developer must consider the process in its entirety (Figure 10.1). It is acknowledged that there is no set order to the process, and therefore we have not produced a step-by-step guide, but have instead described the essential factors to be considered.

All developers will be aware of the costs and expense of simulation activities, both in terms of time and faculty. The initial funding (capital costs) and sustainability (revenue) are obvious concerns; however, finances are equally important on an ongoing basis and provide a valid rationale for employing dedicated managers and/or administra-

tors to consider economic issues relating to sustainability. It is important to identify potential users at an early stage in the planning process as these potential users will probably provide future sources of income. Any business case needs to include projected income from courses that will be offered and specify delegate rates and other income streams (e.g. donations, offers of resources, venues).

The steps in Figure 10.1 are of equal importance and often carried out iteratively as identification of training need, curriculum planning, funding, sustainability and staffing all need to be considered alongside one another. Other activities are necessary at the planning stage for a centre or course to be successful, including quality assurance, governance and ethics, as well as the more practical issues of storage, maintenance and the need to recognize and address the changes in contemporary healthcare delivery.

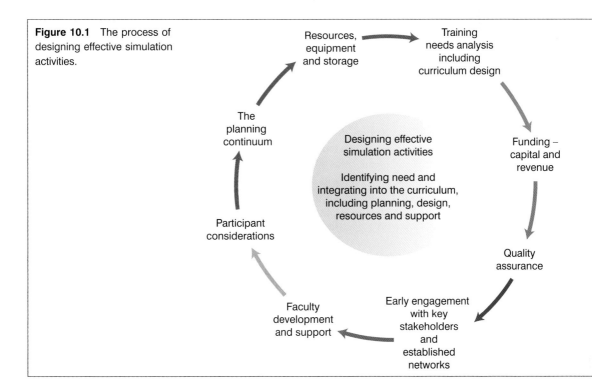

Figure 10.1 The process of designing effective simulation activities.

Resources, equipment and storage

Training needs analysis including curriculum design

The planning continuum

Designing effective simulation activities

Identifying need and integrating into the curriculum, including planning, design, resources and support

Funding – capital and revenue

Participant considerations

Quality assurance

Faculty development and support

Early engagement with key stakeholders and established networks

(Q) Example 1   Funding

In one region within the UK, funding has been provided to support a clinical simulation facility which ensures equity of simulation education across the region as well as across professions. The initial building and equipping of the simulation centre was funded by a legacy (£500 000) left by a businessman to the local hospital where he wanted the money to be spent, to benefit the people who had supported his business for many years.

The running costs of the centre are now met by ongoing government funding with senior management assurance of continued sponsorship based on the stipulation that delegates must be employed by the NHS within the region. This employee status entitles delegates to free training provided by the facility either within the centre itself or at an alternative venue using mobile equipment and simulation centre faculty. For funding to continue, the centre must train 1500 delegates annually and demonstrate this through annual reports detailing simulation activities. The funding also ensures access to the simulation facility for all health care workers.

In healthcare, individuals tend not to work in isolation but in teams whose members rely on one other, especially in a crisis situation. The funding has enabled healthcare workers to be able to come together to train for crisis or complex situations.

Justification for developing a simulation facility

Influencing factors

The rationale for using simulation in clinical education comes from many sources; it is therefore worth noting these when considering setting up a new facility or simply planning to use simulation in an established or new teaching intervention. Initially at the business planning or policy development stage, the developer will need to consider the relevant government, regional, local and professional stance on simulation so as to draw on this in the rationale for bidding for funding. For example in the UK, the Department of Health England (DH) recommendations [1,2], local strategies [3] or curriculum development [4] might be used as justification including Sir Liam Donaldson's (Chief Medical Officer for England 1998–2010) statement, 'Simulation offers an important route to safer care for patients and needs to be more fully integrated into the health service.' [5, p. 49] as he not only stressed the importance of technology enhanced learning but also that simulation-based training needs to be valued and adequately resourced by NHS organizations [6]. These factors are influential, particularly as they have patient safety and improved patient outcomes as their fundamental principles and will therefore appeal to Executive boards and senior managers in healthcare. At the business or policy planning stage however, more detail is required and the more progressive planner will be conscious of the need for establishing a demand to ensure the success of the project. Successful examples of detailed policies established [7] at this early stage of development to support the business case for financial planning and sustainability have led to a long term future and engagement with internal and external partners. Business plans allow a demonstration of the benefits of the centre and therefore the benefits to the organization, be they financial, through increased patient safety behaviours or other healthcare outcome measures [8].

Training needs analysis

Establishing a clinical need, the assessment of how this can be addressed educationally and whether simulation is the best form of pedagogy, are the first steps to take when planning any simulation activity. Only then can developers consider the options and conclude that simulation would be the most suitable to meet learners' educational needs. This process may include undertaking a recognized training needs analysis (TNA) [9] of the prospective delegates as a whole or in specific groups, as part of workforce planning, to support the introduction of a new service or facility or for continuous professional development (Figure 10.2).

All healthcare education should be driven by a clear clinical need for the training and the aim of improving patient outcomes [2] and this is underpinned by sound training needs analysis which informs course development. Once a need has been identified and developed, embedding it into the education curricula not only sustains interest in the training but also attracts ongoing funding. Subsequent training needs analyses are essential to ensure education remains current and meets evolving health requirements. All training providers and facilities must be able to adapt to the changes in demands for courses and new training must be developed as health service and delivery changes [11].

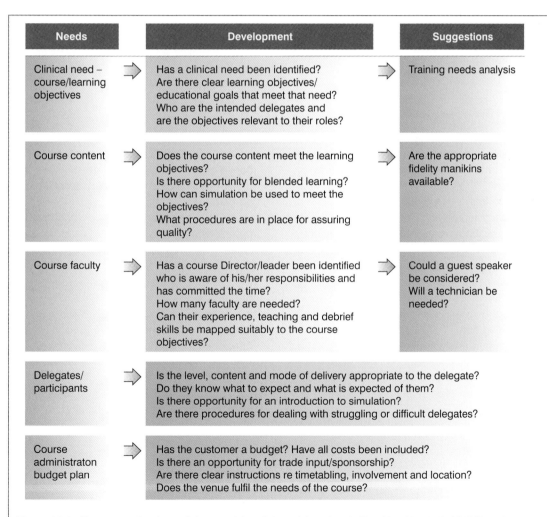

Needs	Development	Suggestions
Clinical need – course/learning objectives	Has a clinical need been identified? Are there clear learning objectives/ educational goals that meet that need? Who are the intended delegates and are the objectives relevant to their roles?	Training needs analysis
Course content	Does the course content meet the learning objectives? Is there opportunity for blended learning? How can simulation be used to meet the objectives? What procedures are in place for assuring quality?	Are the appropriate fidelity manikins available?
Course faculty	Has a course Director/leader been identified who is aware of his/her responsibilities and has committed the time? How many faculty are needed? Can their experience, teaching and debrief skills be mapped suitably to the course objectives?	Could a guest speaker be considered? Will a technician be needed?
Delegates/ participants	Is the level, content and mode of delivery appropriate to the delegate? Do they know what to expect and what is expected of them? Is there opportunity for an introduction to simulation? Are there procedures for dealing with struggling or difficult delegates?	
Course administraton budget plan	Has the customer a budget? Have all costs been included? Is there an opportunity for trade input/sponsorship? Are there clear instructions re timetabling, involvement and location? Does the venue fulfil the needs of the course?	

Figure 10.2 Process to develop training provision. Adapted from Leeds Teaching Hospitals NHS Trust [10].

Embedding simulation into training

It is essential to embed simulation within existing training programmes. In order for this to happen, a training need should be established, followed by an analysis of the curriculum to determine at which point simulation can be encompassed within the programme and ultimately be fundamental to that training. For example, using full body human patient simulators is not appropriate for all clinical training needs and this should be borne in mind when dealing with requests for training. Box 10.1 demonstrates both appropriate and inappropriate uses of such a simulator.

Working proactively with those who require and deliver training (universities, hospitals, post-graduate centres, professional bodies, colleges) and having good communication mechanisms ensures that simulation is embedded appropriately in curricula. In addition these institutional links can help ensure resources are used efficiently and appropriately.

Embedding simulation into the curricula for both undergraduate and postgraduate healthcare professionals is clearly advantageous. Within the nursing sector, there is a recognition in the UK at national regulatory level, of the value of simulation in undergraduate nursing training, due in part to the reduced availability of practice placements, demonstrating a change of mind-set about the value and need for simulation techniques in all aspects of healthcare training [12,13].

Further considerations for the justification of simulation training includes patient expectations, in that it is no longer acceptable to practise on patients

---

Box 10.1   Requests for training

Inappropriate request

Learning outcome: to be able to interpret abnormal cardiac rhythms from rhythm strips

Cohort: Large group of student nurses on undergraduate programme

Request: Transport full body human patient simulator from simulated clinical environment to class room in order to link to ECG machine and produce abnormal rhythm strips

Timing: Request received *five days* prior to training date

Curriculum integration: None.

Faculty: Module leader, untrained in the use of human patient simulator and software as well as theoretical aspects of simulation as a pedagogy

Alternative solution: Utilize ECG simulator in conjunction with monitor

Appropriate request

Learning outcomes: to be able to recognize the acutely ill patient, to be able to lead a team in a crisis situation, demonstrate critical thinking skills, display evidence based practice and identify human factors which could potentially impact on care.

Cohort: Groups of eight nurses on continued professional development module for acute care

Request: Full body manikin in hospital bed in ward setting. Will require monitor, sats probe, oxygen, and appropriate consumables and access to AV kit.

Timing: Request for programme to be developed *12 weeks* prior to delivery

Curriculum integration: Simulation activities incorporated into module specification. Introduction to simulated practice timetabled prior to scenario delivery. Evaluation mechanism i.e. pre and post simulation questionnaires in place

Faculty: Module leader, with no simulation training in partnership with the lead in simulated practice

when there are simulation alternatives [14]. Indeed, the General Medical Council (the UK regulatory body for doctors) recommends that trainee doctors practice on manikins whenever these are available prior to providing direct healthcare to a patient [15]. The general public are increasingly being made aware through media exposure, of high profile serious incidents, where education has been highlighted as deficient [16].

Funding

Following the establishment of need, the next step is to explore the opportunities for funding streams and these may well be the reason for the creation of a facility (Figure 10.3). Legacies, as in the case study, though few and far between, may well fund the internal fittings of the facility. If the organizers are lucky enough to have secured confirmed funding and financial provisions, they also need an awareness of the full economic implications of the service; setting up costs (capital costs) *and* sustainability (revenue) of this type of training. These include the impact on faculty availability and commitment, as well as purchasing and maintaining the equipment. In addition, in order to deliver a quality educational programme, the organizers must identify the best type of simulator

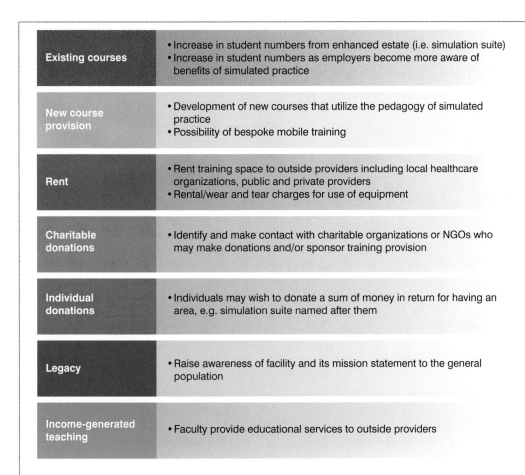

Existing courses	• Increase in student numbers from enhanced estate (i.e. simulation suite) • Increase in student numbers as employers become more aware of benefits of simulated practice
New course provision	• Development of new courses that utilize the pedagogy of simulated practice • Possibility of bespoke mobile training
Rent	• Rent training space to outside providers including local healthcare organizations, public and private providers • Rental/wear and tear charges for use of equipment
Charitable donations	• Identify and make contact with charitable organizations or NGOs who may make donations and/or sponsor training provision
Individual donations	• Individuals may wish to donate a sum of money in return for having an area, e.g. simulation suite named after them
Legacy	• Raise awareness of facility and its mission statement to the general population
Income-generated teaching	• Faculty provide educational services to outside providers

Figure 10.3 Possible funding streams.

or simulation activity that suits the outcomes of the training sessions as opposed to using what is available at the time, or the cheapest/most affordable/readily available manikin (Box 10.1). One issue which is often neglected in the financial planning process are the hidden costs [6] of equipment use, maintenance and replacement. Wear and tear charges and a consumables budget should be incorporated into the overall equipment rental charge as well as the cost of the space and faculty provision. One method of calculating such costs is outlined here [17].

$$5\% \text{ of product cost/replacement}$$
$$\text{cost} + 5\% \text{ of the cost of}$$
$$\text{consumables} = \text{total charge for}$$
$$\text{equipment rental per session}$$
$$\text{(a session being half a day}$$
$$\text{or four hours)}.$$

For example, if one arterial blood gas arm costs £448 (US$706) new, 5% of this is £22.50 (US$35). Replacement skin and veins (consumables) cost £126 (US$198) therefore 5% of consumables is £6.30 (US$10). Add these two costs together and a realistic overall equipment charge for one arterial blood gas arm per session is £28.70 (US$45).

It is paramount to ensure adequate planning has gone into the continued funding of equipment (clinical and audiovisual), consumables maintenance, faculty support (in terms of training and time) and marketing. Paying attention to detail at this stage of development will help secure a continued demand for training and support ongoing delivery [18]. Without such support, staff can quickly become demotivated and students fail to receive maximum benefit from the simulated experience, leading to a poor return on initial investment [19,20]. Figure 10.3 identifies possible funding streams that could be utilized to income generate to support ongoing running costs. Day-to-day running costs can also come from other sources such as the regional or national bodies outlined in the case study at the beginning of this chapter.

Simulation centre managers and developers should keep abreast of changes in training requirements and funding streams (at national and local levels) so that they position themselves to apply for funding to start up facilities and maintain existing provision. To ensure a simulation facility has a share of education and training funding, simulation education must be embedded into medical, nursing and allied health professional curricula. Mandated simulation courses will assist in attracting vital funding streams.

Funding from a sustainable national source is unusual and other streams can be considered such as simulation training for a specific group of students for example, the simulation facility in the case study has an annual service level agreement (SLA) with a nearby university to provide a simulation training day for all two hundred and fifty final year medical students.

Only confirmed revenue sources will sustain and ensure the success of a programme or facility.

Users of the facility

When developing any simulation activity, the numbers of potential students or delegates planning to use the resource must be considered and confirmed. This helps to identify and prepare a space that will accommodate the numbers of users and allow for any expansion that may result following the success of the centre or course. From anecdotal evidence of the benefits of collaboration, it is recommended that this planning includes the involvement of internal and external stakeholders, including the groups planning to use the centre or facilities as trainers or trainees. Examples of external stakeholders might include the local public healthcare providers and commissioners of services, other healthcare providers and non-governmental commissioners such as charitable and independent organizations, emergency services such as the fire service, police, lifeboat or coastguard services, Red Cross, and industry (e.g. occupational health needs). These may well provide valuable income generation for the sustainability of the facility or course. Further examples of possible stakeholders are outlined in Figure 10.4.

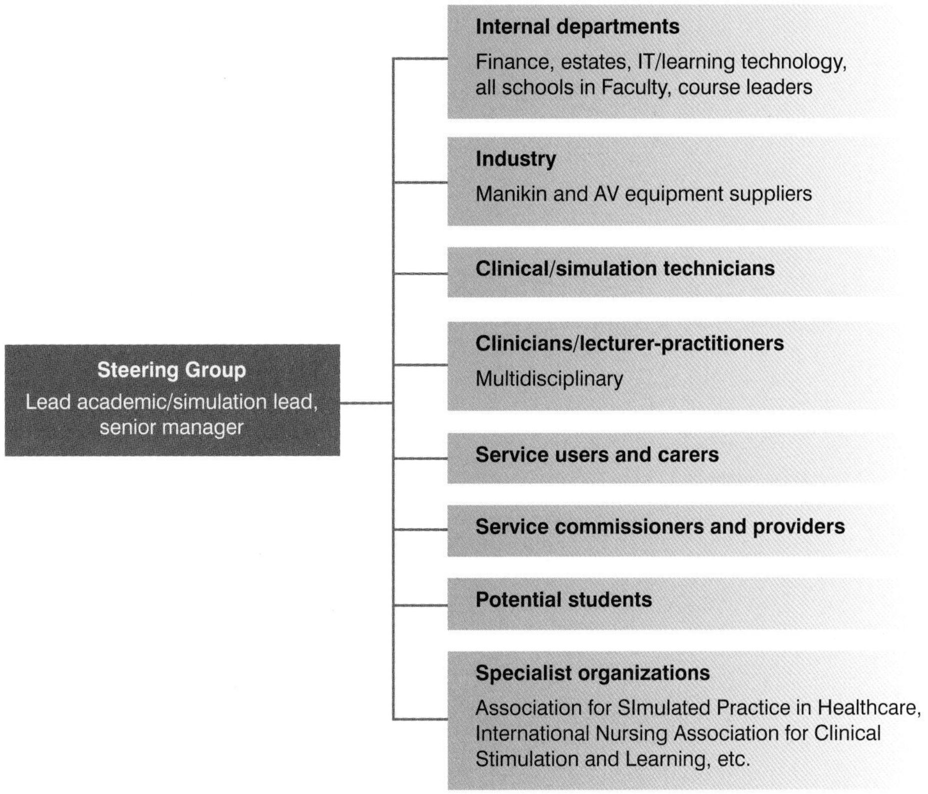

Figure 10.4 Potential stakeholders.

Quality assurance

Once the need and funding has been established, the facility manager or course developer should consider how they will ensure the quality of the training. Using a recognized quality framework [21] or accredited body at the planning stage will underpin and authenticate the training centre or course. Using a proven structured framework will also assist in defining the factors that contribute to high-quality clinical skills and simulation training provision and enable benchmarking against accepted criteria. To support the quality assurance of clinical skills and simulation training, four factors of the continuous improvement cycle (Figure 10.5) form a framework which informs trainers of the requirements necessary to maintain accountability and

contribute to continuous improvement. The four factors identified in the diagram include quality assurance principles – this considers patient safety and is patient centred, supports interprofessional learning and evaluation along with quality assurance based on criteria that are fair, rigorous and transparent, effective and efficient and shared. Quality monitoring is underpinned by benchmarks and quality standards and adherence to evidence-based practice.

The diagram shows the link to patient safety with quality assurance as part of the standards on which all training should be based. When clinical skills and simulation training is quality assured, then the assumption is that the trainee will deliver evidence-based clinical care when back in practice. Training providers are advised to use

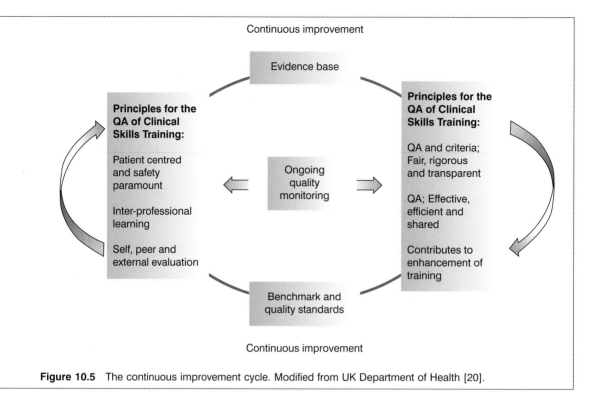

Figure 10.5 The continuous improvement cycle. Modified from UK Department of Health [20].

policies alongside educational quality standards, linking clinical practice and education.

Stakeholder engagement

A fundamental process to developing simulated practice successfully is the early engagement of key individuals and organizations [18,22,23] more often led by an effective steering group [24]. Surprisingly, one of the most difficult groups of people to get to engage with simulation seem to be co-faculty [25] which is probably due to a relatively superficial understanding of what simulated practice can deliver and the perception that it is just an additional 'task' to incorporate into teaching delivery [26]. Successful early involvement in the planning process fosters a sense of ownership

when people recognize that their comments and suggestions will be taken into consideration and acted upon where appropriate [27]. Engagement with simulation may not have any major financial incentive attached, but recognition of such scholarly activity should be included in appraisal and any workforce development planning for all healthcare professionals [27]. Discussing plans and aspirations for future training with key stakeholders not only increases awareness of simulation as a pedagogy, but helps to identify pockets of unmet training needs that may lend themselves to simulated practice [28]. Figure 10.4 lists potential stakeholders, including academics, financial and estates departments, clinicians, service commissioners and providers, specialist organizations, industry and users of healthcare services from the local community, all of whom will have a valuable contribution to make with regards to the planning process [29]. Not all stakeholders will be required in all stages of the planning process but keeping everyone informed of developments enhances the feeling of ownership and encourages continued interest [30].

The planning process can be stratified into three phases [31]:
1. **Conceptualization** – comprehensive brainstorming
2. **Exploration** – obtaining expert opinion
3. **Actualization** – realizing the set concept and translating it into action.

It is often perceived that collaboration is decreasingly important as one moves through these three stages but for optimal success and on-going effectiveness, collaboration (perhaps with different stakeholders at differing stages) should be viewed as equally important in all stages and every effort should be made to foster its continuation [32].

One query that is bound to be raised within the process of discussion and negotiation is the potential cost-effectiveness of simulation. This is often questioned due to high initial set up costs especially for high fidelity simulators [19,33]. However, use of simulation-based education (SBE) in an organization has the potential to attract increased student numbers, aid the development of new and innovative courses as well as enhancing delivery within existing teaching capacity [31] thereby becoming very cost-effective over time. Another aspect to consider is the reduction of clinical errors and increase in patient safety that simulated practice if used appropriately may provide to the local healthcare environment and staff [34], which can be costly in both monetary and health terms [3,35]. Gaba [36] expressed concern that simulation may struggle to become established because of the cost implications despite the current focus on quality and patient safety in healthcare.

With significant initial investment and potential high running costs how does the manager effectively communicate to medical directors and chief executives the added value of simulation training versus the cost? Inviting 'observers' to watch the sessions being delivered can be a useful exercise to demonstrate how this can be achieved through

simulated practice [27]. Cox and Acree [37] summarize this as:

The patient is safer if the trainee first practices on a manikin or some other simulation before attempting to handle their first real case.

and

The intuitive linkage between increasing patient safety and cutting the litigation and settlement costs while improving public image [37, p. 24].

The planning continuum

Once the pedagogy of simulation has been introduced to training, this is not the end of the planning process. With the introduction of both local [38] and international [23,39] standards for simulated practice, ongoing evaluation and monitoring is paramount in order to meet and maintain these recommended benchmarks. Published audit results against these standards have the added benefit of acting as a potential marketing tool [40] but only if they are maintained or surpassed, which requires sustained commitment, leadership and support for training providers [5,20,41]. Figure 10.6 summarizes the process of introducing, integrating, delivering and maintaining standards of simulated practice.

This framework can be applied regardless of where simulation takes place, be it in a brand new bespoke build, a refurbished area of an existing build or in a room in a General Practitioner's surgery. A more individualized approach will be required to develop in-house scenarios or for external bespoke packages to ensure specific learning objectives are met. Initial consideration of location, delegates and availability of equipment will all contribute to and determine the overall process and route the scenario takes (Figure 10.7).

The principles and practices of both Frameworks (Figures 10.6 and 10.7) are generic in nature and can be adapted for use with any form of simulated practice. In the case study at the beginning of the chapter, annual reports are required to clarify the return on investment for the sponsors and consequently fulfil this dimension.

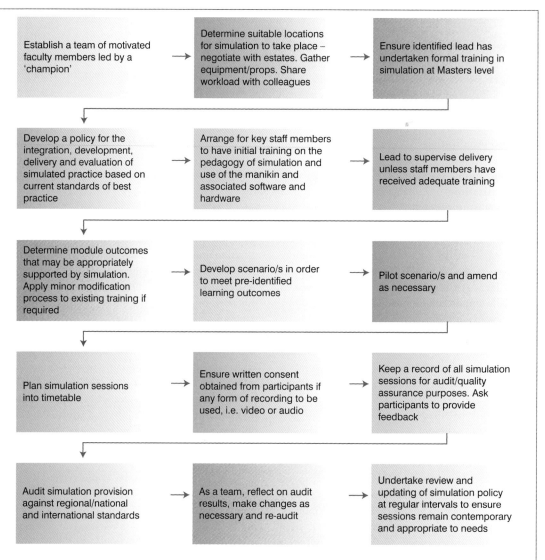

Figure 10.6 A framework for simulation integration and delivery. Adapted from the Simulation Policy and Resource Pack [7].

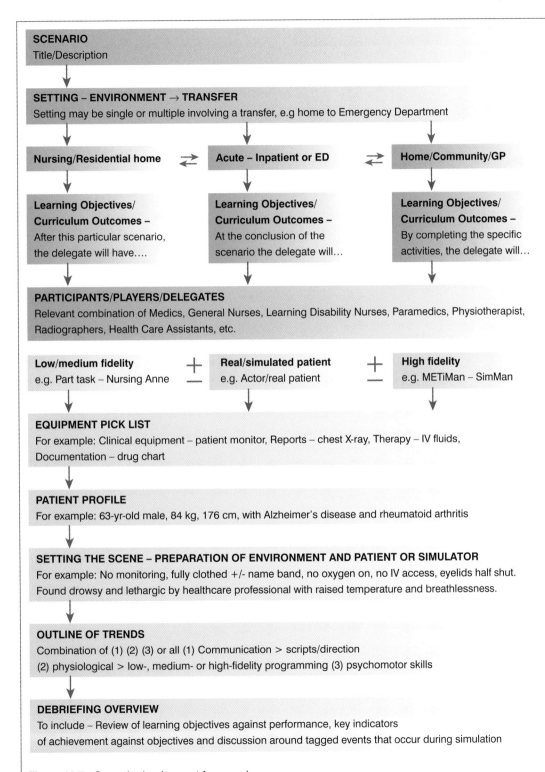

Figure 10.7 Scenario development framework.

ⓘ Top tips

- Discuss your equipment requirements early on with local and national suppliers. Some may be able to offer long term loans of expensive equipment in return for a few days' annual use of your facilities to deliver their own training.
- One simulator cannot be used to teach everything. While it is acknowledged that its utilization is important in order to receive financial return on costs, using a high-fidelity manikin in this way leads to its premature demise. A better strategy is to use less costly task trainers wherever possible and to purchase more than one simulator for running complex scenarios.
- Ensure you join simulation networks/groups. Their pooled knowledge can be invaluable.
- Do not assume that your colleagues have a detailed understanding of simulated practice and what its delivery entails. Running information or taster sessions for staff early in the development process can help to secure understanding and future engagement.
- Develop a faculty resource pack that dovetails the simulation policy. Contents could include attendance sheets, student consent forms, moulage recipes or troubleshooting tips.

Faculty development and support

Before simulation sessions are showcased to interested parties, it is imperative that faculty members feel comfortable developing, delivering, facilitating and evaluating simulated practice sessions. This can be achieved by understanding the pedagogy of simulated practice, ideally via formal study, and supervised practice from experienced faculty [42]. This complex and multifaceted method of teaching requires the investment of time in careful planning of a standardized approach to delivery [36,43,44,45,46,47,48,49,50,51,52,53,54]. As a rough estimation, each hour of simulation delivery will **initially** require twenty hours of preparation and this commitment in terms of time should not be underestimated [55]. Crucial to this process is the identification of a designated coordinator or 'simulation champion,' who has adequate deployment time, enthusiasm, specialist training and a realistic vision for taking simulation forward [20,41]. Implementing a policy for the delivery and ongoing quality assurance of simulated practice is key to its success [25,33,42]. Initial emphasis needs to be placed on providing faculty members with the competencies required to deliver complex scenarios encompassing a range of learning outcomes across the healthcare spectrum [25,33]. Figure 10.8 provides a checklist of inclusions for such training and asks for confirmation from the faculty member/facilitator that this has been received.

This in itself acts as a risk reduction strategy, ensuring that the integrity of the manikin is maintained as well as ensuring a positive learning experience for students [20]. It should be acknowledged that unless delivering simulated practice on a regular basis, academic staff should work with and be supervised by the Lead for simulated practice as it will be difficult to maintain adequate competency of the complex skills required to deliver a high standard of teaching using this pedagogy.

Participant considerations

Participants often worry about performing well in front of faculty and peers [56,57]. Faculty members have an ethical obligation to address and reduce these anxieties as well as any issues that arise relating to safety, competency and knowledge base [58]. A crucial element within this process is the debrief. This is defined as, 'a period of structured reflection and feedback after a simulation exercise that is an essential element of simulation-based education' [58]. Generally carried out immediately after the event in order to support best practice [59], this process is the most important aspect of the entire simulated learning experience [44,60,61,62], a fact that often goes unrecognized. Facilitated well,

---

Confirmation of Simulation Training

Name: _____ **Role:** _____

I, the undersigned, confirm that I have received training in all areas listed below (Please tick to confirm)

Familiarization with simulation policies for both staff and students ☐

Turning the simulator and software on and off ☐

Charging the simulator ☐

Choosing and running a pre-programmed scenario ☐

Altering physiological parameters on the fly ☐

Filling and draining bodily fluids ☐

Use of basic moulage ☐

Use of wireless microphone for voice of simulator ☐

Role of assistant faculty/facilitators ☐

Pre session briefing with students ☐

Debriefing with students ☐

My training has been provided by {insert name} at {name of institution} on {insert dates}.

Signed: _____ Date: _____

This section to be completed by Lead for Simulated Practice

I have peer reviewed the above member of staff running a full scenario on _____
and confirm that they meet the criteria to run simulations unsupervised

Signed: _____ Date: _____

Please note: Separate training is required for the use of audiovisual equipment within the clinical skills and simulation suite

---

Figure 10.8 Extract from a policy and resource document [7].

debriefing will address any emotional baggage following participation in the scenario as well as any other issues raised. It also leads to deeper learning linked with greater knowledge retention that can be enhanced further by the use of video assisted debriefing [58,60]. If facilitated badly, it can cause harm to students in the form of increased anxiety and a reduced confidence [58]. It is therefore crucial that faculty members facilitating simulated practice have received training in the debriefing process [19,60,63,64], especially when the multiple complex competencies required are largely ill-defined [63]. Having a clear framework to guide the process

helps to reduce the chance of negative outcomes [61,65,66], as well being a supportive tool for new facilitators. The detail of facilitating debrief sessions is covered in Chapter 12; however, Table 10.1 outlines a simple three stage framework adapted from Denning [67] and Phrampus and O'Donnell [68] covering the key aspects of a successful debrief.

Audio and video recording of participants during simulation requires their informed consent [27,69]. Consideration of how and when this takes place is again an important part of the planning process. The most favoured method seems to be to obtain written informed consent from participants

Table 10.1   The GAS model of debriefing

Phase	Goal	Actions
Gather	Actively listen to participants to understand their perspectives on their behaviours	Request narrative from team leader Request clarifying or supplemental information from team
Analyse	Facilitate student reflection and analysis of their actions	Review accurate record of events Report observations (correct and incorrect steps) Use advocacy with enquiry to shed light on the thinking process Stimulate reflection and provide redirection where necessary Utilize evidence based guidelines as benchmark for clinical queries/concerns
Summarize	Facilitate identification and review of lessons learned	Verify coverage of all essential teaching/debriefing points Summarize discussions/wrap up session/listen to any comments

Box 10.2   Simulation and Clinical Skills Centre: participant consent for digital audio/video recording

Confidentiality

We, the undersigned, will maintain and keep confidential all information regarding the performance of individuals and details of the simulation scenarios conducted.

Digital/video recording release

We, the undersigned, hereby consent to having our simulation session/s digitally/video recorded for the purpose of education and/or marketing. All recordings become the property of [organization name].

Observers

[Organization name] shares its expertise and experience with those who may occasionally visit to observe the educational, administrative and technical aspects of simulation. We, the undersigned, hereby consent to external professionals observing simulated scenarios in which we participate.

Date:	Session ID:	
NAME		**SIGNATURE**

prior to their first simulation session [70]. If they will be undertaking a number of simulated practice sessions, then the consent form should be worded in such a way as to cover the course of study rather than a particular session. It is also important to insure that consent is obtained for the possible future use/release of any recordings, confidentiality in relation to the simulated scenario and the debrief session and consent for the observation of participants by external observers. Box 10.2 shows an example consent form adapted from two sources [71,72] that captures these aspects.

Sustainability

One aspect of sustainability is the need to create an effective learning environment [73]. Three key mechanisms are required for this to happen:
1. The physical resources – accommodation, equipment, teaching aids and materials.
2. The human component – trainers, learners, programme directors, assessors and managers and most importantly, their availability and capability.
3. The knowledge or cognitive element – the educational programme ethos, faculty motivation and insight into the educational process of learning
All these factors require considerable planning, significant time commitment, faculty participation and industrial/organizational buy-in with an ongoing financial responsibility.

Although funding and investment from external sources may assist in the 'creation' process, it will probably not extend to assisting an organization's ability to sustain not just the state-of-the-art laboratory but the smaller single room training facility. The development and regular updating of a strategic plan is recommended to either help shape a new facility or keep an existing one on track [74]. Global financial constraints and uncertainty around educational and health service configurations is affecting many organizations and key personnel. Planning and reviewing regularly and carefully helps facilities and educational staff stay aware of the challenges ahead and keep senior level management engaged. Be mindful that opportunities will be variable depending on the organizational plan for simulation/ education and differing affiliated tertiary and professional education organizations in countries and regions.

---

① Top tip

Do not aim to grant every request that comes through the door. Once word gets out that you are up and functioning, you will have more requests than you can possibly deal with. Be very careful to choose what you can do well with the people, time, funding, equipment, and experience that you have [75].

It is only through senior management buy-in that you are more likely to acquire the things you need, gain faculty willingness and commitment and as a result, you will have more staff to run your centre. The more senior the people that buy-in, the better the chances of survival and success but it will not be without its challenges [76]. Unlike the case study, many centres and facilities still in their infancy struggle to convince their organization, especially the people holding the purse-strings that simulation is here to stay and needs ongoing investment and robust marketing. Too often the focus in the early days is placed so heavily on financial return that it proves difficult to demonstrate the value of your centre and the educational offerings it has to others when it is not already up and running. As mentioned previously, it is important that course need, approximate numbers and covering of costs are well-researched and planned; learn from the evaluation of courses – remember quality supersedes quantity [75]. Over time, evidence hopefully will suggest that improvements in patient safety arise as a direct result of training using simulation.

However, there are many other innovative ways of providing sustainability, basically the acceptable art of begging or creative procurement [77] (Box 10.3).

Box 10.3   The '10 B's' of creative procurement –

1. **B**orrow hospital-owned clinical equipment from clinical areas, when needed and subject to availability, for example, ultrasound machines.
2. **B**eg your hospitals equipment pool to provide equipment short-term or through a type of 'in active-use storage' [75]. This ensures the hospital's own maintenance and update contract is still valid.
3. **B**ow to the requests of the person. If you are trying to persuade a company to sponsor a room or a piece of equipment, agree to let them use the centre as a showcase or for their training, such a compromise will bring in other companies with similar ideas.
4. **B**udget for using any 'surplus' from hospital stores or equipment discarded as not suitable for the clinical environment, due to damage or redundancy.
5. **B**efriend used medical equipment companies for refurbished items at a fraction of new price.
6. **B**eseech. Use your powers of animation and persuasion. Convey real enthusiasm for your facility/project/training and stimulate people to be willing to give you things.
7. **B**uild up relationships with the larger contracts providing consumables within the organization to provide a proportion of their supplies for training.
8. **B**attle for out-of-date consumables for use in the centre but be prepared to offer a liability release [75].
9. **B**oost the coffers of the facility by opening up (more convenient at weekends) for film companies or the media to help them reproduce realistic clinical environments.
10. **B**id that hospital educators using the facility bring their expired consumables to support their sessions. This is a good way to acquire the expensive items for free, for example, central lines.

Use of space and resources

No two facilities will be the same as regards space, equipment and resources; it is how best it is used that reflects the success of a facility and the ability to build a programme/course around the existing build and/or availability of equipment [74]. Some may opt for designated rooms for specific skills; others will chose to leave rooms minimally furnished to increase versatility of use.

Specific simulated clinical areas within a facility will fundamentally remain the same set-up with the appropriate simulator, paediatric or adult, the prepared scenario with all the furnishings and necessary equipment to replicate the environment for the specific scenario. Such realism can be reproduced quite naturally outside of the facility. *In situ* simulation occurs in the clinical environment. It will identify different learning opportunities from those of a simulation centre and its focus will identify hazards

and deficits in clinical systems, the team and the environment [78]. It is particularly useful in addressing serious untoward incidents [79] through simulation (Figure 10.9). This *in situ* simulation is just as effective as that carried out in a dedicated simulation centre [80]. It is not where the simulation takes place that matters but the fact that it is happening at all that counts [81].

Remember, performance in simulation is related to the perception of realism experienced by the learner [82]. For example, room authenticity could be achieved simply by changing the look instantly by hanging wall life-sized fabric, a floor to ceiling picture or a drape portraying an operating theatre wall, a GP waiting room or a street scene [83] (see Chapter 11 on distributed simulation).

This 'suspension of disbelief' has been found to contribute to whether a student's ability on a simulator transfers successfully to the clinical area [84]. It is quite feasible to produce effective learning and

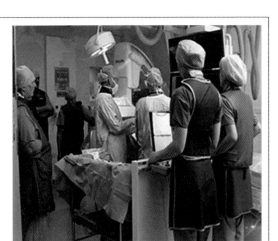

Figure 10.9 *In situ* simulation.

teaching to the required standards using resources that are already available but through a more imaginative and well informed delivery. One such way to suspend disbelief in a participant is to appeal to their senses [85]. Using simulator sounds such as moaning, coughing, vomiting, a telephone ringing, a crash call, a ventilator or suction machine running, all add to the realism. Prerecorded background noises, monitors and pumps alarming, the use of a computerized scent production device or made to order 'smell cube' add to the overall sensory dimension. In order to create authentic simulated clinical areas, the 'must dos' are:

• Remove all equipment that is not relevant to that scenario. Simulation taking place in area resembling a storage cupboard does not convey realism.
• Acquire an extensive selection of props, everything from wigs, books, wash bags to cigarette ends and walking sticks!
• Consider the use of strangers rather than people known to the students for role play activities.
• Have sufficient distractions in the environment so as to replicate the complexity of practice.

In an effort to create realism in a cost-effective manner often expired consumables are used. The centre, faculty and participants should all be fully aware of the risks of using expired consumables, sharps, out-of-date drugs and biological materials for wet labs through adequate risk assessments.

Thought should also be given to their ultimate disposal. There are two caveats:
1. precautions must be taken to ensure that these will never find their way back into the clinical area with the potential for accidental clinical use.
2. actual drugs, even if they have expired, still need to be secured as in real clinical use.
Cleaning staff may well not distinguish between real and/or fake blood coming from a simulated clinical facility; therefore dispose of all such fake waste as if it were real [85].

Equipment

It is important that facilities ensure provision of adaptable, realistic simulation models including both part-task and full-body simulators [3,23]. Knowledge of the various simulation models available and their appropriate use is important to ensure their full potential. The term fidelity is commonly used to describe the realism of the simulation experience and can be defined as, 'the provision of realism through characteristics such as visual cues, tactile features, feedback capabilities, and interaction with the trainee' [86, p. 338]. It is important that users, be they trainers or trainees are familiar with the concept behind fidelity; that of engineering fidelity as opposed to the psychological fidelity. Engineering or physical fidelity is the level to which the device/equipment is able to replicate the physical characteristics of the task, whereas and more importantly, psychological or functional fidelity describes the level to which the skill of the real task is actually captured in the simulated task [87]. Lower fidelity equipment is more appropriate for basic skill acquisition and development [6]. In general a novice practitioner will gain most from a low-fidelity simulator whereas an experienced practitioner requires task refinement and will gain more from a higher-fidelity simulator [88]. Initial purchase of equipment will be strongly influenced by the level of the learner, provision of courses and the expected availability of either experienced or inexperienced faculty. When considering subsequent purchases, especially if there are thoughts of increasing fidelity, do ensure that the benefits of using simulation outweigh the costs of time for faculty, technical support, space and equipment purchases

[89]. Regular audit of equipment use will highlight common problems (Table 10.2).

Staffing

Management

Although not essential, a manager with some clinical knowledge can be an asset for a clinical skill facility [27,55]. Managers need to be able to market the facility and programmes on offer, to engage with and recruit appropriate faculty members and ensure there are enough trainers to deliver all courses, whilst maintaining financial liquidity.

It is always necessary to attract clinical leaders and delegates to use the facility's services and a manager with a clinical background may have more credibility and a greater understanding of the education methodology employed.

Table 10.2 Common problems with equipment use and possible solutions

Problem	Solution
Equipment kept in cupboards between intermittent uses.	Encourage faculty to gain knowledge and experience of simulators through courses, supervised hands-on sessions and/or trade teachings.
Worn out equipment in need of repair or replacement.	Use different approaches to the cycle of replacement and renewal. Ensure that wear and tear costings are included in Course/training charges. Check terms of maintenance contracts. Check asset register information.
Full body simulators used for single procedural skills training.	Review learning objectives of the course. Check rationale for selection of appropriate technology to fit educational needs of learner.
Natural loss of up-to-date trained faculty/technicians/champions.	Ensure regular training and updates are written into equipment manufacturer's maintenance contracts.
Manikins not used to their full potential and/or teaching opportunities not fully utilized due to lack of knowledge of simulator and/or equipment.	Confirm facilitator's depth of understanding of the functionality of specific manikins and their potential uses. Increase knowledge base in order to exploit functionality of the equipment and put to greater use.
Equipment damaged or unkempt, not fit for purpose inappropriately stored	Encourage designated person (technician) to champion equipment, adopt a minimal standard of care for manikins [83] e.g. all tape of any kind should be removed at the end of each day. Provide suitable, catalogued storage containers and/or areas, e.g. mobile shelving system that operate on a single guide track and fits directly to your existing floor needs neither extensive nor costly site work.
Lack of appropriate manikins or insufficient quantity, especially at peak times, e.g. OSCEs	Opportunity for creation of local or regional equipment loan/library. Needs robust infrastructure with clinical/technical and equipment know-how to compete with often discretionary borrowing [89].

Administrative support

Supportive and reliable administrative staff are essential to the smooth running of the facility. Anecdotal evidence suggests delegates who have not had the correct information (an administrative role) prior to their simulation experience can become very hostile to the whole process. The administrator may have many responsibilities including:
• **making** individual bookings/confirmation of booking
• **arranging** course/date bookings
• **preparing** course documentation, e.g. sign in sheets, attendance registers (electronic) certificates, feedback sheets,
• **greeting** delegates/visitors and orientating them to the centre
• **coordinating** availability of refreshments
• **advertising and marketing**
• **maintaining** records with the ability to pull data and run reports on facility use.

Technical support

Really effective skills/simulation facilitators (in common with clinical settings using equipment) have excellent technical support [90,91]. It is important that the level of the technical support is appropriate to the activities of individual facilities with desired skills varying from experienced audio-visual and information technology management, to the 'shifters and the lifters'. Technicians and technician/trainers come from a variety of backgrounds including administration, nursing, operating department practitioners (ODPs), engineers, and the biological sciences. However, although it is not imperative to have a person with an actual technical background, most facilities have found that a clinical background alongside skills and interest in technical tasks benefits the simulation team greatly [91]. The availability of a skilled technician for set-up and sessional support should be routinely costed in to courses and running of the majority of scenarios. Any guarantees that your simulator will be up and running at the beginning of every planned session is dependent upon the quality of the people responsible for using and maintaining it, mainly your faculty and technicians [85]. Box 10.4 outlines

---

> ### Box 10.4 Essential role/skills of the technician
>
> • Caring for and maintaining equipment routinely to ensure quality resources are always available
> • Negotiation and leadership skills – important for the technician to be included in the tendering process for equipment
> • Developing skills in repairing equipment
> • Trouble-shooting – devise inventive solutions for sudden equipment failure and other problems
> • Responsible for inventory and monitoring of equipment and disposables
> • Creating and updating facility policies and procedures (in conjunction with faculty)
> • Devising check lists for equipment/resources/rooms etc. for each course/session
> Training faculty on the technical aspects of the simulator
> • Change set-up in between scenarios
> • Accompanying the educators on external training to set up and operate the equipment
> • Liaising with equipment suppliers

the essential role components/skills for a technician working in a simulation environment [92].

Educators

No two facilities have the same space, equipment, resources or staff and so the specific educational skills required to run the session will vary. The personnel required will be entirely dependent on the professional backgrounds of the participants and what courses are to be offered [21]. To return to the regional simulation centre in the case study, educators from a number of professional groups contribute to process. These include:
• **Clinical/medical educator** – Experienced clinician/senior nurse trained in simulation and debriefing (permanent faculty). Will have varied clinical knowledge and experience to ensure realistic reaction during clinical scenarios with delegates.

• **Simulation fellows** – trainee specialists e.g. anaesthetics/nurse practitioner with an interest in education spending one day a week or more attached to the simulation centre.

• **Visiting specialist faculty** – nurses, doctors, allied health professionals bringing their clinical expertise to the simulation facility for a particular course.

• **ODPs** – medical simulation historically came from anaesthetics [36] and anaesthetic scenarios are widely simulated, requiring an ODP for credibility. They may develop courses for ODPs and other healthcare workers (if funding allows).

• **Simulated patients** – actors trained to 'play' relatives/other roles to maintain realism [93].

Running a facility

The day-to-day operation of any simulation centre is dependent upon 'selling' simulation as a worthwhile educational methodology [94]. In order to entice delegates through the door we have to ensure that what is offered by this approach to education and training cannot be accessed through more traditional (and cheaper) teaching methods. However, we must ensure the simulation activity is not used as an end in itself, i.e. 'simulation for simulation's sake', but should be appropriately integrated in a blended educational approach addressing specific learning and clinical needs [95,96].

Measuring whether simulation education works is very difficult per se as it comes in many guises. It is relatively easy to assess changes in technical competence (e.g. in a procedure or surgical skills) as a result of a simulation event but the impact of simulation on non-technical skills is more difficult to measure. However, many researchers have explored various aspects of the simulation process and what influence it may have for example on patient safety, teamwork, communication, decision-making and competence. Simulation events also vary immensely, however delegates who have been through simulation training in its many forms will often state they feel 'more confident' in their clinical practice after the experience [97,98]. Confidence however is subjective and can be difficult to quantify. One of the more commonly used methodologies to evaluate the impact of simulation on the development of non-technical skills (such as leadership) is through focus groups which are an effective way to gain feedback on participants' experiences and perceptions [99].

SUMMARY

This chapter has highlighted the key issues to be addressed when planning an effective simulation facility or activity, specifically the importance of identifying a need and curriculum planning, capital and revenue cost considerations, early and prolonged engagement with dedicated faculty and key stakeholders, including potential and actual delegates. Bolted on to this is the need to consider quality assurance measures, investing time to establish robust governance frameworks, ethical considerations, as well as more practical elements of planning a facility and course such as equipment procurement, maintenance, staffing, including technicians and administrators for booking delegates onto courses and maintaining data and reporting mechanisms.

Each of the elements within the Framework for Simulation Integration and Delivery (Figure 10.6) are equally important, and although they do not necessarily have to be addressed in any particular order, all must be accomplished for the sustainable delivery of simulation training. Each aspect has been discussed within the chapter and the SOAR analysis [99,100] set out in Table 10.3 summarizes this by highlighting the strengths, opportunities, aspirations and results that arise from the introduction and on-going utilization of simulated clinical practice as a teaching pedagogy.

Table 10.3 SOAR analysis

Strengths	Opportunities
Simulation led by a 'champion'	Collaboration with partner healthcare
Provision of a range of training to meet local	organizations and Universities
clinical needs (as in the case study)	Interprofessional simulations and research
Clear learning objectives stated for each	Increased future funding
simulation exercise	Increased need for enhancing skills within
Tailor training to specific delegate group	the registered and unregistered
Adapt training to changing needs of healthcare	healthcare workforce
workforce [95]	Increased technology enhanced learning

Aspirations	Results
Provide a stimulating but safe learning environment	Provide new research data that helps shape
for students	the future of clinical education
Deliver teaching/enable learning using a pedagogy	Provide a healthcare workforce that is fit for
that is applicable to most preferred learning styles	purpose and keeps the patient at the centre
Provide training that has a direct positive impact on	of care
patient care	

Simulated practice is a rich, complex pedagogy that is labour intensive but undoubtedly provides benefits to both students and patients if introduced and developed in a systematic manner.

 Key points

- Funding needs to be considered early in the process, both capital and revenue to ensure sustainability and maintenance of simulation facilities/programmes.
- Early engagement with all key stakeholders is essential in the process of developing simulation training facilities.
- Quality assurance processes, including governance frameworks and ethical considerations, need to be in place.
- Identifying a need and curriculum integration are key to success.

REFERENCES

1. Department of Health (2008) High Quality Care for All: NHS Next Stage Review Final Report. Available from http://www.dh.gov.uk/prod_consum_dh/groups/dh_digitalassets/@dh/@en/documents/digitalasset/dh_085828.pdf (accessed 19 Feb 2012).

2. Department of Health (2011) A framework for technology enhanced learning. Available from http://www.dh.gov.uk/prod_consum_dh/groups/ dh_digitalassets/documents/digitalasset/dh_131061.pdf (accessed 18 February 2012).

3. Yorkshire and Humber Strategic Health Authority (2010) Clinical Skills and Simulation Strategy. Available from http://www.yorksandhumber.nhs.uk/document.php?o=5371 (accessed 7 February 2012).

4. General Medical Council (2010) Standards for Curricula and Assessment

Systems. Available from http://www.gmc-uk.org/Standards_for_Curricula__Assessment_Systems.pdf_31300458.pdf (accessed 19 February 2012).

5. Donaldson L (2008) 150 years of the Annual Report of the Chief Medical Officer: On the state of public health 2008. Available from http://www.dh.gov.uk/en/MediaCentre/Media/DH_096278 (accessed 18 February 2012).

6. Ker J, Hogg G and Maran N (2010) Cost-effective simulation. In: *Cost Effectiveness in Medical Education* (Walsh K, ed.). Abingdon. Radcliffe Publishing Ltd, 61–71.

7. Sunderland AB (2012) *Simulation Policy and Resource Pack*. Leeds: Leeds Metropolitan University.

8. NHS Litigation Authority (2012) NHSLA Risk Management Standards 2012–13 for NHS Trusts providing Acute, Community, or Mental Health & Learning Disability Services and Non-NHS Providers of NHS Care. Available from http://www.nhsla.com/NR/rdonlyres/6CBDEB8A-9F39-4A44-B04C-2865FD89C683/0/NHSLARiskManagementStandards201213.pdf (accessed 24 February 2012).

9. Care Quality Commission (2010) *The State of Health Care and Adult Social Care in England: Key Themes and Quality of Services in 2009*. Norwich: TSO.

10. Leeds Teaching Hospitals NHS Trust. Prospectus 2012. Available from http://www.medicaleducationleeds.com/assets/Resources/Course-Resources/MEL-amended-Prospectus.pdf (accessed 18 February 2012).

11. Department of Health (2012) Liberating the NHS: Developing the Healthcare Workforce. From Design to Delivery. Available from http://www.dh.gov.uk/prod_consum_dh/groups/dh_digitalassets/documents/digitalasset/dh_132087.pdf (accessed 23 February 2012).

12. NHS Employers (2011) European Working Time Directive. Available from http://www.nhsemployers.org/PlanningYourWorkforce/MedicalWorkforce/EWTD/Pages/EWTD.aspx (accessed 18 February 2012).

13. Nursing and Midwifery Council (2007) Supporting direct care through simulated practice learning in the pre-registration nursing programme. Nursing and Midwifery Council Circular 36. Available from http://www.nmc-uk.org/Documents/Circulars/2007circulars/NMCcircular36_2007.pdf (accessed 18 February 2012).

14. National Health Service Litigation Authority (2012) Clinical Negligence Scheme for Trusts (CNST).Available from http://www.nhsla.com/Claims/Pages/Clinical.aspx (accessed 24 February 2012).

15. Academy of Medical Royal Colleges, Department of Health, Social Services and Patient Safety, Department of Health, NHS Scotland, NHS Wales (2007) The Foundation Programme: Curriculum. Available from http://www.foundationprogramme.nhs.uk/index.asp?page=home/keydocs#c&rg (accessed 24 February 2012).

16. Wardrop M. Nurse caught on CCTV turning off paralysed patient's life support machine. Available from http://www.telegraph.co.uk/health/healthnews/8084841/Nurse-caught-on-CCTV-turning-off-paralysed-patients-life-support-machine.html (accessed: 26 February 2012).

17. Leeds Teaching Hospitals NHS Trust (2011) Calculating the cost of training. [Post graduate medical education meeting].

18. Haworth J, Conrad C (1997) *Emblems of Quality in Higher Education: Developing and Sustaining High Quality Programs*. Boston. Allyn and Bacon.

19. Adamson K (2010) Integrating human patient simulation into associate degree nursing curricula. *Clinical Simulation in Nursing* **6:** 75–81.

20. Brindley PG, Suen GI, Drummond J (2007) Part Two: Medical Simulation – How to build a successful and long-lasting programme. *Canadian Journal of Respiratory Therapy.* **Winter:** 31–34.

21. Yorkshire and Humber Strategic Health Authority (2011) Quality Assurance of Clinical Skills and Simulation Training in NHS Yorkshire and the Humber. Available from http://www.yorksandhumber.nhs.uk/document.php?o=7192 (accessed 18 February 2012).

22. Kearsley G, Shneiderman B (1998) Engagement theory: a framework for technology-based teaching and learning. *Educational Technology* **38:** 20–22.

23. International Nursing Association for Clinical Simulation and Learning (2011) Standards of best practice: simulation. *Clinical Simulation in Nursing* **7**(Suppl): S1–S20.

24. Health and Safety Executive (2011) Managing Standards for Tackling Work Related Stress: Steering Groups. Available from http://www.hse.gov.uk/stress/standards/pdfs/steeringgroups.pdf (accessed 14 February 2012).

25. Baily K (2012) Comprehensive simulation program: a rapid deployment success story (poster abstract). *Clinical Simulation in Nursing* **5:** e129–e155.

26. Anderson M, Bond ML, Holmes TL, Cason CL (2012) Acquisition of simulation skills: survey of users. *Clinical Simulation in Nursing* **8:** e59–e65.

27. Kyle RR, Murray WB (eds) (2007) *Clinical Simulation: Operations, Engineering and Management.* New York: Academic Press.

28. Corbett RW, Miles J, Gantt L, *et al.* (2008) Schools of Nursing, Clinical Partners, and Alumni Collaborate for Senior Nursing Simulation Scenarios: A Theory-based Approach. Clinical Simulation in Nursing. Available from http://www.nursingsimulation.org/article/S1876-1399%2808%2900034-0/pdf (accessed 7 February 2012).

29. Hermann RC, Palmer H, Leff S, *et al.* (2004) *Achieving Consensus Across Diverse Stakeholders on Quality Measures for Mental Healthcare. Medical Care.* Philadelphia: Lippincott Williams and Wilkins.

30. Sapountzis S, Yates K, Kagioglou M, Aouad G (2009) Realising benefits in primary healthcare infrastructures. *Facilities* **27:** 74–87.

31. Lee LYK, Lee JKL, Wong KF, *et al.* (2010) The establishment of an integrated skills training centre for undergraduate nursing education. *International Nursing Review* **57:** 359–364.

32. Kilo CM (1998) A Framework for Collaborative Improvement: Lessons from the Institute for Healthcare Improvement's Breakthrough Series. Available from http://www.chipolicy.org/pdf/5636.Kilo%20CM%20A%20Framework%20for%20Collaborative%20Improvement%2019981.pdf (accessed 18 February 2012).

33. Jeffries PR (2007) *Simulation in Nursing Education: From Conceptualisation to Evaluation.* New York: National League for Nursing.

34. Jeffries PR. (2005) Framework for Designing, Implementing and Evaluating Simulations Used as Teaching Strategies in Nursing. *Nursing Education Perspectives* **26:** 96–103.

35. McCallum J (2007) The debate in favour of using simulation education in pre-registration adult nursing. *Nurse Education Today* **27:** 825–831.

36. Gaba DM (2004) The future vision of simulation in healthcare. *Quality and Safety in Health Care* **13**(Suppl): i2–i10.

37. Cox RC, Acree JL (2008) Guidance for the leader-manager. cost verses value added. In: *Clinical Simulation: Operations, Engineering, and Management* (RR Kyle and WB Murray, eds). Missouri: Academic Press, 19–28.

38. Yorkshire and Humber Strategic Health Authority (2011) Quality Assurance of Clinical Skills and Simulation Training in NHS Yorkshire and the Humber. Available from http://www.yorksandhumber.nhs.uk/document.php?o=7192 (accessed 17 February 2012).

39. Issenberg SB, McGaghie WC, Petrusa ER, *et al.* (2005) Features and uses of high-fidelity medical simulations that lead to effective learning: a BEME systematic review. *Medical Teacher* **27**: 10–28.

40. Yorkshire and Humber Strategic Health Authority (2011) Clinical Skills Online. Available from http://www.qaclinicalskills.co.uk/Login.aspx?ReturnUrl=%2fHomePage.aspx (accessed 8 February 2012).

41. Burns HK (2008) Integrating Simulation into Nursing Curriculum. [Presentation]. Available from http://www.wiser.pitt.edu/sites/wiser/ns08/day1_HB_IntegratSimIntoNursingCurr.pdf (accessed 7 February 2012).

42. Anderson M, Bond ML, Holmes TL, Cason CL (2011) Acquisition of Simulation Skills: Survey of Users. Available at: http://www.nursingsimulation.org/article/S1876-1399%2810%2900147-7/pdf (accessed 11 February 2012).

43. Clapper TC (2010) Beyond Knowles: what those conducting simulation need to know about adult learning theory. *Clinical Simulation in Nursing* **6**: 7–14.

44. Garrett B, MacPhee M, Jackson C (2010) High-fidelity patient simulation: considerations for effective learning. *Nursing Education Perspectives* **31**: 309–313.

45. Howard VM, Englert N, Kameg K, Perozzi K (2011) Integration of simulation across the undergraduate curriculum: student and faculty perspectives. *Clinical Simulation in Nursing* **7**: 1–10.

46. Kardong-Edgren S, Adamson KA, Fitzgerald CA (2010) Review of currently published evaluation instruments for human patient simulation. *Clinical Simulation in Nursing* **6**: 25–35.

47. Lapkin S, Levett-Jones T, Bellchambers H, Fernandez R (2010) Effectiveness of patient simulation manikins in teaching clinical reasoning skills to undergraduate nursing students: a systematic review. *Clinical Simulation in Nursing* **6**: 207–222.

48. Murphy S, Hartigan I, Walshe N, *et al.* (2011) Merging problem-based learning and simulation as an innovative pedagogy in nurse education. *Clinical Simulation in Nursing* **7**: 141–148.

49. Ricketts B (2010) The role of simulation for learning within pre-registration education – a literature review. *Nurse Education Today*. Available from http://www.ncbi.nlm.nih.gov/pubmed/21074297 (accessed 7 February 2012).

50. Swanson EA, Nicholson A, Boese TA, *et al.* (2011) Comparison of selected teaching strategies incorporating simulation and student outcomes. *Clinical Simulation in Nursing* **7**: 81–90.

51. Wagner D, Bear M, Sander J (2009) Turning simulation into reality: increasing student competence and confidence. *Journal of Nursing Education* **48**: 465–467.

52. Weller JM (2004) Simulation in undergraduate medical education: bridging the gap between theory and practice. *Medical Education* **38:** 32–38.

53. Wilford A, Doyle TJ (2006) Integrating simulation training into the nursing curriculum. *British Journal of Nursing* **15:** 604–607.

54. Zulkosky KD (2010) Simulation use in the classroom: impact on knowledge acquisition, satisfaction, and self confidence. *Clinical Simulation in Nursing.* Available from http://www.nursingsimulation.org/article/S1876-1399(10)00142-8/fulltext (accessed 7 February 2012).

55. Jones AL, Hegge M (2008) Simulation and faculty time investment. *Clinical Simulation in Nursing* **4**, e5–e9.

56. Alinier G (2006) Effectiveness of Intermediate Fidelity Simulation Training Technology in Undergraduate Nursing Education. Available from https://uhra.herts.ac.uk/dspace/bitstream/2299/394/1/103694.pdf (accessed 7 February 2012.

57. Whittington Hospital NHS Trust (2010) Simulation Centre. Available from http://www.whittington.nhs.uk/default.asp?c=8427 (accessed 7 February 2012).

58. Flanagan B (2008) Debriefing: theory and principles. In: (RH Riley, ed.) *Manual of Simulation in Healthcare*. Oxford: Oxford University Press, 55.

59. Chickering AW, Gamson ZF (1987) Seven principles of best practice in undergraduate education. *AAHE Bulletin* **39:** 5–10.

60. Chronister C (2011) Comparison of simulation debriefing models. *Clinical Simulation in Nursing* http://www.nursingsimulation.org/article/S1876-1399(10)00204-5/fulltext (accessed 7 February 2012).

61. Neill MA, Wotton K (2011) High-fidelity simulation debriefing in nursing education: a literature review. *Clinical Simulation in Nursing.* Available from http://www.nursingsimulation.org/article/S1876-1399(11)00026-0/fulltext (accessed 7 February 2012).

62. Shinnick MA, Woo M, Horwich TB, Steadman R (2011) Debriefing: the most important component in simulation? *Clinical Simulation in Nursing* **7:** e105–e111.

63. Issenberg SB (2006) The Scope of simulation-based healthcare education. *Simulated Healthcare* **1:** 203–208.

64. Parry MG, Quy S (2011) Simulation for all! [Presentation]. Available from http://www.stfs.org.uk/sites/stfs/files/3.%20Martin%20Parry%20-%20Final%20Sim%20Foundation%20Faculty%20Update%2013%20April_0.pdf (accessed 7 February 2012).

65. American Heart Association (2010) Structured and supported debriefing. Available from http://www.onlineaha.org (accessed 7 February 2012).

66. Anderson M (2008) Debriefing and guided reflection. Available from http://www.sirc.nln.org (accessed 7 February 2012).

67. Denning K (2010) Debrief as a Learning Conversation. Available from www.resus.org.uk/pages/gicDbflc.pdf (accessed 17 February 2012).

68. Phrampus P, O'Donnell J (2008) Debriefing in Simulation Education – Using a Structured and Supported Model. [Presentation]. Available from http://www.wiser.pitt.edu/sites/wiser/ns08/day1_PP_JOD_DebriefingInSimEdu.pdf (accessed 17 February 2012).

69. Riley RH (2008) *Manual of Simulation in Healthcare*. Oxford. Oxford University Press.

70. SimLearn. Clinical Simulation Business Practices for Audio Visual Recordings. Available from http://www.simlearn.va.gov/docs/lib/SimLEARN_Clinical_Simulation_Business_Practices_For_Digital_Recordings_FC_0611.pdf (accessed 20 February 2012).

71. McKeever K, Kimberling B (2010) Capturing Simulations for Better Debriefing. [Conference presentation]. Available from http://www.laerdal.com/usa/sun/pdf/indianapolis/SUN_Capturing_Simulation_for_Debriefing.pdf (accessed 17 February 2012).

72. Boise State University (2011) Confidentiality, Digital Video/Audio, Observer Consent. Available from http://nursing.boisestate.edu/simulation/files/Printversiononly_SimCenter ConfidentialityVideoReleaseForm_FERPASim-06.pdf (accessed 17 February 2012).

73. Curran I (2008) Creating effective learning environments – Key educational concepts applied to simulation training. In: *Clinical Simulation: Operations, Engineering, and Management* (RR Kyle and WB Murray, eds). Missouri. Academic Press.

74. Gantt LT (2010) Strategic planning for skills and simulation labs in colleges of nursing. *Nursing Economics* **28**: 308–313.

75. Alinier G (2008) Prosperous simulation under an institution's threadbare financial blanket. In: *Clinical Simulation: Operations, Engineering, and Management* (RR Kyle and WB Murray, eds). Missouri. Academic Press.

76. Seropian MA, Brown K, Gavilanes JS, Driggers B (2004) An approach to simulation program development. *Journal of Nursing Education* **43**: 170–174.

77. Gillespie J (2008) Creative procurement for your simulation program In: *Clinical Simulation: Operations, Engineering, and Management* (RR Kyle and WB Murray, eds). Missouri. Academic Press.

78. Patterson MD, Blike GT, Nadkarni VM (2008) In situ simulation: challenges and results. In: *Advances in Patient Safety: New Directions and Alternative Approaches*. Vol. 3: *Performance and Tools* (K Henriksen, JB Battles, MA Keyes and ML Grady, eds) Rockville, MD: Agency for Healthcare Research and Quality.

79. Torrance C, Higham H (2011) *Using serious untoward incident (SUI) data to develop team simulation* [Conference presentation]. Cardiff: Association of Simulated Practice in Healthcare.

80. Ellis D, Crofts JF, Hunt LP, *et al.* (2008) Hospital simulation center, and teamwork training for eclampsia management. *Obstetrics & Gynecology* **111**: 723–731.

81. Crofts JF, Ellis D, Draycott TJ, *et al.* (2007) Change in knowledge of midwives and obstetricians following obstetric emergency training: a randomised controlled trial of local hospital, simulation centre and teamwork training. *British Journal of Obstetrics and Gynaecology* **114**: 1534–1541.

82. Gobbi M, Monger E (2008) Using web based multimedia, simulated and virtual practice to assess students' professional practice skills. Higher Education Authority and University of Southampton. Available from https://docs.google.com/viewer?a=v&q=cache:mpdLg8U340sJ:www.hsaparchive.org.uk/rp/publications/projectreports/marygobbi.pdf+HEA+Gobbi,+M+and+Monger,+E.+(2008)+Using+web+based+multimedia,+simulated+and+virtual+practice+to&hl=en&gl=uk&pid=bl&srcid=ADGEESh UZUQkdSLdIw_oTAwnnrWOM3E 7A2050fyGIi68hm0YW5g922i_ 2OeogaHffsQQioGcq09JL0RWqzBK6x GUabyxgPCnp9PQicCm_ehuCEaSwIk-ZzMLartl6fMwO_gpsRMElWQM&sig= AHIEtbQ9SH1I6JKhxS4g2fAuRK2 IViHC0Q (accessed 11 February 2012).

83. Hwang JCF, Bencken B (2008) Integrating simulation with existing clinical educational programs: dream and

develop while keeping the focus on your vision. In: *Clinical Simulation: Operations, Engineering, and Management* (RR Kyle and WB Murray, eds). Missouri. Academic Press.

84. Jha A, Duncan B, Bates D. (2001) Simulator-based training and patient safety. In: *Making Health Care Safer: A Critical Analysis of Patient Safety Practices.* Evidence Report/Technology Assessment Number 43. Rockville, MD: Agency for Healthcare Research and Quality, 510–517.

85. Stern PA, Harz CR (2008) *Serious Games for First Responders: Improving Design and Usage with Social Learning Theory.* Malibu: Pepperdine University.

86. Hammoud MM, Nuthapapaty FS, Goepfert AR, *et al.* (2008) To the point: medical education review of the role of simulators in surgical training. *American Journal of Obstetrics and Gynecology* **199:** 338–343.

87. Maran NJ, Glavin RJ (2003) Low to high-fidelity simulation – a continuum of medical education? *Medical Education* **37**(Suppl)**:** 22–38.

88. Aggarwal R, Mytton OT, Derbrew M, *et al.* (2010) Training and simulation for patient safety. *Quality and Safety in Health Care* **19**(Suppl)**:** 34–43.

89. London Deanery (2012) Faculty Development. E-Learning for Clinical Teachers: Using Simulation in Clinical Education. Available from http://www.faculty.londondeanery.ac.uk/e-learning/using-simulation-in-clinical-education (accessed 24 February 2012).

90. Du Boulay C, Medway C (1999) The clinical skills resource: a review of current practice. *Medical Education* **33:** 185–191.

91. Vollmer J, Monk S, Heinrichs W (2008) Staff education for simulation: train-the-trainer concepts. In: *Clinical Simulation: Operations, Engineering, and Management* (RR Kyle and WB Murray, eds). Missouri. Academic Press.

92. Yorkshire and Humber Clinical Skills Network (2011) *Role of the technician. [Workshop discussion].* Leeds: Clinical Practice Centre.

93. Dudley F (2012) *The Simulated Patient Handbook.* London. Radcliffe Publishing Ltd.

94. Patillo RE, Hewett B, McCarthy MD, Molinari D (2010) Capacity Building for simulation sustainability. *Clinical Simulation in Nursing* **6:** e185–e191.

95. Department of Health (2003) Streamlining quality assurance in healthcare education: purpose and action. Available from http://www.dh.gov.uk/prod_consum_dh/groups/dh_digitalassets/@dh/@en/documents/digitalasset/dh_4072931.pdf (accessed 21 February 2012).

96. Department of Health (2008) Safer Medical Practice: Machines, Manikins and Polo Mints. Available from http://www.dh.gov.uk/prod_consum_dh/groups/dh_digitalassets/documents/digitalasset/dh_096227.pdf (accessed 18 February 2012).

97. Nishisaki A, Keren D, Nadkarni V (2007) Does Simulation improve patient safety? Self-Efficacy, competence, Operational performance and patient safety. *Anaesthesiology Clinics* **25:** 225–236.

98. Howitt D (2010) *Introduction to Qualitative Methods in Psychology.* Harlow, England. Prentice Hall.

99. Slack T (2009) Learning from the Military: Developing an A1-Based Project Debrief Toolkit. Available at http://www.appreciatingpeople.co.uk/images/stories/aipfeb09article8.pdf (accessed 12 February 2012).

100. Hill T, Westbrook R. (1997) SWOT Analysis: it's time for a product recall. *Long Range Planning* **30:** 46–52.

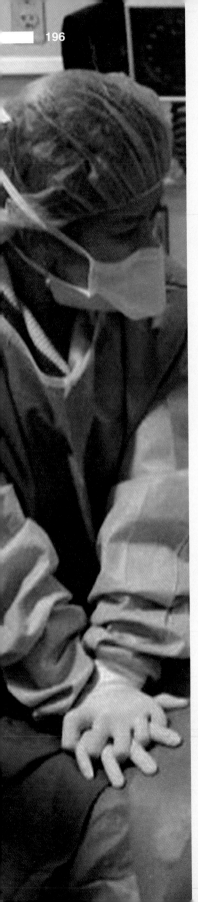

CHAPTER 11
Distributed simulation

Jessica Janice Tang, Jimmy Kyaw Tun, Roger L Kneebone and Fernando Bello   Imperial College London, London, UK

Overview

In this chapter, we present an overview of the concept of distributed simulation (DS) – low cost, portable simulation that is 'sufficiently immersive'. DS is a novel approach to conducting simulations, aiming to address some of the challenges currently faced by simulation practitioners in trying to establish best practice in simulation-based medical education (SBME), particularly with cost and limited access.

We present the philosophical and theoretical underpinnings of the concept, and some ongoing research and development that we are currently undertaking. In addition, we also discuss the technological developments of the key components of DS (such as its physical components and design process), which have allowed us to develop and conduct simulations based on this innovative approach.

The research and development strategy of DS is introduced in terms of empirical studies designed to explore and validate the use of DS for SBME in order to provide evidence to support and refine the concept. This work sets out to provide practical examples of how DS can be utilized to conduct simulations in a range of clinical specialities, including surgery, emergency medicine, intensive care and cardiology.

Finally, we discuss our experience and ongoing work on the potential applications of DS outside medical education. Although DS was conceived through the need to provide cost-effective accessible SBME, this novel approach to simulation has other applications, such as translational research, care pathway modelling and public engagement.

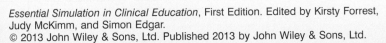

Introduction

The importance of immersive simulation is increasingly recognized across all disciplines in response to widespread changes in the training of healthcare professionals over the last couple of decades. These changes have partly resulted in a drive from time-based outcomes to competency-based training and include reductions in training opportunities as a result of reduced working hours and an increasing emphasis on patient safety. At the same time, it is no longer ethically acceptable to practise and train on patients without prior development of skills. The importance of simulation is becoming embedded in major healthcare education policies around the world, for instance the 150 Years of the Annual Report of the Chief Medical Officer has an extensive section discussing the applications and benefits of simulation [1]. Although the need for simulation is widely accepted, issues remain on how medical educators should use it most effectively. In 2009, McGaghie *et al.* presented a synthesis of the current healthcare simulation literature, identifying 12 key features and best practice for simulation-based medical education (SBME) [2]: (1) feedback; (2) deliberate practice; (3) curriculum integration; (4) outcome measurement; (5) simulation fidelity; (6) skill acquisition and maintenance; (7) mastery learning; (8) transfer to practice; (9) team training; (10) high-stakes training; (11) instructor training; and (12) education and professional context. Effective SBME requires knowledge of suggested best practice, interpreted in the light of local values and priorities. However, current approaches to simulation in healthcare settings do not always address these features.

The implementation of simulation takes two main approaches. The first relates to the top-down implementation of simulation in healthcare settings. Top-level stakeholders have the power to allocate resources to facilitate the development of healthcare simulation. A good example is the recent, rapid establishment of dedicated static facilities for immersive simulation training. Although such centres achieve many good educational outcomes, they are scarce, relatively expensive and inaccessible to many learners. Clinical practice and training involve management of dynamic relationships between clinicians, patients and complex environments with multiple variables. Simulation in healthcare setting, therefore, should be user-orientated and more sensitive to individual needs. Top-down implementation of simulation activities may also result in resistance to SBME because learners do not have a sense of 'ownership' of their training.

The second approach draws comparisons between healthcare and high technology/high risk professions in simulation design. For example, aviation professionals are trained to work in a highly standardized simulated environment where the interaction between the pilots and the aeroplane is explicit, with pre-set instructions [3]. Such an approach may not be appropriate in healthcare settings, where clinicians are faced with complex and varied human anatomy, physiology and diseases. Attempts to base healthcare simulation on other high-risk professions may contribute to a mismatch of simulation (and/or simulator) design and pedagogy in clinical training. Moreover, there is no 'one size fits all' in clinical training; a high-tech manikin may create a highly engaging experience for anaesthetists when the response is seen through traces on monitor screens, but a live simulated patient (SP) is more effective than any manikin for recreating the subtleties underpinning consultation dynamics.

Best practice in SBME requires simulation stakeholders to explore other ways of designing and conducting simulation to complement current methods. Distributed simulation (DS) represents a novel approach to conducting immersive simulations.

Distributed simulation: conceptual and theoretical foundations

The aim of the DS concept is to provide cost-effective, versatile and accessible immersive simulation for training and assessment. This flexibility allows DS to support a wide range of learning needs without being unduly prescriptive. Key to this flexibility is being able to tailor the level of fidelity of simulation scenarios, including the simulated environment.

The specifications of DS include:
• a self-contained immersive environment which can be closed off from its surroundings, allowing

any available space to be converted into a convincing 'clinical' setting for the duration of the simulation;

• minimum necessary cues (visual, auditory and kinaesthetic) to recreate a realistic 'clinical' environment (including clinical equipment and sounds);

• simple, user-friendly equipment for observing, recording, playback and debriefing, similar to that used in static simulation centres;

• practical, lightweight and easily transportable components which can be erected quickly by a minimal team;

• the flexibility to recreate a range of clinical settings according to individual requirements.

In the following sections, the conceptual foundations of DS are discussed further.

Optimized level of fidelity

Current immersive simulation activity aims to reproduce real clinical environments as closely as possible. Yet it is recognized that simulation fidelity is only one of a multitude of factors affecting effectiveness. At the same time, trying to reproduce all the elements of a real clinical environment can incur high costs.

A key feature of DS is optimizing the level of fidelity by designing simulation through the eyes of the participants. Instead of faithfully *reproducing* all aspects of a clinical setting, DS *selects and recreates* only salient features that provide key cues which engage participants and achieve educational outcomes.

The design concept of DS draws on theories of attention in cognitive psychology, which suggests that visual attention is selective in nature and that the processing capacity of our visual system is limited. Concentrating resources on a particular spatial locus is a key strategy in overcoming this limit. Two influential models describing how this mechanism works in our visual attention systems are the Spotlight Model and the Zoom Lens Model.

The Spotlight Model [4] proposes that a shift of visual attention corresponds to a shift in processing resources among several analysed locations, like moving a spotlight. This model describes attention in terms of focus, fringe and margin. The *focus* is an area that extracts information selectively from a

visual scene: the centre is where visual attention is directed and where resolution is highest. By contrast, the area surrounding the centre of focus, known as *fringe*, extracts information in a rougher manner, hence visual images have lower resolution. The fringe extends to a specific area that reaches the attentional limits, the cut-off of which is called *margin*.

The Zoom Lens Model [5] utilizes the properties of the Spotlight Model, but also includes the property of changing size in visual attention. This property was inspired by the zoom lens function on a camera in which there is a trade off between the size of the visual attention region and processing efficiency. Since fixed attentional resources are distributed over a larger area when the centre of focus is larger, the mental processing is slower in that area of focus. Both models illustrate a phenomenon in visual perception, whereby focusing one's attention on a task results in peripheral images being blurred. A practical example would be map reading, when trying to find a street name (e.g. Bond Street) on a London map, your visual attention will scale down to a specific area of the map, allowing the identification of specific details of the street names near Bond Street Tube Station. Hence, your peripheral images, such as other street names in area further away from Bond Street maybe blurred, which restricts you from perceiving the details of other streets (e.g. the exact location of Old Queen Street near St James's Park Tube Station).

The application of these visual attention models were embedded in the idea of 'optimized level of fidelity' in DS. DS designers carefully selected the key features of a clinical environment from the participants' perspective in order to reproduce the clinical learning environment cost-effectively. During an immersive simulation, through the eyes of the participants, all 'blurred' regions need not be recreated by real clinical elements (e.g. the drug trolley in an operating theatre) because the participants are cognitively unable to perceive the details of them.

Memory also plays a significant role in attention and awareness; working memory allows clinicians to shift their primary focus of attention to other tasks [6]. Likewise, we theorize that participants within a simulation do not give equal attentional

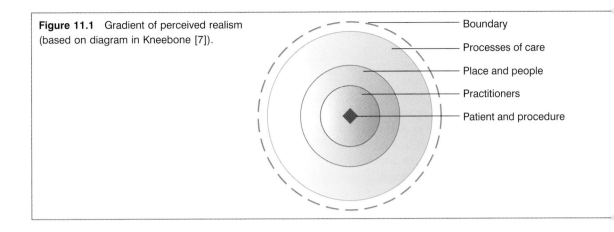

Figure 11.1 Gradient of perceived realism (based on diagram in Kneebone [7]).

Boundary

Processes of care

Place and people

Practitioners

Patient and procedure

weighting to all the elements within the simulated environment. Previously, Kneebone [7] proposed the notion of 'circles of focus', a theoretical model which forms the basis of simulation design in DS. This model describes the concentric nature of participants' selective perception, awareness, and attention to the different elements that make up a clinical setting within a simulation, whereby there is a 'gradient of perceived realism' (Figure 11.1).

Kneebone illustrated this model using the example of a simulated surgical operation. In the surgeon's primary focus, the attention is on the operative field, with surgical instruments, anatomy and movements well defined in the clinician's view. Around the centre of attention the context of the procedure plays its role, though at a lower level of awareness. Within this layer, a clinician's general sense of being in the operating theatre comprises sights, sounds and sensations, for instance the beeping of the anaesthetic monitor. These two layers are embedded within the wider picture of the clinical scenario, such as the circulating nurse fetching some drugs to the surgical team. All these circumstances happen outside the primary focus of the surgeon. This gradient of perceived realism in the 'circle of focus' assists designers to create an effective simulation experience through the process of traversing different layers in the model (see Design process and anatomy of the distributed simulation system).

Low-cost, portable and versatile: widening access to meet users' needs

It is generally acknowledged that successful simulation-based training requires delivery through a robust curriculum, whereby training is distributed and integrated into a range of different teaching modalities (including work-based learning). However, dedicated simulation centres are unable to support this relationship between learning in real clinical practice and simulation-based training due to their static nature. At the same time, the high-cost of dedicated simulation centres can restrict many learners' access to simulation-based training resulting in short and often disconnected courses, not embedded into a coherent curriculum or training programme.

These issues have been addressed previously by using other simulation methods. For example, LeBlanc [8] described 'in-situ' simulation whereby simulations, equipment and technology are brought to the real clinical workplace. This offers a high level of contextual richness, providing a stronger relationship between work-based learning and simulation-based training. However, there are drawbacks in terms of feasibility. As a consequence of global recession, many countries have massively reduced their public service budgets, while demands on healthcare services continue to rise. With the difficulty in accessing space in hospitals, lining up 'in-situ' simulations in existing healthcare settings becomes challenging. Also, the needs of clinical service provision may not easily allow for use of the real workplace to conduct simulations which may disrupt existing clinical activities.

DS widens access to simulation facilities, emphasizing the importance of accessibility and flexibility of the simulation system to meet needs of individual users which can be achieved through three principles. First, simulation should be tailor-made for learners to attain specific educational goals, supporting simulation's role of strengthening clinical practice. Second, simulation must be widely accessible to learners in order to fully address their training needs, which include time and geographical constraints. Third, simulation design and implementation should be cost-effective. The modular design of DS allows simulations to be set up in any suitable space – for example in an office, gymnasium or hospital training room – overcoming some of the usual constraints of simulation centres and in situ simulation. Costs of setting up and maintaining the simulation facilities should match training outcomes. The relative low cost of DS compared with more conventional static simulation centres is another major benefit which is achieved as a result of its selective fidelity design discussed earlier.

What's the evidence?

Kneebone R, Arora, S., King, D., Bello, F., Sevdalis, N., Kassab, E., Aggarwal, R., Darzi, A., Nestel, D. Distributed simulation – accessible immersive training. *Medical Teacher* 2010;32: 65–70.

This conceptual paper introduces the DS concept. It describes the key elements of DS that can be provided within a lightweight, low cost and self contained setting which is portable and accessible to wide range of clinicians. The paper also presents the design process of DS and the domains in recreating a simulated operating theatre.

Kneebone R. Simulation, safety and surgery. *Quality Safety Health Care* 2010;19(Suppl 3): 47–52.

This paper explores the place of simulation in contemporary healthcare education and training. It also highlights the key challenges to recreate clinical environment for clinical education. The author suggested the importance of selectively identifying key features of a clinical setting in order to reproduce the essentials in simulation development. The paper introduces the conceptual framework of 'circles of focus' and its theoretical and practical implications on surgery and other craft specialties.

Design process and anatomy of the distributed simulation system

The following section describes how our group at Imperial College London has developed the concept of DS, outlining key stages in the design process. A multidisciplinary group of professionals, including clinicians, educationalists, psychologists, design engineers and computer scientists, provides specialist input into all areas of design, using an iterative process of continual development. See Figure 11.2 for the design cycle of DS components.

In the design process, industrial designers and engineers provide expertise in physical and electronic design and use of materials to ensure low cost and portability. A crucial component of their role is to determine which cues and stimuli needed to be recreated to provide an authentic clinical environment. Computer scientists create bespoke software to support the simulation activities, such as audio and video interfaces as discussed later or customized computer-based simulators. Clinicians, educationalist and psychologists provide expertise to ensure the designs meet the educational requirements and are clinically accurate.

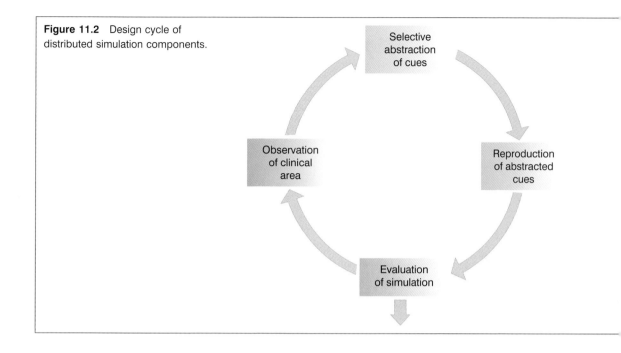

Figure 11.2 Design cycle of distributed simulation components.

A crucial step is to select the right elements from the gradient of realism (as suggested in the model of 'circle of focus' described earlier) to recreate the necessary cues for an effective simulation experience. We have termed this process 'selective abstraction'. During initial development, design engineers (newcomers to the clinical world who until then were wholly unfamiliar with the surgical environment) spent extended periods of observation in the operating theatre. This was followed by extended in-depth discussions with clinicians, engineers and psychologists, in order to identify key components constituting a simulation setting. Referring again to the 'circles of focus' model, maximum realism was achieved in the central layer through prosthetic expertise, using silicon models to create anatomically accurate models with high levels of perceived authenticity. To recreate more peripheral cues, recorded background noise and a suitably coloured portable enclosure provided the context layer of realism.

Details of the main components of the DS system fall into three main categories: DS *environment*, DS *audiovisual technology* and DS *simulators*.

The distributed simulation environment

The key elements of the DS environment are a self-contained, enclosable space, furnished with pull up backdrops representing key items of equipment (Figure 11.3); a lightweight, custom-designed operating lamp; and small loudspeakers. The self-contained, enclosable space creates a boundary in clinical training, establishing a context for education and professional practice by supplying important visual cues for the participants.

Initially, we used self-standing 'pop up' banners imprinted with operating theatre or emergency room scenes (Figures 11.4 and 11.5). These were able to recreate a clinical space that worked well for those participants facing the scenes, but did not provide a good level of immersion for those facing out towards the surroundings. The next design iteration resulted in a 360 degree inflatable 'igloo' that can be erected in 3 minutes with minimum effort (Figure 11.6), and that can effectively block participants away from the surrounding environment (e.g. normal office setting or assembly hall). An alternative to the inflatable enclosure suitable for recreating smaller clinical spaces is provided by

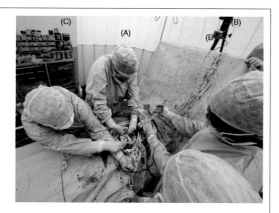

Figure 11.3 Distributed simulation (DS) surgical environment. (A) A self-contained and enclosable space, (B) a portable operating lamp (stand only shown), (C) pull-up banners, (D) video-cameras (part of AV system) mounted on enclosure wall and operating lamp stand.

wheeled partitions imprinted with high resolution photographs and graphics (Figure 11.7). Depending on specific training requirements, these portable assessment environments (PAEs) may be populated with a variety of scenarios, faculty members and simulators.

The pull-up backdrops used inside the inflatable enclosure are printed with high-resolution photographs of clinical equipment, such as trolleys or instrument cupboards (Figure 11.8). They can effectively recreate various components within the clinical space at minimum cost and may be tailored to the requirements of a specific centre.

Our observation of various clinical areas highlighted the importance of adequate audio cues. These are recreated in the DS environment through small loudspeakers playing back a variety of clinical sounds (e.g. heart monitor, ventilator and clinical background noise).

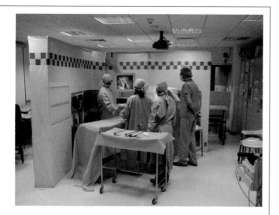

Figure 11.4 Operating theatre self-standing 'pop-up' banners.

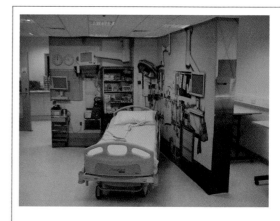

Figure 11.5 Emergency room self-standing 'pop-up' banners.

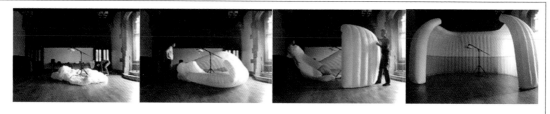

Figure 11.6 The inflatable 'igloo'.

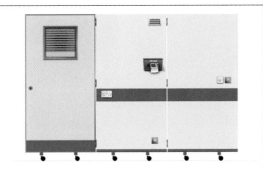

Figure 11.7 Distributed **s**imulation partitions.

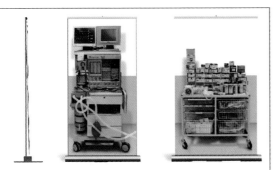

Figure 11.8 Distributed **s**imulation pull-up backdrops.

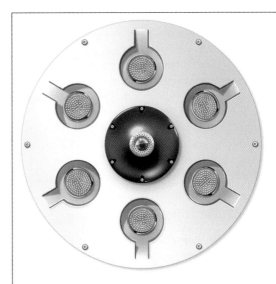

Figure 11.9 Distributed **s**imulation lamp.

A tripod-mounted portable operating lamp represents another crucial component of the DS system (Figure 11.9). This lamp is moulded from lightweight plastic and uses low-voltage light emitting diodes (LEDs). Although much smaller and lighter than a normal operating lamp, its circular shape, adjustable position and bright lights recreate the presence of an actual operating lamp while providing adequate illumination. The DS lamp is also equipped with a video camera and microphone integrated in the central handle, providing quality recording of the interactions in the operative field. This function is crucial to clinical skills feedback, debriefing and assessment, and an important part of retaining best practice in SBME.

The importance of context on learning, practice and assessment is well established in medical simulation literature [9,10]. McGaghie *et al.* [2, p. 60] commented that 'SBME that ignores its educational and professional context for teaching, evaluation or application in clinical practice is misdirected'. Therefore, the idea of creating a dedicated space for participants to experience an appropriate level of realism during simulation training is significant. Pawson *et al.* [11,12] discussed the difficulties in creating a variety of key elements in clinical education interventions which can be overcome by the portability and flexibility of the DS environment's simple and flexible design allows simulation users to refine and adapt the elements into a variety of simulations.

Distributed simulation audio and visual interface

A key component of any static simulation centre is a control room from which activities within the simulation can be observed and managed without disrupting activity. DS uses wireless cameras, a laptop computer and customized software to provide a 'portable control room' which can be located remotely from the simulation. In addition to the video recording features of the DS lamp, off-the-shelf wireless high image quality cameras and clear sound recording microphones allow for the recording of team interaction and team performance. The wireless cameras are portable, lightweight and can be positioned within the DS enclosure (i.e. the 'igloo' or PAE partitions), according to individual learning and teaching needs. A bespoke software interface presents and records in real time the various video feeds from the DS lamp and wireless cameras. The DS software interface is particularly useful for debriefing and post-analysis to provide assessment and evaluation of clinical skills training, again at a fraction of the cost of fully equipped static installations.

Distributed simulation simulators

The DS environment provides selected visual cues to secure participants' engagement in their simulation experience. To achieve this effect, we applied the DS concept of selective abstraction to a number of elements that are critical to surgical and anaesthetics training and assessment.

Realistic physical interface: instruments and synthetic models

During the active design process, our design team identified the importance of details in the clinicians' central focus of attention in the 'gradient of realism'. Anatomical structures, surgical instruments and hand movements of the surgical team are all prominent components of the central field of visual awareness. Real instruments, real clinicians and trained actors are therefore employed in DS simulations in order to maximize realism. Since real human tissue can seldom be used in simulations due to practical and ethical constraints, we built on expertise from prosthetic design and technology to produce realistic models (Figures 11.10 and 11.11) for medical training and assessment purposes. These prosthetic models can be adapted to a range of clinical settings according to learning requirements, and may be attached to a simulated patient played by a trained professional actor to provide authentic interactions to the scenario participants.

Simulated anaesthetic machine

The simulated anaesthetic machine (SAM) is a simulated anaesthetic interface that aims to provide immersion for anaesthetists by providing key sen-

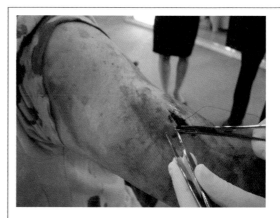

Figure 11.10 Synthetic model for suturing.

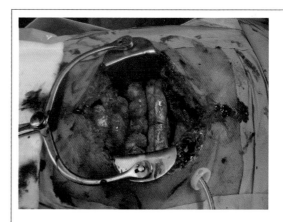

Figure 11.11 Synthetic model for open surgery.

sory cues and interactions. Currently, immersive anaesthetic simulations typically utilize real anaesthetic machines, which are very expensive (Figure 11.12)

At the core of the SAM is a trolley with a coloured moulded plastic panel giving clinicians appropriate visual cues of the clinical context. A breathing bag and ventilation circuit is attached to a balloon with variable compliance providing the cues necessary for manual ventilation. The anaesthetic monitor is represented by two iPads®. Custom written software provides accurate representations of visual and audio cues. One iPad® displays basic physiological monitoring data, such

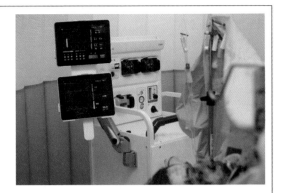

Figure 11.12   Simulated anaesthetic machine.

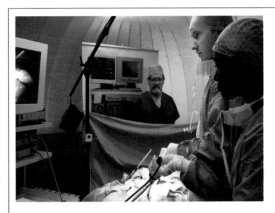

Figure 11.13   Distributed simulation laparoscopic cholecystectomy setting.

as blood pressure, heart rate and oxygen saturation, whilst the second iPad® shows ventilator settings and allows adjustment via a touch sensitive screen. Clinical parameters on the iPads® are remotely controlled by an independent controller (via an iPod Touch® device) using Bluetooth® technology. This set-up allows faculty to control a patient's physiological status, while at the same time recreating many of the important cues for anaesthetics training and assessment.

Exploring and investigating the distributed simulation concept

So far we have discussed the conceptual and design principles of DS and how it draws on theories in psychology and education. However, as with all new simulation methods and technologies, systematic evaluation is needed to demonstrate if, why and how the DS concept and its various components work. In addition, as part of this process and our own research interests, we have developed various practical uses of DS for educational activities.

Our initial focus was to explore the feasibility of DS in providing contextual richness to simulation training in General Surgery. This was followed by an investigation into the use of DS in various contexts, such as Emergency Medicine, with an integration of simulated clinical challenges. Finally, the feasibility of DS in science communication was explored through a series of public engagement activities.

Validation of distributed simulation

Preliminary validation of DS used a surgical setting [13]. Twenty surgeons were recruited to perform a laparoscopic cholecystectomy on a porcine model in order to study the face, content and construct validity of the DS concept. A counterbalance approach was adopted, half of these participants were novices with fewer than 50 laparoscopic cholecystectomies performed, and the other half were experts with more than 50 laparoscopic cholecystectomies performed. One half was randomly assigned to start with the DS session, while the other half started with a part-task session on a decontextualized bench-top box trainer. The DS session required participants to attend a full team immersive simulation in which they needed to review a set of patient notes, scrub up and perform the procedure with a draped box trainer. As in a normal operating theatre, there was an anaesthetist, a scrub nurse and an assistant to work with the participants. The DS environment used for the DS session of this study consisted of the inflated igloo, pull up banners, DS lamp and lightweight speakers playing background noise recorded from the real operating theatre (Figure 11.13). Also, the DS AV interface was used to record and playback the clinical performance of the participants for outcome assessments.

Face and content validity of the DS simulations were assessed using post-scenario questionnaires with Likert-type items evaluating realism and comprehensiveness. Construct validity of the simulation was determined by comparing performance of experts and novice surgeons. Surgical performance was assessed by two independent expert raters using Objective Structured Assessment of Technical Skills (OSATS), a previously validated rating tool [14]. Semi-structured interviews were also conducted to explore the participants' perceptions and experience of the DS simulations in depth.

The results demonstrated a strong face and content validity, with significant differences in performance between experts and novices in the DS session. The full team immersive simulation experience offered in the DS session was authentic enough for the objective raters to distinguish levels of performance. Significant differences between experts and novices in teamwork performance added further evidence in support of the holistic approach of SBME, avoiding overemphasis on part-task training. In this first DS empirical study, the DS system demonstrated that it offers an accessible, cost-effective and authentic simulation concept underpinned by a philosophy and key components that have wide potential application as a surgical training tool.

What's the evidence?

Kassab E, Kyaw Tun J, Arora S, King D, Ahmed K, Miskovic D, Cope A, Vadhwana B, Bello F, Sevdalis N, Kneebone R. 'Blowing up the barriers': exploring and validating a new approach to simulation. *Annals of Surgery* 2011;254(6): 1059–1065.

This paper studies the face, content and construct validity of DS. Twenty participants (10 novice and 10 expert surgeons) performed a laparoscopic cholecystectomy in the DS environment and on a standard surgical box trainer and their performance was being compared with objective measures. The results demonstrate a strong face, content and construct validity and the study concludes that DS offers a valid, low cost, accessible environment for training and assessing surgeons.

Context augmented surgical training (CAST)

This initial DS empirical study showed that the performance of expert surgeons in a full team immersive simulation was significantly better than that of novices. To further explore the differences between 'contextualized' and 'decontextualized' surgical performance, 11 novice surgeons were recruited from a surgical skills training course organized by the London Deanery (the body responsible for postgraduate medical training across London). The participants ranged from third year to sixth year general surgery speciality trainees (STs) (i.e. residents) who performed a small bowel anastomosis on a porcine model. As with the first validation study, participants were asked to perform the procedure in the DS environment and on a decontextualized part-task bench top-model. The part-task bench top model consisted of cadaveric pig bowel pinned to a cork pad, with no attempt to provide a clinical context. In the DS session, a segment of porcine intestine was dyed with simulated blood (to provide a natural colour) and presented within a silicone model representing the surrounding abdominal organs. The whole model was covered with drapes to simulate the operative field. This prosthetic model was designed to achieve maximum fidelity in the central attentional field. Together with the DS environment adopted from the previous study, participants were asked to go through the normal surgical process (i.e. checking patient notes, scrubbing, and interacting with other surgical team members). After all simulations, participants took part in a semi-structured interview and a questionnaire survey in order to compare their simulation experiences in the DS session and the part-task session and to rate the content and realism of the environment. Preliminary results further demonstrate the value of DS in surgical training, with participants rating the DS system as a better tool for junior surgeon to practice their skills before operating in a real operating theatre compare with bench top model. The immersive simulation offered by the DS system allowed the participants to experience some of the typical pressures and challenges in a real operating theatre.

These studies provided initial validation of the DS concept in the context of surgery. The consistently higher scores in the DS sessions on different surgical procedures (e.g. laparoscopic cholecystectomy and small bowel anastomosis) for experts compared to novices, and the preference of participants for the DS sessions over the part-task sessions, demonstrate reliability and acceptability. Participants also valued the level of fidelity within the DS environment. The DS AV interface was useful in recording the performance for post-simulation assessments and debriefings. During these studies, the DS system was set up in different locations at the participants' convenience (i.e. where they were available), thus demonstrating the portability and flexibility of the DS system.

What's the evidence?

Kassab E, Kyaw Tun J, Kneebone R. A novel approach to contextualized surgical simulation training. *Simulation in Health* 2012;7: 155–161.

This paper explores surgeons' views on training in a contextualized, novel high-fidelity simulation environment DS, in comparison to the traditional bench-top model. Eleven novice surgeons performed a small bowel anastomosis on a bench model and in DS. Their perceptions were measured by questionnaire and interviews. The results demonstrate that DS was perceived as a better training tool than the bench top model for clinical education. Surgeons believed that contextualized simulation should be integrated after bench-top training and before practising in a real OR, while DS allows junior surgeons to gain confidence before practising in a real operating theatre.

Simulating clinical challenge in procedural skills simulation

Effective SBME should allow a range of difficulty and challenge for the participant to match their level of education and training. Some procedures are intrinsically more challenging than others. For instance, a lumbar puncture can be thought to be more difficult than a venepuncture. However, the challenge of a given task can be affected by many other factors including patient, environment and learner factors, all of which may affect the perceived difficulty of a task even if the task itself is seen as straightforward – performing venepuncture on a fit healthy patient is quite different from performing the same procedure on an intravenous drug user, a needle-phobic patient or a patient suffering cardiac arrest. Clinical procedural competence therefore requires trainees to demonstrate not only technical ability in a range of contexts, but also a range of other professional skills in an integrated fashion.

Despite this, much of the current simulation of procedural skills focuses on technical skills without taking into account this wider clinical context. Previously, Kneebone *et al.* [15] described the use of hybrid simulation, multimodal simulation combining simulated (actor) patients (SPs) with part-task trainers, allowing clinicians to demonstrate the technical and non-technical skills in an integrated fashion. We hypothesized that hybrid simulation within a realistic clinical environment can allow adjustment of the level of challenge of the same procedure by simulating different clinical contexts. We aimed to investigate this hypothesis by systematically designing and validating simulations of different levels of clinical challenge using the principles of DS and hybrid simulation. Two hybrid simulation (HS) scenarios of low and high clinical complexity (HS1 and HS2 respectively) were designed to assess emergency doctors' competence in the management of traumatic skin laceration. Cognitive task analysis was used to define the procedure, drawing on the experience and expert opinion of senior emergency medicine clinicians [16]. The HS1 and HS2 simulation scenarios were designed to reflect what was expected of a Foundation Year 2 doctor (intern) and Emergency Medicine ST3 (third year resident) respectively would be capable of performing. Clinical challenge was achieved by adjusting the patient's behaviour and medical history (as portrayed by a trained actor) (see Case study 11.1).

🔍 Case study 11.1   Simple and complex hybrid scenarios

Hybrid simulation 1 (HS1) – simple scenario

A 30-year-old pleasant and compliant female city worker, who was previously fit and well, sustained a laceration to her anterior mid right thigh following a fall from her bicycle at low speed. She sustained no other injuries and is stable on admission.

Hybrid simulation 1 (HS2) – complex scenario

A 50-year-old intoxicated and disruptive city banker, with known hypertension and penicillin allergy, but otherwise fit and well, sustained a laceration to the medial aspect of his mid right upper arm due to a fall over a metal railing. Patient is not compliant and does not stay still during treatment (wound closure). He sustained no other injuries and is stable on admission.

We identified perceived realism as a crucial requirement for engagement with this innovative approach to simulation. Our early hybrid simulations combined existing part-task trainers (e.g. suture pads) with simulated patients. Scenarios had to be stage managed by 'pre-draping' the wound to make it appear to be part of the patient. This limited our ability to provide an authentic scenario. Such scenarios were limited to the act of wound suturing itself, while in reality a full history and neurological assessment needs to be performed prior to wound closure.

To create effective hybrid simulations, realistic, 'wearable', yet reproducible wound prosthetics were designed by experts from the film and television industry. These models, made from high-grade silicon, were applied by stockinettes to create the illusion of being part of the patient. Experienced simulated patients adopted standardized roles using semi-structured scripts. Simulations took place in the DS environment portraying a cubicle in an Emergency Department, furnished with clinical equipment normally used in the workplace. This setup was in line with the circles of focus concept, emphasizing realism in the centre through the patient and wound within an enclosure (the inflatable igloo).

In summary, this study demonstrated that, by systematically designing simulations using the principles of DS and hybrid simulation, clinical challenge can be effectively incorporated into the simulations, which is an important attribute of simulation-based assessments.

Public engagement

The studies described earlier demonstrate the validity and reliability of DS in the context of surgery and of learners and teachers within the clinical world. Our exploratory work on DS continues in the field of education and public understanding of science. In recent years, public engagement has become a key agenda of research institutes, research councils, government departments and universities [17]. In the medical field, many universities made an explicit commitment to public engagement in order to raise awareness of medical issues. The versatile nature of DS allows medical professions to 'communicate' with the public in a very effective and attractive manner through simulation activities. By providing highly realistic, immersive portrayals of clinical situations, lay people are able to observe and participate in a world which would otherwise be inaccessible.

For a number of years we have been taking part in immersive public engagement events. At a major London science festival (Royal Society Summer Science Exhibition 2007) our event entitled 'How Good a Surgeon Are You?' made use of the pop-up banners described in the section The distributed simulation environment (Figures 11.4 and 11.5) to recreate an operating theatre (where a laparoscopic cholecystectomy took place using a virtual reality simulator) and a consultation room (used as a lipoma removal station). The event generated widespread interest and a few years later led to participation at the Cheltenham Science Festival's Wellcome

Trust Operation! Live [18]. Here, a simulated laparotomy for a stab wound was presented, giving members of the public opportunities to participate as surgical assistant, helping the primary surgeon to find an internal bleeding point. A range of related activities established DS as a powerful means of introducing non-clinicians to the closed world of the operating theatre. More recently, a series of high profile events in major museums and galleries in London, national science and engineering fairs, and coverage on television and radio has highlighted the potential of DS as a powerful tool for public education.

Based on the experiences mentioned earlier of public engagement, the potential for DS as a gateway into the world of healthcare for the general public seems highly significant. Applying the DS concept outside the core medical field further demonstrates its flexibility, portability and cost-effective nature, providing a platform for the public and medical research teams to appreciate different perspectives through simulation.

Future work on distributed simulation

Following these empirical research projects, the DS team has further explored DS in other domains of medicine, such as emergency medicine and interventional cardiology.

Trauma team training

The versatile nature of the DS platform offers much potential. In Emergency Medicine, there is a global need for simulation-based training in trauma assessment and team management. The most well-established trauma support training is the Advanced Trauma Life Support (ATLS®), but the concept of ATLS® assumes a lone provider or minimal support team; however, the range of specialties responsible for clinical care is diverse, and team work is essential. Our group has developed a multi-specialty trauma team training scenario, based upon observational work in our Emergency Department. This hybrid simulation involves a human simulated patient, highly realistic silicone wounds, a full trauma team played by real clinicians and adjustable physical parameter monitoring inside the

DS system. The resuscitation bay was simulated by adapting the DS environment using pull-up banners with graphics of a standard resuscitation bay. The SAM was employed to represent and manipulate the physical parameters of the simulated patient. This approach illustrates the versatility conferred by a modular simulation approach, allowing components of a clinical environment to be selected and combined as required.

Care pathway modelling

An emerging concept in simulation is the ability to simulate key elements in a patient's care pathway rather than focusing on a single element of care (such as a consultation or operation) [19]. By selecting representative components of a clinical trajectory and linking them together, this *sequential simulation* (SqS) can sample across different sectors of a healthcare system (e.g. community, hospital and paramedic services) and different time frames (condensing an extended pathway into a few minutes).

This has a number of potential applications. First, from the perspective of assessment, it is recognized that an effective clinician must be competent across a range of different domains. For example, the CanMEDS framework dictates that a competent clinician must be an expert scholar, communicator, collaborator, health advocate, professional and manager, on top of being a medical expert [20]. Current immersive simulations have a tendency to focus on limited clinical encounters, e.g. clinic consultation or performing procedural skills, which may not be able to provide the necessary information about a clinician's other abilities. By simulating the different components of a patient's care pathway, a clinician's skill set across different domains can be assessed. Using the assessment and training of competencies related to performing a clinical procedure as an example, care pathway simulation can allow for sampling skills such as decision-making prior to performing the procedure, communication skills during consent taking, technical and other non-technical skills when performing the procedure, and after care.

This sort of care pathway modelling can be challenging, particularly in creating multiple environments to simulate different components of the

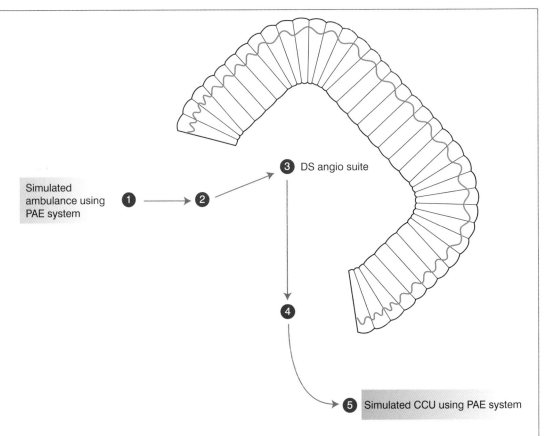

Figure 11.14 Overview of simulation. DS, distributed simulation; PAE, portable assessment environments; CCU, cardiac care unit.

pathway simultaneously. The DS concept, by means of its flexible, modular nature, can allow simulation of multiple clinical environments in a suitable sized space. Currently, the DS team is investigating the use of such a simulated care pathway. An initial pilot care pathway simulation has been developed based on the context of acute coronary care, simulating the care pathway of a patient who had sustained a myocardial infarction and requires primary percutaneous coronary intervention.

In our experience, it is not practicable to simulate every component of a patient's journey. However, by drawing on the principles of selective abstraction outlined earlier (Figure 11.2), key components of the pathway to be simulated can be determined though a series of observations of real clinical practice. Such selectivity has allowed us to simulate only key components of the pathways for purposes of assessment and training while maintaining authenticity. Figure 11.14 shows an overview of the different environments developed for this pathway, and how they are used sequentially to recreate the scenario of a patient requiring primary percutaneous coronary intervention for acute myocardial infarction.

In summary, DS provides a promising means for simulating entire care pathways. Future work will investigate the validity and utility of this form of simulation for research and education.

Conclusion

Simulation is playing an increasingly central role in contemporary clinical training and education but there is a tension between widely available but decontextualized bench-top simulators, and the immersive but relatively scarce and costly facilities of static centres. The concept of DS offers an innovative alternative to existing approaches which overcomes many of these limitations. The flexibility of DS provides high levels of individual control over how simulation facilities are used, while the portability and relatively low cost of the concept brings immersive simulation within reach of a wide constituency. This offers the possibility of sophisticated simulation becoming an everyday resource in all clinical settings rather than remaining the province of specialized centres alone.

In this chapter we have drawn upon our own experience in developing an innovative approach, which uncouples the educational benefits of simulation from the need for elaborate and costly inbuilt facilities. We have shown that a selective approach can create high levels of immersion using minimal cues at relatively low cost. For the purposes of illustration, we have drawn upon our recent experience with inflatable environments and photographic backdrops. However, we describe these in order to illustrate a principle. A key characteristic of DS as a concept is its flexibility and the opportunity it affords to align simulation activity with the educational aims that underpin it.

Under the constraints of a resource limited healthcare system, clinicians should be flexible and creative in designing authentic simulation which matches all the designated outcomes. Simulation should not be an end in it itself, but rather should allow clinicians to function authentically and to develop their skills and insight so as to improve patient care delivery.

We believe that DS offers a valuable additional perspective in the simulation debate, providing further opportunities to augment and support the clinical experience, which must always lie at the heart of healthcare education.

This chapter presents a philosophical overview of the concept of DS with its underlying design and development principles, describing in detail the key components of DS and how the concept has been explored and validated in the context of surgery. Potential applications of DS are explored in relation to ongoing and future projects in medicine, such as trauma team training and care pathway modelling. The chapter concludes by discussing how DS might contribute to achieving best practice in medical education.

SUMMARY

✓ Key points

- The need for simulation is widely accepted across all disciplines in medical training, but there remain issues of cost and effective utilization – DS offers a novel alternative.
- DS is a concept of simulation that can provide a cost-effective, accessible and versatile approach to teaching and learning tailored to the needs of individual groups at the right level of fidelity.
- The key components of the DS platform are DS environment, DS audiovisual technology and DS simulators. Their development involves an iterative process of active design that draws on expertise from a multidisciplinary group of professionals.
- The preliminary exploration and validation work of the DS was conducted in a surgical setting with clinicians at different levels of experience and different surgical procedures.
- Future work on DS includes investigation of relevant concepts, such as sequential simulation and care pathway modelling in different domains of medicine and in different hospital settings.

REFERENCES

1. CMO (2009) *150 Years of the Annual Report of the Chief Medical Officer (CMO): On the State of Public Health.* London: DH.

2. McGaghie WC, Issenberg SB, Petrusa ER, Scalese RJ (2010) A critical review of simulation-based medical education research: 2003–2009. *Medical Education* **44:** 50–63.

3. Grote G, Zala-Mezo E, Grommes P (2004) The effects of different forms of coordination in coping with workload. In: *Group Interaction in High Risk Environments* (R Dietrich, and TM Childress, eds. Aldershot: Ashgate, 39–55.

4. LaBerge D (1983) Spatial extent of attention to letters and words. *Journal of Experimental Psychology: Human Perception and Performance* **9:** 371–379.

5. Eriksen C, St James, J (1986) Visual attention within and around the field of focal attention: a zoom lens model. *Perception & Psychophysics* **40:** 225–240.

6. Cowan N (1998) *Attention and Memory: an Integrated Framework.* Oxford: Oxford University Press.

7. Kneebone R (2010) Simulation, safety and surgery. *Quality Safety Health Care* **19**(Suppl)**:** 47–52.

8. LeBlanc D (2008) Situated simulation: taking simulation to the clinicians. In: *Clinical Simulation: Operations, Engineering and Management* (R Kyle and W Murray, eds). Burlington: Elsevier, 553–557.

9. Kneebone RL, Kidd J, Nestel D, *et al.* (2005) Blurring the boundaries: scenario based simulation in a clinical setting. *Medical Education* **39**: 580–587.

10. Kneebone R (2009) Simulation and transformational change: the paradox of expertise. *Academic Medicine* **84:** 954–957.

11. Pawson R, Greenhalgh T, Harvey G, Walshe K (2005) Realist review – a new method of systematic review designed for complex policy interventions. *Journal of Health Services Research & Policy* **10**(Suppl)**:** 21–34.

12. Pawson R (2006) *Evidence-based Policy: a Realist Perspective.* Thousand Oaks, CA: Sage Publications.

13. Kassab E, Kyaw Tun J, Arora S, *et al.* (2011) 'Blowing up the barriers': exploring and validating a new approach to simulation. *Annals of Surgery* **254:** 1059–1065.

14. Martin JA, Regehr G, Reznick R, *et al.* (1997) Objective structured assessment of technical skill (OSATS) for surgical residents. *British Journal of Surgery* **84:** 273–278.

15. Kneebone R, Nestel D, Vincent C, Darzi A (2007) Complexity, risk and simulation in learning procedural skills. *Medical Education* **41:** 808–814.

16. Johnson S, Healey A, Evans J, *et al.* (2006) Physical and cognitive task analysis in interventional radiology. *Clinical Radiology* **61:** 97–103.

17. Ward V, Howdle P, Hamer S (2008) You & Your body: a case study of bioscience communication at the University of Leeds. *Science Communication* **30:** 177–208.

18. ISSUU (2010) The Times Cheltenham Science Festival 2010 brochure. Available from http://issuu.com/cheltenhamfestivals/docs/the-times-cheltenham-science-festival-2010 (accessed 6 March 2013).

19. Kneebone R (2010) Simulation, safety and surgery. *Quality Safety Health Care* **19**(Suppl)**:** 47–52.

20. Frank JR, Danoff D (2007) The CanMEDS initiative: implementing an outcomes-based framework of physician competencies. *Medical Teacher* **29:** 642–647.

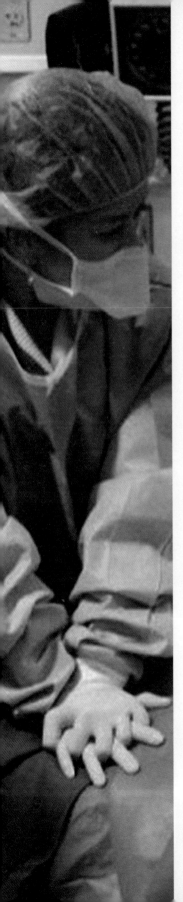

CHAPTER 12
Providing effective simulation activities

Walter J. Eppich[1], Lanty O'Connor[2] and Mark Adler[1]
[1]Ann & Robert H. Lurie Children's Hospital of Chicago, Chicago, USA; [1,2]Northwestern University Feinberg School of Medicine, Chicago, USA

Overview

A host of interdependent factors play an essential role in the effective design and delivery of simulation-based learning activities. Robust curriculum development processes, including needs assessment, selection of relevant educational targets, use of various modes of simulation and development of assessment methods, are addressed elsewhere in this book. Our emphasis here is the practical implementation of simulation-based training with a primary focus on those aspects of the learners' course experience that promote learning.

The purpose of this chapter is to provide practical guidance for the implementation of simulation-based training in healthcare. We endeavour to translate the theoretical frameworks presented in other chapters into pragmatic strategies for implementing simulation as an educational strategy. We use the simulation setting model outlined by Dieckmann [1] as a framework to address (a) setting the stage for high-impact educational sessions, (b) establishing rapport with learners and creating a safe learning environment, (c) orienting participants to the simulated learning environment, (d) implementing simulation scenarios, (e) facilitating debriefings that stimulate reflection and performance improvement, (f) promoting engagement and meaningful learning and (g) leveraging technology to augment educational outcomes. Throughout, we emphasize the inherent learner-centeredness of simulation as an educational strategy.

Essential Simulation in Clinical Education, First Edition. Edited by Kirsty Forrest, Judy McKimm, and Simon Edgar.
© 2013 John Wiley & Sons, Ltd. Published 2013 by John Wiley & Sons, Ltd.

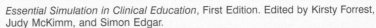

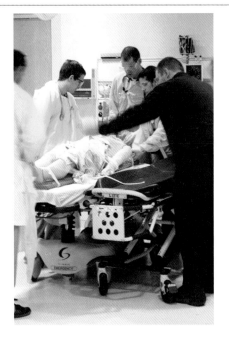

Figure 12.1 Trauma team simulation. Photo by Laura Seul, copyright Northwestern Simulation.

Case background

You are preparing to serve as faculty on a 2-day trauma team-training course for a multiprofessional and interdisciplinary group of healthcare providers (Figure 12.1). In scanning the participant roster, you note that the 14 participants have different clinical and educational backgrounds and variable years in practice. Several of the nurses signed up for the course have less than 1 year of clinical experience. Eight participants are from a variety of different institutions while six are from your own hospital. Participants comprise both emergency medicine and surgical staff. Key attendees include the emergency department (ED) medical director who is coming to the course 'to see what simulation is all about' and the ED nurse educator who wants to learn more about how simulation can help her meet the educational needs of her nurses.

Several thoughts go through your mind:
• How am I going to deal with such a mixed group of learners?

• How will I help less experienced providers feel comfortable performing in front of their clinical supervisors?
• How are experienced clinicians going to engage in simulation scenarios that are not real?
• How will I give them feedback when they make mistakes? I don't want to step on anyone's toes or make anyone look bad in front of the group, especially the more experienced clinicians.
• How am I going debrief clinicians with more experience than myself? How will I promote their learning?
• Not everyone can participate in every simulation scenario. How can I keep the observers engaged so that they don't get bored?

Introduction

In order to implement a successful simulation session or course, simulation instructors have to accomplish several specific goal-oriented tasks in addition to the simulation scenario and debriefing. Dieckmann [1] describes the 'simulation setting' as the interrelated elements of a simulation-based course. This useful model deconstructs a simulation course or session into its component parts, each of which plays a specific role in concert with other course elements (Table 12.1). For example, familiarizing trainees to the simulated learning environment promotes their later engagement during the simulation scenario and may help avoid defensive reactions about realism during the debriefing.

Each element of the simulation setting requires specific attention and skills; collectively they contribute to the success of the educational session. Not all courses include all these elements while some elements may occur multiple times in a given course or session. For example, if learners are familiar with the simulated learning environment from participation in many prior sessions, this step may be abbreviated or even skipped, and the focus might be on participation in multiple scenarios and debriefings.

Simulation-based educators assume many roles during an educational session [2], including that of instructor and facilitator [3,4]. In a purist sense, instruction denotes the imparting of knowledge and

Specific elements	Purpose
Pre-briefing before the course	Prepare learners for the session, clarify expectations in advance, provides logistical information
Setting/course introduction	Develop rapport between course faculty and participants Clarify course/session goals and objectives Establish ground rules Promote psychological safety
Theory inputs	Didactic instruction to promote learner success in the simulation, e.g. theory about crisis resource management May be formal theoretical input or brief 'just-in-time' teaching to close knowledge gaps that have been identified during the debriefing
Simulator briefing/ orientation	Orient participants to the simulation environment and the simulator
Case briefing	Provide participants with the information they need to successfully engage with the simulation (Who they are, where they are, who else is in the simulation is, what is going on)
Scenario	Provides an experience that serves as the basis for the subsequent debriefing
Debriefing	Express feelings, clarify key events and actions during the scenario Analyse the performance and especially the participant's rationale for their actions/inactions Discuss strategies to close performance gaps; provide feedback Begin integrating and applying lessons learned from the case for the future
Course end	Generalize, apply and integrate lessons learned from the course for the future

Table 12.1 Interrelated elements of the simulation setting (modified after Dieckmann [1])

facilitation the making of learning easier through promotion of self-discovery. Here, we refer to the simulation instructor/educator as one who moves easily between these various roles. In each role, the instructor's function is to identify gaps in learner performance, knowledge, and skills and help them to improve future performance through targeted instruction, facilitated reflection, and deliberate practice of essential skills.

As an educator, accompanying a group of undergraduate students or practising healthcare professionals through a simulation-based course has many similarities with other types of small group teaching and many recommendations from that literature base apply here [5,6]. Some course participants may be anxious, unsure of what to expect; others may ask themselves how their knowledge and skills compare to their peers. They may also have

preconceived notions about simulation: 'They will point out all of your mistakes!' or 'They make you take care of a fake dummy!' It may be the first time they have engaged in a simulated learning environment and it may feel potentially threatening. However, several deliberate strategies implemented before the course, during the course introduction and as the course proceeds can help set the tone for collaborative work, especially for those sessions in which most participants do not know each other at the outset.

Pre-briefing

The *pre-briefing* occurs in the days or weeks preceding the course (Table 12.1), at which time the instructor and or instructor team communicate with participants (e.g. email, mailed documents) to

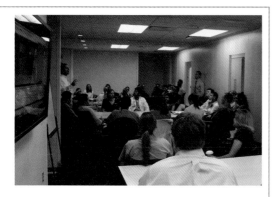

Figure 12.2 Setting ground rules and fostering a supportive yet challenging learning environment is a key success factor. Photo by Laura Seul, copyright Northwestern Simulation.

provide a course description. This helps generate initial expectations and outline essential participation information, including when to arrive, how long the course will run, where to park as well as initial preparatory reading. These initial interactions – and how participants' questions and concerns are addressed – set the tone for each individual participant.

Course/setting introduction

During the *course/setting introduction* (Figure 12.2), educators seek to develop rapport with participants and establish a safe learning environment [1,5,7,8,9,10,11,12]. Some methods to achieve this goal:

• **Begin by fostering informal discussion** – Provide an opportunity for informal conversations between faculty and course participants before the official course starts as participants arrive and settle in.

• **Start with introductions** – Once the course officially begins, both faculty and participants should have an opportunity to introduce themselves to the group and share and clarify hopes and expectations for the course.

• **Consider an *icebreaker activity*** – Investing the time in an icebreaker activity may be especially helpful in settings in which participants may be

uncomfortable talking about themselves in front of the group or when the group composition is very heterogeneous. As an example, instead of having participants introduce themselves, ask the group members to pair off with a course participant they do not know well and spend three to five minutes getting to know them. *State up front that after the introductions are finished, each course participant will have an opportunity to comment for themselves on their hopes and expectations for the course.* Request that participants present to the group from memory – this prevents reading from extensive notes when brevity is the goal. Typically, the participants are asked to introduce their partner's name, background and simulation experiences, and perhaps some personal interest, hobby or aspiration [7]. Course instructors may also participate in order to promote a flat hierarchy between faculty and participants. Inevitably this approach allows one or several participants and faculty to interject some humour; judicious, savvy, and well-timed use of humour goes a long way in helping the participants feel comfortable.

• **Encourage a level playing field among instructors and within the group** – Consider asking for agreement from participants to address faculty, and each other, on a first name basis, even if only for the duration of the course. This informality should be balanced with cultural and language norms.

• **Learn and use participant's names** – Nametags can most helpful in this regard. Referring to participants by name and linking their comments and expectations to active discussions later in the course shows you were listening and demonstrates your authentic interest in their learning.

• **Provide a well-organized session overview** – Include goals and learning objectives, the course schedule, as well as ground rules for working together during the course. Instructors should clearly address several key issues, including (a) confidentiality of the participants' performance during the scenario and comments during the debriefings, (b) the importance of mutual respect in interactions with other participants and faculty, (c) the significance of specific, honest feedback in helping everyone improve, (d) the importance of the debriefing to reflect on and explore one's own rationale for action during the simulation and (e) the role of error in learning, and that learning – not the performance – is the focus of the sessions when assessment is *not* the explicit emphasis.

• **Providing clear ground rules** about acceptable ways in which participants and facilitator(s) should interact are an important component of the social practice in simulation [1,2]. Instructors can solicit active agreement from the participants such as a head nod or a statement of 'yes' to convey understanding and acceptance of these conditions as a learning contract. Contributing to the development of safety is the articulation of a basic assumption [8] or essential premise that underlies the faculty – participant and participant – participant interactions during the course and forms the basis for honest and critical conversations: participants in the course are 'intelligent, capable, care about doing their best and want to improve' [8]. This basic assumption was introduced to the simulation community by the faculty of the Center for Medical Simulation, Cambridge, MA, and it is posted on the walls of many simulation centres worldwide. All participants should be asked to actively agree to this basic premise as part of course introduction. Achieving this explicit agreement a priori can be helpful later in the course if a participant acts out or becomes highly critical of his/her peers. A reminder about the basic assumption to which everyone had agreed may aid redirection in these difficult situations.

• **Foster psychological safety** – Creating a challenging yet supportive learning environment is essential especially in simulation-based contexts since participants put their knowledge and skills on display for all to see and critique [8,9,13,14]. Edmondson [15] discusses psychological safety within teams; the participants of a simulation-based course can also be viewed as a team working together to promote individual and group learning. Edmondson characterizes team psychological safety as 'shared belief that the team is safe for interpersonal risk taking' that arises from a 'sense of confidence that the team will not reject, embarrass, or punish someone for speaking up' [15, p. 354]. Mutual respect and trust among team members both play an essential role. In a practical sense, this sense of safety helps support honest self-appraisal during the debriefing since it 'alleviates excessive concern about others' reactions to actions that have the potential

for embarrassment or threat' [15, p. 355]. In addition, a psychologically safe learning environment creates an atmosphere in which genuinely difficult conversations about important issues are possible, such as when participants make seemingly critical errors during the scenario. The simulation instructor, functioning as a group facilitator, has the important role to develop and maintain this supportive yet challenging learning environment on an individual and group level. This important factor in particularly important for multi-day courses. Participant-participant interactions usually promote learning, but at times they can be a threat to the safety we are striving to achieve. Effective simulation instructors monitor and foster beneficial group processes; the explicit discussion of ground rules as discussed earlier contribute greatly to psychological safety.

Time and energy invested in the course/session introduction coupled with close attention to group dynamics lays the foundation for a supportive yet challenging learning environment in which participants feel psychologically safe for interpersonal risk taking [15].

Orientation to the simulated learning environment

Given the tangible differences between the simulated and actual clinical environments, as well as the substantial differences between some modes of simulation (partial task trainer, full-scale simulation manikin) and a human patient, simulation educators should properly orient learners to the simulated environment, thus providing them with the tools they need to engage more fully. The purpose of the simulator briefing is to orient the learner clearly to the environment in which they will be working, what types of resources and equipment are available to them, and if manikin-based simulation, how the simulator functions and its simulator's limitations.

Several components of the simulation environment contribute to learning: the physical space and equipment, the simulated patient itself and the personnel in the room who are not participants. Each aspect of the environment has an impact on the participants' experience and should be

---

Box 12.1   Key elements of the orientation to the simulated environment

Features of the simulation room
- Location and operation of essential equipment, including crash cart, airway equipment, etc.
- Issues related to participant safety (e.g. use of real electricity with defibrillator, disposal of sharps)

Manikin
- When discussing the simulator, it can be helpful to talk about a patient needing care and how the patient responds in various clinical states, etc., rather than talking about the simulator as mechanical device
  Explain which physical signs can be elicited on the simulated patient
  - Explain the features and physical examination findings of the simulator and then offer participants an opportunity to examine the patient, listen to the breath sounds, palpate pulses, determine blood pressure, assess pupils, etc.
  - Explain how to access information about the patient that is not evident on physical examination (e.g. abdominal findings such

as tenderness or organomegaly, temperature of the skin, capillary refill)
- Explain how to get information from the monitor, how the display is set-up, including colour of the tracings and values
  - Heart rhythm
  - Vital signs

Role of simulated or standardized patients, role of confederates
- How to interact with these individuals during the scenarios and what role they play, such as providing information
- How to interpret these individuals' responses – they will strive to stay 'in character' when offering responses

Rules of engagement during the simulation
- How to call for help during the scenario (calling a code, calling for a consult)
- How to perform interventions on the simulator
- How to give treatment to the simulator (e.g. will participants actually infuse intravenous fluids? Will they administer nebulizer treatment, etc.?)

---

considered thoughtfully in the planning process. Box 12.1 provides an outline of key topics to include in an orientation to the simulated learning environment.

The *physical space* is generally non-clinical (e.g. simulation laboratory, conference room or other space temporarily transformed into a self-contained simulation environment [16,17]) or clinical (patient room on a ward, emergency department, intensive care unit or operating theatre). In non-clinical space, we can manipulate the environment as needed and avoid the pressures of competing with clinical needs. This space can be altered to represent a broad variety of clinical settings. Patient monitors, crash carts/trolleys and resuscitation equipment can be placed in the space as needed to meet scenario objectives. Having a dedicated space offers certain

conveniences: the simulator equipment can be set up and ready to go, audiovisual recording equipment can be permanently installed, conference room space for debriefing or didactic sessions is often nearby and the clinical equipment used is dedicated for simulation training. However, a dedicated physical space can be costly and all of the medical equipment that would be needed for a given scenario must be purchased or borrowed. While it is tempting and sometimes necessary to use outdated equipment to fulfil a need, the potential for negative learning (unintentional learning with potentially negative implications) on such non-standard equipment exists, especially if this equipment differs in its functionality from that used in the clinical space. In particular, it can most helpful – especially for *in situ* simulations – to coordinate monitor set-up and colour of the tracings (e.g. oxygen saturation) to match the monitors in clinical use. Recent work in the area of distributed simulation has explored the use of temporary self-contained simulation environments that can be set up on demand for the duration of the educational event [16,17] (see Chapter 11).

The *simulated patient* itself (either standardized patient or manikin based) provides the participants of a simulation with a host of cues and triggers for action. In certain instances, such as events that focus on interpersonal communication or on physical examination, the use of a trained individual as the simulator may be preferred over a manikin. These *standardized or simulated patients (SPs)* can be helpful toward creating realism [18,19] (see Chapter 6). For manikin-based simulation, running the simulator itself is a unique skill. It requires sufficient clinical knowledge to react to participants' actions, especially if they deviate from an expected path, and to manipulate the vital signs and other key features of the simulator in a physiologically realistic way. If instructors are not running the simulator themselves, they must provide simulation technicians with sufficient information about the case. This step allows the technicians to manipulate the simulator in order to generate the critical scenario events that trigger the targeted behavioural responses. The technician benefits from reviewing the learning objectives and having a flow sheet of the critical events, anticipated learner actions, appropriate simulator responses to those actions and any anticipated alternate pathways that trainees might take.

Given that it can be difficult to predict how learners will react to a scenario or what steps they might take once immersed in the simulation, it is important to provide them with a sufficiently generalized orientation that would include equipment or resources (consultants, information such as labs or images) that they might request [20]. For simulations done in an actual clinical environment (*in situ*), an orientation to the simulator is equally essential and should emphasize any aspects of the simulation that deviate from actual clinical practice. For example, rules for accessing the code cart or crash trolley for resuscitation drugs may be different during simulations that take place in actual clinical settings. In many institutions, the 'real' code cart/crash trolley may not be used for *in situ* simulations to avoid using costly medications or equipment needed for patient care; a specially designated 'training' crash trolley may be used instead. Trainees need to be oriented to these alterations in the clinical environment that impact their participation in the simulation scenario.

The facilitator should also establish the 'fiction contract' with the participants [21,22]. The fiction contract captures the interdependent relationship that both the instructor and the trainee have to contribute equally to the success of the simulation. The trainees agree to engage in the simulation to the best of their ability; the instructors/facilitators do their best to construct an appropriate environment to promote that engagement. It is also most helpful to let participants know up front that despite their best efforts to act in the simulation scenario as if they would in real life, they may act differently. This single statement often leads to visible relief especially from those trainees anxious about participating in their first scenario.

Perceived realism plays a central role in simulation-based training. As simulation-based educators, our goal is to facilitate participants' getting into and out of the reality of the simulated experience; our hope is that they will sufficiently engage in the scenario. Several authors have written in great detail regarding the issue of realism in simulation [1,21,22,23,24]. Realism and reality and not the same; realism is the degree to which something (in the simulation) is a similar to the original (actual clinical practice); 'reality' is related to whether something exists [1]. Realism has three components [21,22]:

1. the realistic physical properties of the simulator and/or simulated equipment (e.g. plastic, cold)
2. the elements of the actual simulation environment including simulator and medical equipment respond as they should (e.g. oxygen saturation improves when adequate oxygen therapy is administered)
3. Those emotional or psychological components of realism that lead participants to engage in scenario enough to say, 'that *felt* so real!' (e.g. stress reaction to a deteriorating patient, sadness when delivering bad news).

All three modes of thinking about realism during simulation are critical to success of the endeavour [1,21].

The terms 'fidelity' and 'realism', while subtly different, are often used interchangeably. We explore these terms further here since they directly impact scenario execution. Fidelity refers to the 'accuracy of the details' [25] represented. It is common to hear the terms 'high fidelity' and 'low fidelity' in the context of discussions surrounding realism during simulations, which leaves the impression that fidelity is unidimensional: the more fidelity the better. Interestingly, perfectly realistic scenarios are not necessarily the gold standard [21,23,26]. A scenario may have low fidelity in a physical sense but may be highly realistic for participants at an emotional or psychological level. Realism is important to the extent that *enhancing realism is relevant for the particular learning objectives of the case*. Well-titrated degrees of realism help learners better engage in the simulated environment in a meaningful way. It is important to consider the learning goals of each scenario in order to help guide the degree to which relevant enhancements in simulated realism will promote engagement and learning [1,22,24,26]. For example, physical aspects of the simulation may need to be more highly realistic for certain types of procedural skills training or for certain audiences, whereas emotional or psychological components of realism are more critical for team training [22,26].

It can be an advantage to use the simulation to augment learning experiences since it allows instructors to include aspects or features that would not be possible in real life, such as contracting or expanding time [1]. Indeed, a distortion of reality can be helpful toward meeting training objectives; from a cognitive perspective, a higher degree of realism is not always necessary [27]. A distortion of reality in the simulated experience can reduce a trainee's cognitive load and promote their information processing. For example, critical components for disease recognition can be amplified, such as a low oxygen saturation or blood pressure. As a trainee progresses and becomes more accustomed to recognizing critical diagnostic features, the degree of distortion can be lessened in an effort to promote detection of more subtle but critical cues. **Selective abstraction**

is another key concept described by Kneebone [16] that highlights the notion that elements of a given scenario need to be recreated with greater or lesser degrees of authenticity to heighten perceived realism depending on how central a certain element is to the case. For example, the beeping sounds of a monitor in the operating theatre that change as oxygen saturation falls requires higher authenticity; the appearance of the suture cart may even be represented by a poster since this element does not fall within an operating team's circle of focus [16].

Scenario briefing

The scenario or case briefing occurs immediately before the simulated scenario begins. The goal is to provide the participants with enough information to understand the situation they are about to encounter so that they may respond to the best of their ability; it 'establishes the here and now of the scenario' [1, p. 107]. Although the amount of information provided will depend on the learning objectives of the case, the person performing the scenario briefing should offer the scenario participants at minimum the following facts:

• The participants' roles: '*You are the members of a rapid response team*'.
• The situation: '*You are called to assess a patient because he is having trouble breathing*'.
• If there are to be other people besides the participants in the simulation, what these roles these people will be filling, such as simulated parents or nurse: '*The patient's wife and daughter are in the room with him*'.
• Where the simulation takes place and what resources are available: '*You are responding to an inpatient ward in a district hospital with a full complement of subspecialty services*'.
• When the simulation takes place, if relevant: '*It is 3 o'clock in the morning*'.

When providing information during the scenario briefing, one should keep in mind that participants are often anxious about the upcoming scenario. They can easily be overwhelmed with too much information, which can lead to difficulties during the scenario. This problem is most clearly seen when participants make comments such as 'Who am I?' or 'Where are we?' during the scenario. Providing participants with written information, a paper chart or an electronic health record can be helpful; another strategy would be to check understanding at the end of the scenario briefing by asking participants to summarize the key elements of the case they are about to encounter.

Simulation scenario

The simulation scenario provides learners with the experience that forms the basis for discussion in the debriefing and serves as an entry point into the experiential learning cycle [28]. Our aim here is not to consider the intricacies of scenario design, however, as it relates to bringing simulation scenarios to life, the event-based approach to training (EBAT) [29,30] informs scenario design as well as execution and may well be a useful additional resource. EBAT is a general methodology that links critical scenario events with targeted behavioural responses based on explicitly defined knowledge, skills, behaviours and attitudes necessary for performance in clinical settings. As the simulation scenario unfolds, it is critical that the simulation educator enacts predetermined triggers for specific actions at the right time. The triggers may be obvious (cyanosis and very low oxygen saturation) or subtle (slowly falling blood pressure over time) depending on the scenario objectives and participants' level of training or sophistication.

There are several approaches for planning and executing the scenario in line with the principles of EBAT. From a technical perspective, two main approaches exist: (a) educators can map out and program scenarios in great detail in the manikin's software or (b) scenarios can be run on-the-fly with little or no pre-programming (Figure 12.3).

Programming the scenario ahead of time provides a high degree of consistency across participants and instructors but less flexibility to adapt if trainees do not follow a particular treatment path. Additionally, pre-programming the scenario often prescribes transition times from one condition to another. It can be challenging to modify dynamically these pre-prescribed times to adapt to different learners' needs – there is the risk is that the key triggers for action are missed; participants may become confused because their 'patient' is not

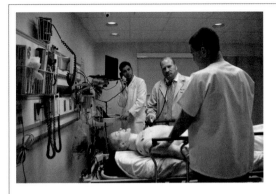

Figure 12.3 Manikin-based simulation: note the integration of telephone conversations into the scenario. Photo by Laura Seul, copyright Northwestern Simulation.

responding to their interventions in a way they expect. Participants interpret all cues as intended triggers – if oxygen is applied for low oxygen saturation, the response (or non-response) of this value to the application of oxygen will drive the group's next actions. If the response or non-response is due to operator (or simulator) error, the scenario will not proceed as intended. Therefore, it is imperative that the instructor team conducting the scenario understands the learning goals and objectives so they share a common mental model about how the scenario should proceed.

Such inconsistencies in scenario implementation threaten learner engagement and represent a disadvantage of relying on a heavily programmed scenario. One advantage, however, is that the individual running the simulator does not need significant medical expertise (Figure 12.4).

In contrast, running a scenario on-the-fly provides much more flexibility to adapt dynamically to the participants' performance and allows for better synchronization between triggers and target behaviours. Without pre-programming, greater case-to-case variability may result. This variability in how the scenario unfolds can be problematic since different groups may experience the same scenario in completely different ways. This is a particular issue in high-stakes testing environments or research settings that demand highly consistent delivery of the

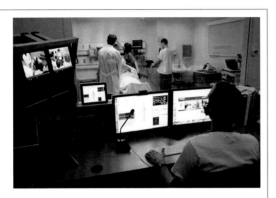

Figure 12.4 Bringing a scenario to life: the view from the control room. Photo by Laura Seul, copyright Northwestern Simulation.

simulation scenarios. In most cases, the ability to run a scenario on-the-fly requires either substantive clinical expertise or an experienced simulator technician who is well versed in the scenario flow.

In addition to the simulator or simulated patient, other strategies can both serve as triggers for action and promote realism in the scenario:

• **Vocal cues** – For manikin-based simulation, the addition of a patient's voice can be particularly helpful to help participants engage with the simulation. Learners can gather relevant information for clinical decision-making and management as well as assess the patient's mental status. It is important to have pre-planned, standardized responses to expected questions to provide consistency, especially if the voice actor of the patient is less clinically experienced. Given the impact of the patient's 'voice' on the participants' experience, it is recommend that the voice actor play to role as 'straight' as possible and avoid the temptation to employ humour or engage in informal comments that may 'break' the emotional realism of the case. In paediatric simulations, judicious use of age-appropriate vocalizations (crying, cooing) alerts participants to the infant or young child's level of responsiveness and mental status. Such cues are particularly important; in our experience, participants tend towards more aggressive interventions when their perception is that the mental status is deteriorating. Vocal cues can counteract these trends if they

are in line with the scenario design and learning objectives.

• **Moulage** – Applying make-up and other products to the simulator can augment the realism of a scenario in a relevant way by creating physical manifestations of disease (a rash) or injury (abrasions, lacerations, burns, or other trauma). The moulage only needs to be sufficiently realistic to trigger a target response. For example, a 'bruise' on the abdomen of trauma patient with low blood pressure should prompt investigation of abdominal trauma even if it does not look perfectly real. Moulage is not limited to make-up; wigs or medical supplies such as an ankle wrap or cast can help enhance the trainees' understanding of the case.

Other personnel are often used to augment a simulated scenario. These actors, or *confederates*, can promote realism as well as facilitate the evolution of the scenario [20]. Confederates, as the name implies, are team members who are 'on the inside' of the training event. They are placed in the simulation to play specific roles, usually a clinical (nurses, emergency medical technicians, or other healthcare provider) or family member role. In some instances, these actors are used to fill out a team that does not have all its members – a simulation scenario for a group of residents or junior doctors would be improved if an actor assumed the role of simulated nurse rather than one of the participants 'pretending' to be a nurse. In paediatric (or geriatric) simulations, an actor can play the parent/guardian who provides both information and cues to the patient's status. ('Why are his hands so cold?' or 'She isn't acting right – what's wrong with her?'). The confederate should be properly attired to 'look the part'. Often, the confederates will need orientation and training [19]. In particular, we have observed that inexperienced confederates tend to switch over to a participant role thereby interfering with the other participants' ability to experience the simulation as intended. Finally, the actions a confederate may or may not perform and what triggers they are permitted to give should be planned ahead by the simulation team. In more sophisticated simulation set-ups, the confederate wears an earpiece, allowing the instructor to provide real-time information and cues to facilitate the scenario dynamically as needed. For example, if a scenario starts to veer off the anticipated trajectory, a confederate nurse could be advised to provide a critical piece of information that helps get the scenario back on track [20].

Operationalizing the theoretical concepts outlined earlier requires planning and practice. Table 12.2 shows a checklist that highlights the key steps of running a course and implementing a scenario.

Engaging observers in the learning is a key consideration since on many courses, not all attendees of a session or course will be active participants in the simulation scenario. During the scenario, inactive participants may observe from different vantage points (e.g. in the room or in an adjacent room through a one-way mirror or via audiovisual equipment). They may keep track of certain elements of performance such as specific aspects of clinical management or teamwork. In the debriefing, observers can be particularly helpful in providing peer to peer feedback once active participants have had a chance to offer comments. Vicarious experiential learning [31] plays a role in most institutions since observers are typically present due to the number of learners attending simulation sessions.

Table 12.2 Simulation event checklist

	Item
Pre-event planning	Confirm space availability for both simulation and debriefing
	Confirm faculty and staff availability
	Send announcement or invitation to participants
	Meet with simulation team to review plans
	Order supplies (food, special SIM equipment, etc.)
Pre-briefing	Send readings and event details to participants and faculty
Pre-course instructor team meeting	Arrive ahead of time to setup and test all technology (simulator, audio-visual equipment)
	Prepare dry erase boards or flipcharts as needed
	Set up event welcome space (snacks, coffee)
	Prepare name tags, course manuals
	Review course flow
	Review faculty and staff responsibilities
Course setting and introduction	Mingle with course participants as they arrive
	Begin on time with group introduction
Orientation to environment	Discuss with group the space, equipment and simulators to be used
	If features of simulator are novel, allow participants to interact with simulator (e.g. listen to normal breath sounds)
	Introduce confederates and explain their roles
Simulated event	Provide scenario briefing (who they are, where they are, what they will be doing)
	Ensure that instructor team on the same page about case, learning objectives, key triggers
	Start recording (optional)
	Start simulation program
	Debriefer (ideally) is watching events without needing to fulfil another role
	End event and transition to debriefing, ideally immediately after the scenario ends
	Reset room for next event, ensure return to correct simulator and environmental states

Using audiovisual equipment

Capturing performance with video recording and playback is not absolutely necessary but in skilled hands can be useful for video-assisted debriefing [32]. When deciding on an audiovisual system several key considerations inform the complexity of the system used, including price and familiarity with the technology.

Your set-up

When considering an audiovisual capture and playback system, it is important to understand how you will use this resource in your programme and identify a budget; various considerations for this needs analysis will be discussed here. There are three levels of systems: minimalist, moderate and high end.

Option 1

A minimalist system will consist of a computer (laptop or desktop), audiovisual capture software and a camera that can send the image to the computer. A most basic design uses a laptop with a built-in video or attached USB video camera utilizing a computer's built-in software to capture video. This system can be quite flexible for smaller scale simulation and debriefing.

Option 2

A moderate system will go further and begin to incorporate multiple cameras and a higher quality microphone to enhance quality. Multiple cameras can be used to capture multiple simulations or multiple angles of a single simulation. Depending on what capture software is used, a computer for each camera may be required. Incorporating a separate camera can be an effective method of enhancing the audio that is captured. This can be as simple as purchasing an external microphone that is designed to work with the cameras that are being used.

Option 3

A high-end system will go further yet and begin to incorporate networking, audiovisual routing options

to change camera feeds on-the-fly, matrices to create picture-in-picture output, DVRs to capture audiovisual in a central location, and a mechanism to route the centralized, captured video to a playback location.

Simulation educators can adapt each of these options depending on different priorities. For example, if high-definition (HD) quality video is important, a budget-conscious HD camera can be purchased for a minimalist system and a more fully featured HD camera can be purchased for a moderate or high-end system. If clear audio is important, an external microphone system can be incorporated to each system and various price points.

Budget considerations are one important aspect, but so is the environment in which audiovisual capture will be needed. Will the audiovisual equipment be in one space permanently? Will this equipment need to be mobile? Will an audiovisual solution need to be used in an *in situ* environment? In what ways might this system need to be expanded upon in the future? The answers to these questions will guide your equipment needs.

Several manufacturers make audiovisual systems for simulation centres that have a multitude of features. These systems are flexible and expandable, and most will fall under the category of 'high-end systems.'

Further considerations

A few further items to consider when planning audiovisual capture for an upcoming simulation include: camera angles, capturing audio, capturing movement from one location to another, routing video and environmental considerations.

It is important to give some thought to camera angles before beginning the simulation. Where will the participants be standing? Is it important to capture a wide-angle? Do you need to clearly see them interacting with the equipment? Do you need to capture the vital signs of the manikin? How many camera angles will you need to meet your goals? Keep in mind that not only can the camera equipment be manipulated to give you the appropriate view, but the setup of the room itself can be manipulated to fit different pieces into the view of the camera. By setting up the room in a particular way, it will force the participants to engage with much of the equipment and the patient in a way that best allows you to capture the scenario.

Audio quality and clarity are important considerations. It's very hard to review trainee performance with muffled or unclear audio. Audio can be dramatically improved by purchasing a camera that allows for an external microphone to be connected. Often attaching a 'shotgun' microphone to a camera will allow the camera to clearly pick up a conversation among several people who are all concentrated around a central location (such as when trainees gather around a manikin). Other options include placing a wireless microphone on the manikin, a patient actor, or on the trainee who is leading a particular scenario. Another option is to suspend a microphone from the ceiling above the patient. There are a variety of options to allow for high-quality audio capture at all budget levels. The use of an external microphone will enhance both the clarity of the audio as well as the outcomes for the learner during video-assisted debriefing.

Capturing movement from one location to another, either in the simulation lab or in an *in situ* setting, can be a challenge. Most cameras are tethered to their capture system, and it can be challenging to find cables that are long enough for the job. Often, cables that are too long will degrade the quality, increase the delay of the video, or not work due to maximum length limits of different technologies. Two possible solutions to these restrictions exist. One is to purchase accessories that allow audiovisual to be transmitted wirelessly. Often these technologies will permit audiovisual to be transmitted over 30 metres. Another solution is to purchase cameras that are small enough to be mounted to an intravenous pole attached to the patient cart or can be attached to a participant or a confederate. For example, participants fitted with cameras on helmets can yield useful images. They are small, record to an SD card, allow for external microphones and have batteries that can last several hours. Other solutions include the use of the high-quality cameras that are built into many modern smartphones.

These can be creatively mounted to intravenous poles, carts and other accessories. Their main limitation will be the quality of the audio.

When working in an in-situ environment, it's helpful to have a light and adaptable audiovisual kit. Often, time is limited when working in an *in situ* environment and there is often little time to set up or take down simulation equipment. Small, wireless cameras are best in this environment. audiovisual can be stored on a memory card in the camera (as is the case in the aforementioned helmet cameras) or can be transmitted wirelessly to an audiovisual capture location in another room. The wireless solution is often the best for quick, post-scenario debriefing because transferring data from a memory card to a computer for debriefing can take some time.

Thinking through where the video will be routed and viewed from is often overlooked. Does the video feed need to be viewed from another location in real time? Is it important that more than one person have access to the audio feed as the scenario unfolds? Depending on the number of observers, there may be limited access to watch the scenario as many people crowd around one screen. One elegant solution to this problem is to simulcast the video feed online so that it can be viewed from other computer terminals. This need not be expensive: there are several free solutions for this including Skype™, UStream™, and Apple's FaceTime™. This will allow multiple people to watch the simulation from multiple locations.

If you plan to capture video in high-definition, in real time, it is recommended to purchase a computer that supports Firewire™ peripherals. Many companies make equipment that can take an HDMI signal and convert it to Firewire for real-time recording on a laptop or desktop computer. These exist in wired and wireless forms.

Debriefing

Many authors have highlighted the role of debriefing in critical incidents [33,34], in experiential learning contexts [4, 35–37] and notably in healthcare simulation [3,8,9,10,11,12,14,38,39,40,41,42,43]. At its core, debriefing promotes the transformation

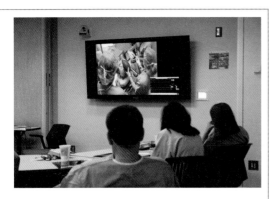

Figure 12.5 Video-assisted debriefing – while not essential, the skilled integration of video into debriefings can provide feedback and promote reflection. Photo by Laura Seul, copyright Northwestern Simulation.

of experience into learning [28] through reflective practice [22,38,44]. In this section we will use the term debriefer to refer specifically to the person leading the debriefing (Figure 12.5).

Even before the debriefing begins, multiple course or session elements lay the foundation for a supportive yet challenging learning environment that is conducive for effective debriefings [1,14,43]. These include the course or session introduction, the orientation to the simulation environment and an adequate scenario briefing. We have discussed the components of establishing rapport and creating psychological safety; these come to bear in the debriefing itself. During the actual simulation scenario, the debriefer observes the participants' performance, identifies performance gaps and begins generating debriefing points.

The terms 'feedback' and 'debriefing' are both important concepts for simulation-based educators, but they should not be used interchangeably. On the one hand, *feedback* is the specific information about the comparison between the observed performance and a standard, given with the intention of improving performance [45]. On the other hand, *debriefing* is the facilitated reflection in the experiential learning cycle [39] that is embedded in a conversation with the express purpose of helping learners identify and close performance gaps in

knowledge and skills [46]. That simulation and debriefing is a social practice [1,2] is a key consideration since some of the greatest obstacles to sharing critical performance feedback are concerns about 'stepping on someone's toes', 'hurting someone's feelings', being 'overly judgmental' or 'too harsh' [13,14].

Skilled debriefers aim to help trainees identify their own learning needs, promote reflective practice, and augment future performance on both individual and team levels. By giving feedback based observed performance gaps and then using specific facilitation strategies to uncover the participants' rationale for action, debriefers can tailor the discussion and teaching to individual and team learning needs in a variety of domains [8]. Effective debriefings maximize the reflective component of experiential learning cycles [10,39] and provide a forum for critical feedback that is essential to performance improvement [45,47,48,49]. Accurate feedback in learning is also a key feature of the deliberate practice model that links performance feedback based on standards and opportunities for repetitive practice as key drivers for the development of expertise [49,50,51,52,53,54,55].

While there is widespread acceptance about the importance of accurate performance feedback and debriefing in experiential learning contexts such as simulation, little empirical data informs the pragmatic approach simulation-based educators should take [46,56], this is changing [13,14,57]. Although further scholarly work is needed, a significant body of literature both within healthcare and from other disciplines offers guidance that informs common approaches to debriefing.

Although several debriefing frameworks exist, a widely applied model of healthcare debriefing is known as 'Debriefing with Good Judgment'. Debriefing with Good Judgment was developed and refined by simulation educators at the Center for Medical Simulation in Cambridge, MA [40,41]. Effective debriefers are able to uncover ('surface') learners' mental models or rationale for action by embodying a debriefing stance that combines both curiosity and respect for trainees with the explicit sharing of their own point of view and valuable perspectives. By sharing their own point of view, debriefers allow these perspectives to become part of the conversation. In practice, Debriefing with Good Judgement operationalizes these notions through a specific communication strategy called advocacy–inquiry [40]. By surfacing the trainees' mental models, instructors encourage self-reflection and deep learning, while helping learners identify strategies for improved future performance.

Specifically, advocacy–inquiry presents one model of conversation in which educators state an observation and share their point of view or judgement about it prior to inquiring about the trainees' perspective [40,41]. Let's take a scenario in which a team leader assists a less experienced clinician manage a patient's airway; during the intubation attempt the oxygen saturation falls to 70%. Instead of asking 'Why did you keep your back to the monitor?', the debriefer might use advocacy–inquiry to ask:

- Observation: 'During the intubation I noticed you standing with your back to the monitor'.
- Instructor's point of view: 'I was worried that you couldn't see that the oxygen saturation was falling'.
- Inquiry: 'How did you see it?'

The specific observation could also be related to something the participant said. Instead of asking the team leader, 'Do you think summarizing promotes teamwork?' using advocacy–inquiry, the debriefer might ask:

- Observation: 'After the intubation was done, I heard you say 'let's take a second to summarize what we've done so far'.
- Instructor's point of view: 'I thought that was great'.
- Inquiry: 'What were you trying to accomplish?'

The rationale for advocacy–inquiry is several fold: (a) to anchor the discussion in objective observed elements of the performance or results of the performance, (b) for the debriefer to state explicitly his/her point of view about the performance, thus allowing it to become part of the conversation and (c) for the debriefer to formulate a simple inquiry or question designed to solicit trainees' perspectives. A guiding principle here is the notion of performance gaps [8]. A performance gap is the discrepancy between desired performance and the actual observed performance. These gaps, equally representing both suboptimal and excellent performance, form the basis for individual units of

inquiry that collectively comprise the majority of the debriefing. At the heart of this model is the notion that debriefers can, in many instances, best promote learning and reflection by surfacing trainees' rationale for their actions, thus better diagnosing their learning needs and providing for more targeted educational solutions. When we keep in mind that our trainees are trying to do their best and do not intend to harm patients, we become curious to explore their motives for action or inaction. Indeed, learners value an honest yet non-threatening approach to debriefing [13].

Components of a debriefing

From a pragmatic point of view, the debriefing has several components:

Preparing the physical space

This includes modifying it as participants arrange themselves. This can be done with the participants standing around the manikin or ideally away from the simulator or in another space with participants and debriefers sitting in a circle or around a table with participants in the scenario (or 'hotseats') and the debriefer(s) within the circle. Observers who were are part of the session or course but were not active in the scenario may be sitting outside the circle. The debriefer should avoid standing over a group to promote a flatter hierarchy (Figure 12.6).

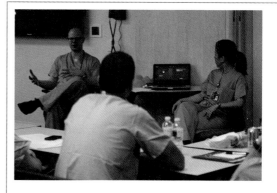

Figure 12.6 Effective debriefing is a critical component of simulation-based education. Photo by Laura Seul, copyright Northwestern Simulation.

Structuring the debriefing

The debriefing should be structured so that each component is matched with key functions:

• **Setting the stage and clarifying expectations**, especially for the first debriefing of a course, should include an clear description of the debriefing structure, timeframe, an expectation that everyone is encouraged to participate and to reflect on their actions and what was going through their minds, on what went well and what challenges they faced [3,14,43].

• Allowing for **initial reactions** [8], venting [9], emotional washout [3], defusing [10] and managing learner reactions [13] helps participants step out of ('de-role from') their part in the simulation and prepare for the learning to follow [58]. Indeed, some of these initial reactions will become evident as soon as the scenario is over. Participants often vent on the way to the debriefing room; it can be helpful for the debriefer to listen carefully to any comments that surface during this time. These potentially rich, emotionally laden comments are a primary reason to begin the debriefing as soon as possible after the scenario ends otherwise the group will begin debriefing themselves.

Once the stage for the debriefing has been set, an opening question of 'how did you feel during the scenario?' or 'first thing that comes to mind?' may also yield initial emotional reactions can help identify particular areas of interest, need or concern for learners. At times, the debriefer will need to manage learners who are confused or unhappy [13]. It may be appropriate and even advised to incorporate some topics into the later portions of the debriefing [8]. At times, an enthusiastic participant interprets the opening question as a request for a detailed cataloguing of events or actions that need to be improved. Acknowledgement of these comments and redirection can be achieved by thanking the participant for their comments, indicating that those areas will be addressed later in the debriefing, and indicating a desire to hear a response from everyone involved before discussing specific details. During the initial phase of the debriefing, it can be helpful to inquire specifically if the scenario felt real [3,9]. Participants may have varied perceptions about the realism they experienced. In dealing with realism issues, it is important to acknowledge to the participants that simulation is not real rather than entering a lengthy discussion.

• **Description of the main events** of the case and **primary issues** the participants needed to address; this reality check is important for debriefer and participants to ensure everyone is on the same page and is a non-threatening start to the debriefing. Example questions might include: 'Can someone summarize what the case was about from a medical perspective so that we are all on the same page about what happened?' or 'What were the main issues you had to deal with?' A key challenge here is to strike a balance between a description of major events and focusing on too much detail up front. Later in the debriefing, during the analysis of specific events, it might be appropriate and even essential to describe specific events more precisely.

• The majority of the debriefing will be spent analysing the aspects of participants' performance that were done well and those that need improvement (Figure 12.3). Strive for balanced discussions about positive aspects and opportunities for improvement; very rich dialogue can follow a scenario in which the team performed exceedingly well. Although most of the discussion will focus on components of the performance that relate to the pre-established learning objectives, it may serve the learners' needs to incorporate a key topic they identified during their initial reactions after the simulation scenario. In order to gauge the participants' frame of mind, it can be most helpful to solicit and explore participants' perspectives at the beginning of the analysis portion of the debriefing. Asking what they think went well and why, and then repeating the same question probing for the performance elements they believe did not go so well or what they found challenging can help promote reflection. It can be helpful for the debriefer to share their own perspective, which can encourage contributions from the participant group, e.g. 'I think there were many aspects of the case you managed well, but I am keen to hear your impressions first.' It is most valuable for debriefers to put aside their assumptions about why participants did what they did during the simulation. Indeed, inexperienced debriefers frequently assume that insufficient knowledge is the reason for what appears to be suboptimal performance; exploring participants' rationale for action reveals valuable insight into their mental models.

Another common pitfall is to leave an important mental model unexplored – digging deeper and probing beyond the surface may yield important insights that lead to the heart of the matter. If available, several brief video segments can promote recall of events and help participants assess their own performance. Before playing the video recording, it can be most helpful if the debriefer focuses participants' attention on the important elements in advance, e.g. 'I'd like you to focus on the basic life support' or 'I'd like you to pay close attention to how the team is communicating during the intubation'. Box 12.2 summarizes essential techniques and strategies to promote discussion as well as some

---

Box 12.2 Debriefing: facilitation techniques and strategies to promote discussion

(Note: All example questions relate to a simulation scenario in which a team manages the airway in a patient with traumatic brain injury)

Do's
- Help participants reflect on their experience in way that promotes meaningful learning for their own clinical practice setting
- Use open-ended questions
- Use honest yet non-threatening language (14)
- Listen carefully; allow participants to answer completely before formulating your next question; use participants' responses to help formulate your next question/comment
- Use specific facilitation techniques (4)
  - Use active listening techniques (echoing, reflecting, expanding)
  - Turn questions back to the group
  - Use silence liberally; it gives participants time to craft a response and encourages engagement
- Tell participants what you would like to talk about in order to frame the discussion
  - For example: 'I'd like spend a few minutes talking about intubation and maintaining oxygen levels during the intubation attempt'
- Pose questions for which multiple answers are possible – if one learner responds, others can still contribute in a meaningful way
  - For example: 'What is your approach to managing the airway in a patient with traumatic brain injury?'
- Use specific observations to anchor the discussion
- Use your honest point of view to your advantage; it lets participants know where you are coming from. Not infrequently, participants are eager to discuss challenging aspects of patient management; they are just waiting for the time to do so.
  - For example: 'As I was watching it seemed to me like you had a hard time with the intubation. . . .'
- Use advocacy-inquiry (32)
  - Use specific observations to anchor the discussion; then explicitly state your point of view or personal reaction about what you saw; finally invite the participants to respond. For example: 'During the intubation attempt I saw the oxygen saturations fall to 60% before you successfully intubated the patient. I felt uncomfortable that oxygen levels fell so low, especially in a patient with traumatic brain injury, since preventing hypoxia is an important part of management. How did you all experience that?'

Continued

- Use several short video segments to focus attention as well as promote discussion and self-reflection

Don'ts
- Avoid closed questions
- Avoid interrupting participants with your next question before they have had a chance to finish
- Avoid speaking more than the participants
- Avoid adhering to a rigid agenda
- Avoid questions that suggest an answer
  - For example: *'Do you think it would be important to avoid a drop in oxygen saturation during an intubation attempt, especially in a patient with traumatic brain injury?'*
- Avoid many questions with a single answer since they limit the discussion

- Avoid 'read my mind' questions; a clue that you have posed this type of question is a query from participants 'do you mean. . . . ?'
- Avoid questions that include phrases such as, 'Do you remember what you said?' or 'Do you remember what you did next?' Simply describe what you saw/heard and ask the participant(s) to comment
- Avoid questions that begin with a compliment BUT then criticize
- Avoid asking multiple questions in sequence; it can lead to confusion especially if each question has a slightly different twist
- Avoid blaming or accusing
- Avoid inappropriate humour

common traps to avoid. When important mental models and rationale for action are identified and explored, debriefers can facilitate a discussion that helps learners' close performance gaps or promote strategies to sustain excellent performance in the future. Near the end of the analysis of performance, debriefers should help learners generalize lessons learned to their own practice environment and identify strategies for overcoming potential barriers to change

- **Application and summary** – Near the end of the debriefing, the debriefer should indicate that the debriefing is moving to an end, but inquire if any burning issues remain. This question can avoid the sometimes awkward ending to a debriefing when a participant brings up a completely new issue after other participants have already stated their major take home messages. This ending phase of the debriefing is forward looking and ideally should not represent a rehashing of the simulation, but rather how participants will integrate and apply what they have learned. After the participants have had an opportunity to offer their key learning points, the debriefer may wish to provide a brief

summary to highlight a critical element of the case, although this final step may not always be necessary or desired. The debriefer may actively end the debriefing by thanking the participants for their hard work.

Course ending

Once the cycle of simulation scenarios plus debriefings or other course elements have been completed, the course approaches its end. An active ending to a course represents an opportunity to encourage participants to share big picture take home messages. Even more important is to help participants generalize lessons learned and articulate concrete next steps when they return to their clinical practice. Facilitating a discussion of barriers to implementation as well as strategies to overcome can be fruitful. Finally, in the spirit of ongoing curriculum development and revision, inquiring what participants liked about the course, what helped them, and what they would change can help guide curriculum revision.

SUMMARY

Several separate but interrelated elements comprise a simulation course or session, including course introduction, orientation to the simulation learning environment, case briefing, designing and running simulation scenarios and debriefing. The relative emphasis on each element depends on the target audience, their familiarity with instructor team and local simulation environment, and finally the course learning objectives. Close attention to factors that establish psychological safety and a clear statement of ground rules for participation, promote engagement during the simulation scenarios and honest reflection in the debriefings.

Briefing participants before a scenario with key information is essential. An event-based approach to training informs not only scenario design but execution as well. Realism for realism's sake is less important than matching degrees of fidelity to case learning objectives and using selective abstraction to promote efficient learning. Post-scenario debriefing plays a central role in simulation-based education as a forum to provide critical performance feedback, promote reflection and augment learning in a way that strives meet the needs of individuals and the team. When resources allow, video playback can support debriefing efforts.

Key points

- Healthcare educators must master several essential skills in order to implement simulation-based training effectively.
- Several interrelated elements of a simulation-based learning encounter contribute to the effectiveness of the educational experience.
- Developing rapport with participants of a simulation course begins to establish psychological safety; clear ground rules for simulation-based training promotes engagement during both simulation scenario and debriefing.
- High-quality scenario execution brings clinical cases to life in a manner relevant for the target audience and ensures that learning goals of the case are met.
- Effective debriefings are organized, create a challenging yet supportive atmosphere in which participants can reflect on their performance, and incorporate critical feedback to help learners achieve and maintain clinical knowledge and skills.

REFERENCES

1. Dieckmann P (2009) Simulation settings for learning in acute medical care. In: *Using Simulations for Education, Training, and Research* (P Dieckmann, ed.). Lengerich: Pabst.

2. Dieckmann P, Molin Friis S, Lippert A, Ostergaard D (2009) The art and science of debriefing in simulation: ideal and practice. *Medical Teacher* **31:** e287–294.

3. Dieckmann P, Reddersen S, Zieger J, Rall M (2008) Video-assisted debriefing in simulation-based training of crisis resource management. In: *Clinical Simulation: Operations, Engineering, and Management* (RR Kyle and WB Murray, eds). Burlington: Academic Press, 667–676.

4. McDonnell LK, Jobe KK, Dismukes RK (1997) *Facilitating LOS Debriefings: A Training Manual.* Washington, DC:

National Aeronautical and Space Administration.

5. Walton H (1997) Small group methods in medical teaching. *Medical Education* **31:** 459–464.

6. McCrorie P (2010) Teaching and leading small groups. In: *Understanding Medical Education: Evidence, Theory, and Practice* (T Swanwick, ed.). Chichester: Wiley-Blackwell, 124–138.

7. Buskist W, Saville BK (2001) Rapport-building: creating positive emotional contexts for enhancing learning and teaching. Association for Psychological Science. Available from: http://www.psychologicalscience.org/teaching/tips/tips_0301.cfm (accessed 6 March 2013).

8. Rudolph JW, Simon R, Raemer DB, Eppich WJ (2008) Debriefing as formative assessment: closing performance gaps in medical education. *Academic Emergency Medicine* **15:** 1010–1016.

9. Flanagan B (2008) Debriefing: theory and techniques. In: *A Manual of Simulation in Healthcare* (RH Riley, ed.) New York: Oxford University Press, 155–170.

10. Zigmont JJ, Kappus LJ, Sudikoff SN (2011) The 3D model of debriefing: defusing, discovering, and deepening. *Seminars in Perinatology* **35:** 52–58.

11. Gururaja RP, Yang T, Paige JT, Chauvin SW (2008) Examining the effectiveness of debriefing at the point of care. In: *Simulation-Based Operating Room Team Training Advances in Patient Safety: New Directions and Alternative Approaches.* Vol. 3: *Performance and Tools* (K Henriksen, JB Battles, MA Keyes, ML Grady, eds). Rockville MD: Agency for Healthcare Research and Quality.

12. Rall M, Manser T, Howard SK (2000) Key elements of debriefing for simulator training. *European Journal of Anaesthesiology* **17:** 516–517.

13. Ahmed M, Sevdalis N, Paige J, *et al.* (2012) Identifying best practice guidelines for debriefing in surgery: a tri-continental study. *American Journal of Surgery* **203:** 523–529.

14. Arora S, Ahmed M, Paige J, *et al.* (2012) Objective structured assessment of debriefing: bringing science to the art of debriefing in surgery. *Annals of Surgery* **256:** 982–988.

15. Edmondson AC (1999) Psychological safety and learning behavior in work teams. *Administrative Science Quarterly* **44:** 350–383.

16. Kneebone R, Arora S, King D, *et al.* (2010) Distributed simulation–accessible immersive training. *Medical Teacher* **32:** 65–70.

17. Kassab E, Tun JK, Arora S, *et al.* (2011) 'Blowing up the barriers' in surgical training: exploring and validating the concept of distributed simulation. *Annals of Surgery* **254:** 1059–1065.

18. Barrows HS (1993) An overview of the uses of standardized patients for teaching and evaluating clinical skills. *Academic Medicine* **68:** 443–451

19. Kassab ES, King D, Hull LM, *et al.* (2010) Actor training for surgical team simulations. *Medical Teacher* **32:** 256–258.

20. Dieckmann P, Lippert A, Glavin R, Rall M (2010) When things do not go as expected: scenario life savers. *Simulation in Healthcare* **5:** 219–225.

21. Dieckmann P, Gaba D, Rall M (2007) Deepening the theoretical foundations of patient simulation as social practice. *Simulation in Healthcare* **2:** 183–193.

22. Rudolph JW, Simon R, Raemer DB (2007) Which reality matters? Questions on the path to high engagement in healthcare simulation. *Simulation in Healthcare* **2:** 161–163.

23. Beaubien JM, Baker DP. The use of simulation for training teamwork skills in

health care: how low can you go? *Quality and Safety in Health Care* 2004;**13** (Suppl 1): i51–6.

24. Kneebone R (2010) Simulation, safety and surgery. *Quality and Safety in Health Care* **19** (Suppl 3): i47–52.

25. Merriam Webster Online Dictionary. Merriam Webster. Available from: http://www.merriam-webster.com/dictionary/fidelity (accessed 6 march 2013).

26. Scerbo MW, Dawson S (2007) High fidelity, high performance? *Simulation in Healthcare* **2**: 224–230.

27. Dror I, Schmidt P, O'Connor L (2011) A cognitive perspective on technology enhanced learning in medical training: great opportunities, pitfalls and challenges. *Medical Teacher* **33**: 291–296.

28. Kolb D (1984) *Experiential Learning: Experience as a Source of Learning and Development.* Upper Saddle River, NJ: Prentice Hall.

29. Fowlkes JE, Dwyer DJ, Oser RL, Salas E (1998) Event-based approach to training (EBAT). *International Journal of Aviation Psychology* **8**: 209–221.

30. Rosen MA, Salas E, Wu TS, *et al.* (2008) Promoting teamwork: an event-based approach to simulation-based teamwork training for emergency medicine residents. *Academic Emergency Medicine* **15**: 1190–1198.

31. Roberts D (2010) Vicarious learning: a review of the literature. *Nurse Education in Practice* **10**: 13–16.

32. Savoldelli GL, Naik VN, Park J, *et al.* (2006) Value of debriefing during simulated crisis management: oral versus video-assisted oral feedback. *Anesthesiology* **105**: 279–285.

33. Mitchell JT (1983) When disaster strikes . . . the critical incident stress debriefing process. *Journal of Emergency and Medical Services* **8**: 36–39.

34. Mitchell JT (1988) Stress. Development and functions of a critical incident stress debriefing team. *Journal of Emergency and Medical Services* **13**: 42–46.

35. Steinwachs B (1992) How to facilitate a debriefing. *Simulation Gaming* **23**: 186–195.

36. Lederman LC (1992) Debriefing: Toward a systematic assessment of theory and practice. *Simulation Gaming* **23**: 145–160.

37. Dismukes K, Smith G. *Facilitation and Debriefing in Aviation Training and Operations.* Aldershot, UK: Ashgate; 2000.

38. Dreifuerst KT (2009) The essentials of debriefing in simulation learning: a concept analysis. *Nursing Education Perspectives* **30**: 109–114.

39. Fanning RM, Gaba DM (2007) The role of debriefing in simulation-based learning. *Simulation in Healthcare* **2**: 115–125.

40. Rudolph JW, Simon R, Dufresne RL, Raemer DB (2006) There's no such thing as 'nonjudgmental' debriefing: a theory and method for debriefing with good judgment. *Simulation in Healthcare* **1**: 49–55.

41. Rudolph JW, Simon R, Rivard P, *et al.* (2007) Debriefing with good judgment: combining rigorous feedback with genuine inquiry. *Anesthesiology Clinics* **25**: 361–376.

42. Dismukes RK, Gaba DM, Howard SK (2006) So many roads: facilitated debriefing in healthcare. *Simulation in Healthcare* **1**: 23–25.

43. Simon R, Raemer DB, Rudolph JW (2009) *Debriefing Assessment for Simulation in Healthcare: Rater Version.* Cambridge, MA: Center for Medical Simulation.

44. Schön D (1987) *Educating the Reflective Practitioner: Toward a New Design for Teaching and Learning in the Professions.* San Francisco: Jossey-Bass.

45. van de Ridder JM, Stokking KM, McGaghie WC, ten Cate OT (2008) What is feedback in clinical education? *Medical Education* **42**: 189–197.

46. Raemer D, Anderson M, Cheng A, *et al.* (2011) Research regarding debriefing as part of the learning process. *Simulation in Healthcare* **6** (Suppl)**:** S52–57.

47. Issenberg SB, McGaghie WC, Petrusa ER, *et al.* (2005) Features and uses of high-fidelity medical simulations that lead to effective learning: a BEME systematic review. *Medical Teacher* **27:** 10–28.

48. McGaghie WC, Issenberg SB, Petrusa ER, Scalese RJ (2010) A critical review of simulation-based medical education research: 2003–2009. *Medical Education* **44:** 50–63.

49. Ericsson KA (2008) Deliberate practice and acquisition of expert performance: a general overview. *Academic Emergency Medicine* **15:** 988–994.

50. Ericsson KA (2004) Deliberate practice and the acquisition and maintenance of expert performance in medicine and related domains. *Academic Medicine* **79** (Suppl)**:** S70–81.

51. McGaghie WC (2008) Research opportunities in simulation-based medical education using deliberate practice. *Academic Emergency Medicine* **15:** 995–1001.

52. Siassakos D, Bristowe K, Draycott T, *et al.* (2011) Clinical efficiency in a simulated emergency and relationship to team behaviours: a multisite cross-sectional study. *British Journal of Obstetrics and Gynaecology* **118:** 596–607.

53. Hunt EA, Fiedor-Hamilton M, Eppich WJ (2008) Resuscitation education: narrowing the gap between evidence-based resuscitation guidelines and performance using best educational practices. *Pediatric Clinics of North America* **55:** 1025–1050, xii.

54. McGaghie WC, Issenberg SB, Cohen ER, *et al.* (2011) Does simulation-based medical education with deliberate practice yield better results than traditional clinical education? A meta-analytic comparative review of the evidence. *Academic Medicine* **86:** 706–711.

55. Ericsson KA, Krampe RT, Tesch-Romer C (1993) The Role of deliberate practice in the acquisition of expert performance. *Psychological Review* **100:** 363–406.

56. Eppich W, Howard V, Vozenilek J, Curran I. Simulation-based team training in healthcare. *Simulation in Healthcare* 2011;**6** (Suppl)**:** S14–9.

57. Brett-Fleegler M, Rudolph J, Eppich W, *et al.* (2012) Debriefing assessment for simulation in healthcare: development and psychometric properties. *Simulation in Healthcare* **7:** 288–294.

58. Stafford F (2005) The significance of de-roling and debriefing in training medical students using simulation to train medical students. *Medical Education* **39:** 1083–1085.

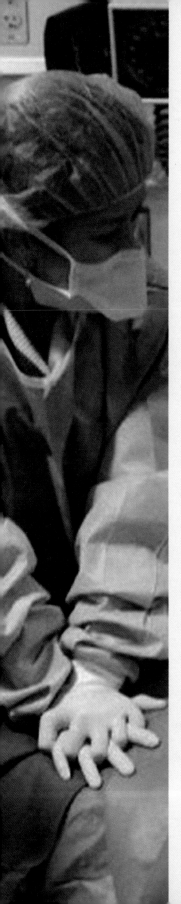

CHAPTER 13
Simulation in practice

Jean Ker   University of Dundee, Dundee, UK

Overview

Learning consistent with high standards of clinical skills is core to both the development of safe healthcare practitioners and the delivery of quality care for patients. This chapter focuses on the practical applications of simulation and brings some exciting and varied case examples from experts across the world which share the challenges and opportunities that the use of simulation in healthcare education can bring. They are excellent illustrations of how complex healthcare practice can be analysed for improvement and how simulation-based education can be effectively and efficiently used to enhance standards and standardize the practice of healthcare practitioners. The case studies cover the wide uses of simulation using different modalities of fidelity and are intended to provide triggers for considering how simulation can be used to develop cognitive, psychomotor and safe behavioural skills.

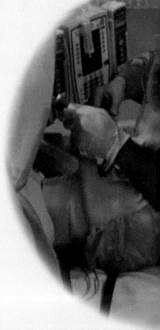

Many examples are cited of the excellent use of simulation to enhance standards of clinical practice for both novice and experienced practitioners. Simulation can be used to rehearse management of common events or those events that clinicians rarely see in their professional clinical lifetimes. Included in this chapter are reports and examples from around the world; from Australia, the Netherlands, the USA, Africa and the UK and from both primary and secondary care.

Each worked example reports their experience using the following broad structure:
- Background/Context
- What was done
- Results and outcomes
- Take-home messages
- Hints and tips

Essential Simulation in Clinical Education, First Edition. Edited by Kirsty Forrest, Judy McKimm, and Simon Edgar.
© 2013 John Wiley & Sons, Ltd. Published 2013 by John Wiley & Sons, Ltd.

Simulation for learning cardiology

Section contributor: Ross J. Scalese University of Miami, Miami, USA

Background

While there is universal agreement that physical examination and bedside diagnosis are fundamental clinical skills, research has demonstrated deficiencies in the ability of healthcare professionals – not only those in training but also those in practice – to identify important cardiac physical examination findings and to diagnose corresponding clinical conditions [1,2]. Changes in healthcare delivery (including trends in managed care towards shorter hospital stays for patients with higher acuity of illnesses), especially at academic medical centres (with trainee work hour restrictions and pressures for faculty to increase research and clinical productivity), compound the problem by limiting both the availability of real patients as educational opportunities and the time for faculty to teach essential skills at the bedside. Simulation-based training offers solutions to many of these challenges: simulators can be available at any time and reproduce a wide variety of (even rare or critical) clinical conditions on demand. Many simulators have built-in feedback functions and are well-suited for independent learning, thereby saving faculty time. Because of their programmability, simulators do not become tired or embarrassed or behave unpredictably, and thus provide a standardized educational experience for all learners.

Dr Michael Gordon at the University of Miami School of Medicine led an international consortium of clinicians, educators and engineers in developing the 'Harvey' simulator, which can reproduce with high fidelity the bedside physical examination findings of almost all cardiac conditions; these include blood pressure, venous and arterial pulses, precordial movements, and cardiac and pulmonary auscultatory findings. More than 300 institutions worldwide – comprising not only medical schools, but also postgraduate teaching hospitals, nursing schools, physician assistant training programmes, etc. – currently use this life-sized manikin for teaching and assessing fundamental cardiac clinical skills. Accompanying Harvey is a comprehensive cardiology curriculum, based on 30 clinical cases programmed into the simulator, detailing not only the salient historical and physical examination findings, but also important aspects of the diagnostic work-up and treatment for patients with these conditions.

What was done

An exemplary case illustrating simulation-based training for learning cardiology is the implementation of the Harvey system throughout the training programmes in Miami. In keeping with recent trends towards vertical integration within the curriculum, medical students train with Harvey in all 4 years of the (graduate-entry) programme: the first two 'basic sciences' years are organized around organ system modules, and during the longitudinal 'Doctoring' course when students are initially taught to perform physical examinations, they first encounter Harvey when they learn about the 'normal' cardiac examination (Figure 13.1). When they later study pathophysiology in the cardiovascular module, they examine Harvey programmed with important (left-sided) valvular lesions (aortic stenosis/regurgitation and mitral stenosis/regurgitation). During third-year clinical clerkships, students have weekly sessions during the required 2-month Internal Medicine block, again revisiting valvular abnormalities and also examining 'patients' (Harvey) with cardiomyopathy, pericarditis, myocardial infarctions and other conditions of importance in this

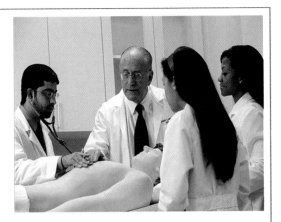

Figure 13.1 Harvey simulator in use.

specialty. In the fourth year, students may elect to take 2- or 4-week courses in cardiology that feature the entire Harvey programme. One station of the annual summative Objective Structured Clinical Examinations (OSCE) employs Harvey to assess final-year students' competence in demonstrating these cardiology clinical skills.

Results and outcomes

Harvey is perhaps one of the best studied manikin simulators, with numerous trials demonstrating significant increases in knowledge, skills and confidence related to cardiac physical examination technique, identification of findings and ability to make clinical diagnoses at the bedside. Such research (including several multicenter studies) has been conducted with medical students [3], residents in various specialties [4], pre-licensure and advanced practice nurses, and physician assistants [2], all showing similar positive results. Additionally, some of the studies with medical students demonstrated that skills learned with the simulator transferred to

clinical settings when examining real patients with cardiac conditions [5].

Take-home messages

Various interventions using Harvey share certain features that seem to have contributed to their educational effectiveness, including provision of feedback (either from instructors or accompanying e-learning modules); opportunities for deliberate practice of skills [6] (especially, in this case, hands-on examination of Harvey); integration of simulation activities as required (not optional or 'just for fun') with components of the overall curriculum; presentation of a broad range of clinical scenarios (with gradual increase in level of case difficulty according to achievement of clearly defined outcomes); active engagement in the simulation, rather than passive learning (as bystanders); and individualization of instruction (adapting various strategies for different learning styles). A Best Evidence Medical Education (BEME) Collaboration systematic review found that these features were frequently cited among educational programmes in various domains that have likewise demonstrated effectiveness of simulation-based training [7].

ⓘ Hints and tips

Simulators *per se* are just tools; they may enhance training if their use is aligned with learning objectives. Educators should pay careful attention to integration of simulation methods within the overall curriculum, provision of feedback and opportunities for deliberate practice of skills, and other evidence-based features of simulation to improve educational practice and, ultimately, patient care.

Assessing leadership skills in medical undergraduates

Section contributors: Helen O'Sullivan, Arpan Guha and Michael Moneypenny
University of Liverpool, Liverpool, UK

Background

'Our clear view is that doctors have for 25 years, perhaps longer, been failing to give the leadership of which they are eminently capable, and which society rightly expects of them' [8]

This quotation sums up the recently developed consensus that doctors need to take and develop leadership and management roles. It is becoming widely accepted that a logical consequence of this requirement is the need to make leadership and management development much more explicit in the undergraduate curriculum. This view is endorsed by the UK's General Medical Council, [9] whose outcomes and standards on undergraduate medical education states:

'Medical students are tomorrow's doctors. In accordance with Good Medical Practice, graduates will make the care of their patients their first concern, applying their knowledge and skills in a competent and ethical manner and using their ability to provide leadership and analyse complex and uncertain situations.'

In response to the need for doctors to be more actively involved in the review, planning, delivery and transformation of health services, the Academy of Medical Royal Colleges and the NHS Institute for Innovation and Improvement with a wide range of stakeholders established a UK-wide project: 'Enhancing Engagement in Medical Leadership'. One of the project outcomes was the Medical Leadership Competency Framework: the MLCF [10]. The MLCF describes the skills and competencies

that medical students and doctors need in order to contribute to running successful services. The Framework has five domains: Demonstrating Personal Qualities, Working with Others, Managing Services, Improving Services and Setting Direction (Figure 13.2).

The MLCF rightly recognizes that not all of these will be perceived as important to medical students and therefore has a separate section for undergraduate medical education. Finding opportunities to develop leadership skills in the medical undergraduate curriculum is relatively straightforward. What is much more difficult is assessing them. This case study outlines the development of an assessment tool that can be used formatively and summatively to assess these important skills.

What was done?

A series of focus groups were held with medical undergraduates to establish the key attitudes, behaviours and skills that they thought were important in leadership and team working in the medical context. These factors were supplemented by a critical evaluation of the relevant literature. A short, simulated scenario was designed at the Cheshire and Merseyside Simulation Centre (CMSC) that involved an emergency and a scripted conflict point during its management, where a senior colleague attempted to deliberately make a potentially fatal mistake. An assessment tool was designed to assess leadership and team-working skills in this scenario. The tool was piloted on a small sample of the full cohort and then validated through assessing a sample of volunteers from the MBChB final year cohort at Liverpool.

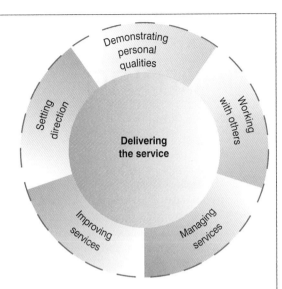

Figure 13.2 The five domains of the the Medical Leadership Competency Framework. © NHS Leadership Academy and Academy of Medical Royal Colleges, 2010. All rights reserved.

Results and outcomes

Each volunteer was briefed and then carried out a videotaped scenario. Each participant watched back the videotape immediately after the session and used a think aloud technique to explain what they had been thinking and feeling at each stage. Finally, the student received formative feedback on their leadership and teamworking skills. Intraclass correlation was used to determine inter-rater reliability and a two-way mixed model to estimate the intraclass correlation coefficient (ICC). Internal consistency of the scoring system was tested for using Cronbach's Alpha. High internal consistency suggests that the elements are measuring the same characteristic, e.g. teamwork or leadership. All tests showed that the tool was reliable, reproducible and valid. In addition, students were given a questionnaire after the experience and these results of this confirmed that the students found the assessment to be authentic.

Take-home message

Simulation provides an opportunity for students to develop leadership and teamworking skills in a safe environment while emphasizing the importance of these skills in providing good clinical care and safe patient care. This assessment tool provides a way to summatively assess these skills in a valid, reliable and authentic way.

What went well/worked well

Introducing a conflict point produced some very interesting and unexpected results. A small number of students did not challenge the potentially fatal actions of their senior colleague, even though they acknowledged in the 'think aloud' session that they knew the mistake was being made. This mirrors some widely reported real-life clinical incidents where more junior members of the team have not been able to summon up the various leadership skills needed to challenge an established clinical hierarchy, even though their actions may have led to a safer outcome. This led us to speculate on the nature of culture and hierarchy in medicine and on the potentially negative impact of these on patient safety.

The students appreciated the opportunity to get formative feedback on their leadership and team working skills. Given the validity of the tool, it could be used in both a formative and summative context.

What would you do differently?

In rolling this out to the whole cohort, we would not repeat the think aloud session with each student as this was part of the research into the validity of the tool.

> ⓘ **Hints and tips**
>
> Involving the students in the design of the assessment tool helps in establishing authenticity with the students. When you are assessing skills and behaviours that the students also believe are important, we predict that there will be less cynicism about the assessment and less strategic behaviour in preparing for the assessment.

Simulation for interprofessional learning

Section contributor: Stuart Marshall   Monash University, Melbourne, Australia

Background

Airway management is a high-risk intervention outside the operating theatre. Studies suggest the risks of death or hypoxic brain injury associated with airway management in the Emergency Department (ED) or Intensive Care Unit (ICU) are up to 70 times the incidence in the operating theatre environment. The main concerns are the required urgency of the interventions and physiological instability of the patient cohort. Although these patient factors cannot easily be controlled, some of the difficulties may be minimized. The medical staff involved in these cases are often junior, inexperienced and working with nursing staff that may be ill at ease with airway management techniques. When anaesthetic nurses and doctors are called to assist, the unfamiliar equipment and environment outside theatre can be unnerving and lead to errors and poor patient outcomes. We have developed and delivered an airway management course for ICU, ED and anaesthetic nurses and doctors to standardize education, equipment and procedures across four large metropolitan teaching hospitals: the Team Response to Airway Crises (TRAC) course.

What was done

Following a learning needs analysis, review of critical incidents and a pilot course of emergency physician trainees and nursing staff, a one-day interprofessional course was designed. The course outlined the skills of effective airway management outside the operating suite and was aimed at anaesthetic, ED and ICU nurses and trainees. Technical skills workshops on bag–valve–mask ventilation, supraglottic devices and safe endotracheal intubation were augmented by discussions about non-

technical skills such as situation awareness, triggers to change technique and assertiveness. Discussions of teamwork aspects were triggered by videos of common teamworking errors such as social rather than clinical communication and failure to adequately assign roles. Attention was also paid to standardized approaches to dealing with a difficult airway and performing emergency surgical airway techniques. Short immersive scenarios followed the skills workshops. The scenarios were designed to reinforce the material through repeated practice and feedback in a team setting. Feedback was sought at the end of the course and at 6 months following the course to determine reported transfer of the learning into clinical practice.

Results and outcomes

Fifty-seven medical (n = 21) and nursing staff (n = 36) completed the course in its first 6 months. Participants were almost evenly split from Anaesthetic (n = 20), Emergency Department (n = 21) and ICU (n = 16) backgrounds. The majority of responses (80.3%) immediately following the course listed non-technical aspects as the most important covered. The most common free text responses when asked to describe key messages from the day were methods for effective communication, planning and prevention of fixation during crises. Participants reported that many previous myths about airway management and tracheal intubation had been dispelled. One key message reported by the majority of respondents was that that oxygenation rather than intubation is the priority in all cases.

In addition to the individuals' learning outcomes, there were unexpected effects on the organization's processes. In parallel to the standardization of the education, the critical care areas of the four hospitals standardized the equipment and guidelines for emergency surgical airway management, and made plans to further align equipment and processes. In keeping with other educational interventions, changes in clinical patient outcomes can rarely be directly attributed to the training. Anecdotal evidence of improved management of airway difficulties has already been forthcoming. Even if hard data are not easily attained, the shared understanding of airway emergencies and team training has at least improved the confidence and decision-making of clinical staff in dealing with these cases in unfamiliar environments.

Take-home messages

Investigating where expertise can be shared between and across professions can ensure best practice is disseminated through an organization. Such sharing of expertise results in meaningful and productive interprofessional learning. By involving multiple departments and professional groups, we were able to demonstrate best practice to a larger audience and leverage system change and standardization. This standardization should further reinforce the learning in the clinical setting and ensure transference of practice to actual patient care.

ⓘ Hints and tips

Learner engagement with interprofessional simulation-based learning appears to be higher when simulation educators with clinical experience from those professions are represented in the teaching faculty. Providing senior clinicians as instructors from the same backgrounds as the participants allows not only role modelling on the individual instructor, but an appreciation that senior professionals can teach as well as learn together.

Use of *in situ* simulations to identify barriers to patient care for multidisciplinary teams in developing countries

Section contributor: Nicole Shilkofski John Hopkins University, Baltimore, USA

Background

Teams and individual clinicians caring for ill children in resource-poor settings often function poorly due to unfamiliarity with the environment, equipment, available resources, language and cultural barriers, and the unique needs and presentations of paediatric patients. Few educational aids or programs exist to remediate this problem and to reduce the cognitive load associated with caring for paediatric patients in resource-challenged environments. To optimize the design of educational aids for use in this context, it is important to understand from an emic (i.e. from a person living in the culture) perspective the barriers that exist to provide adequate care for children in resource-poor settings, and to understand the naturalistic decision-making processes of clinicians inherent in caring for children in these environments.

Of the nearly 10 million annual deaths occurring in children under 5 years of age in developing countries, over 80% are potentially avoidable [11]. By understanding the barriers that exist to efficient teamwork in resource-constrained settings, an educational intervention and cognitive aids can be designed that focus clinicians on those tasks or routes of decision-making that result in more favourable outcomes for patients and reduce barriers to care. The removal of barriers to teamwork and efficiency of decision-making processes becomes even more salient in resource-constrained settings within the developing world, where clinicians may often have to rely on intuition, empirical thought and macro-cognitive functioning rather than testing to assess, diagnose and treat paediatric patients.

The goal of the study undertaken was to use qualitative methodology to identify from an emic perspective the team-based factors and environmental factors that pose barriers to patient care within unfamiliar settings by teams with members from different countries, practice settings and cultural backgrounds.

What was done

A qualitative phenomenological study was conducted in 14 different countries in Africa, Asia, South America, the Caribbean and Eastern Europe. Data from observations of 42 simulated emergencies were coded for thematic analysis. Key

informants representing different training backgrounds, practice settings and cultures were interviewed regarding the perceived benefit of acute care scenarios as well as their process for naturalistic decision-making within the simulated scenario. Simulations utilized low- and medium-fidelity simulation manikin and focused primarily on:
1. fluid resuscitation in a child with dehydration/hypovolaemic or haemorrhagic shock
2. emergent management of a critically ill child with respiratory distress and subsequent dysrhythmia.

In keeping with qualitative methodology, data analysis was approached by axial coding and open coding through analysis of interview transcripts and researcher observations recorded via field notes during simulated emergencies. Subsequently, thematic coding categories were developed over time with repeated interviews and observations.

Results and outcomes

Coding of observations yielded common themes: impact of culture on team hierarchy, communication and language barriers impacting on situational awareness, identification of equipment and logistic barriers, lack of systematic emergency procedures, differences in organizational norms, lack of clear role delineation, improvement in shared cognition through simulations and improvement in resource awareness via simulations.

Take-home messages

The results of our study suggest that culture and nationality of origin have an impact on conceptualization of team constructs, including hierarchy, leadership/followership models and role delineation within teams during emergency situations. In teams with members from different cultures and nations such as those in our study, dichotomy within team models can create barriers to communication and effective patient care. However, participation in team simulations helped to improve communica-

tion and create a shared mental model that reached beyond cultural boundaries for teams in our study. As a form of experiential learning, simulation can appeal to diverse types of learners. Our results support the idea that simulation can improve several areas of team functionality, including membership, role, context, process and action-taking by focusing intentional learning effort on each of these areas. Simulation can also provide a means of identifying barriers to patient care resulting from latent threats in the environment. These include identification of faulty or missing equipment as well as awareness of resource limitations, with a resulting plan for systematic workarounds to address these limitations.

What went well/worked well

In a resource-limited setting, what worked well was the utilization and impact of low or medium fidelity simulators. The use of these types of inexpensive simulators also promoted local sustainability and propagation of our curriculum, given the local availability of equipment and resources. In addition, it proved critical to design scenarios using the local epidemiological burden of disease in order to create buy-in from participants and improve realism. Engaging interdisciplinary teams in the simulations was also successful in bringing together groups of individuals who frequently learn in educational silos.

What would we do differently

While this study had local stakeholders identified from pools of local physicians, there was usually a lack of champions within local pools of nursing and allied health staff. Identifying pre-established local stakeholders at each institution in various disciplines would have been helpful. This would facilitate the dissemination of curricula using simulation, ensuring commitment to use simulation in the long term and promote interdisciplinary team working and education.

Clinical skills assessment for paediatric postgraduate physicians

Section contributor: Joseph O. Lopreiato Uniformed Services University of the Health Sciences, Bethesda, USA

Background

The clinical skills of postgraduate physicians can be assessed by direct observation of trainees and other workplace-based assessments (WPBAs). However, a recent study of paediatric trainees in the UK noted that WPBAs are difficult to accomplish and may not always be accompanied by immediate feedback [12,13,14,15]. To address this problem, a structured clinical skills assessment (CSA) using standardized (simulated) patients in an OSCE station format for paediatric postgraduate physicians was created by the Uniformed Services University of the Health Sciences in the USA. This CSA is a practicable and feasible exercise and provides immediate direct feedback to trainees.

What was done

First and third year paediatric postgraduate physicians rotated through five standardized patient stations and one human patient simulator station where their clinical skills in history taking, physical exam, counseling, and emergency management were assessed (Figures 13.3 and 13.4). Immediate feedback after each case was provided by paediatric faculty who observed the encounter on closed-circuit television. The cases were chosen based upon topics already presented in didactic lectures and after experience with patients in the paediatric clinic. The purpose of this assessment was to compare physician performance in various clinical scenarios with faculty expectations at the end of the first and third postgraduate training year.

Results and outcomes

Overall, the clinical skills of paediatric a postgraduate physicians met the expectations of faculty. However, some skills, for example the musculoskeletal examination of an adolescent were scored at less than expected in half of the trainees. This suggests a problem at the programme level rather than an individual trainee problem. Changes in the curricula were instituted the following year and assessed with another clinical skills assessment.

In some cases, trainees who scored well on standard written tests performed less well in direct observation of their clinical skills and vice versa, suggesting that a CSA measures behaviours not captured by knowledge tests. Trainees were given direct feedback by faculty immediately after each simulated case; this was the most appreciated aspect of the assessment among trainees.

Take-home messages

Assessing the clinical skills of postgraduate paediatric residents is a valuable exercise to obtain programme level and individual level assessment data.

What went well/worked well

Immediate feedback by faculty at the completion of each case.

What would we do differently

Ensure some standard-setting among faculty who are assessing postgraduate physician clinical skills. This can be done in short training sessions before the clinical skills assessment session.

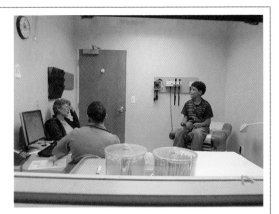

Figure 13.3 A first year paediatric postgraduate trainee interviews a mother and her child about school problems as part of a comprehensive clinical skills assessment using standardized (simulated) patients. Faculty view the encounter through closed circuit television and give direct feedback to the trainee at the end of the encounter.

ⓘ Hints and tips

If the assessment is to be used for high-stakes decisions, choose cases for assessment that reflect topics in the curriculum and with which trainees have had some exposure before the onset of the clinical skills assessment.

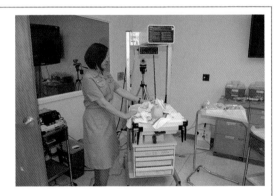

Figure 13.4 Paediatric postgraduate trainees experience a delivery room scenario as part of their clinical skills assessment.

The challenge of doctors in difficulty:

using simulated healthcare contexts to develop a national assessment programme

Section contributors: Kevin Stirling, Jean Ker[1] and Fiona Anderson[2] [1]University of Dundee, Dundee, UK; [2]NHS Education for Scotland, UK

Background

A small number of newly qualified doctors will experience behavioural, performance or educational difficulties early in their postgraduate training and may benefit from additional help [16]. The UK NHS needs to find effective and practical methods for assessing the performance of trainee doctors and then provide effective support and remediation to those individuals who have been identified with performance issues [17].

Educators need to be provided with methods to guide supportive interventions to identify and access the most appropriate remediation resource that meets the educational requirements of the junior doctor. The Postgraduate Ward Simulation Exercise (PgWSE) provides direct evidence of performance using simulation-based education. It lasts for twenty minutes and during the exercise the doctor receives timed interruptions while dealing with a new admission, an emergency situation and a specific communication issue. These reflect both the clinical content and context of the doctor's workplace practice. The doctor has the support of a qualified nurse and a senior healthcare professional.

What was done

The ward simulation exercise was developed at the University of Dundee [18] in collaboration with the postgraduate deanery responsible for the monitoring of postgraduate doctors. In 2008, a management group was established to coordinate the development of the PgWSE as a national resource in Scotland. Since this time the management group has worked to standardize the processes of the PgWSE in following key areas.

Ensuring the standardized processing of candidates

As the national centre for the doctors in difficulty programme, trainee doctors can be referred from any of the four postgraduate deaneries in Scotland.

To ensure consistency, a national advisory group was established to coordinate and advise referring deaneries on the best course of remediation for a trainee doctor. A dedicated website was created that trainee doctors could access as a preparatory resource prior to their PgWSE.

Ensuring standardized training of assessors

The management group has recruited a diverse bank of assessors for the PgWSE. All assessors are consultants practising in a wide range of specialties. The management group has recruited assessors from across Scotland to ensure that there is minimal local bias. Three consultants assess each PgWSE. Each consultant must attend a 1-day introductory training day prior to become an assessor. As an assessor a consultant must conduct two assessments per year and attend an annual update.

A standardized process of assessment has been created:
1. Each assessor conducts an individual assessment of a trainee doctor's performance while observing the PgWSE (Figure 13.5).
2. The assessors then make a consensus judgement based on their individual judgement. This includes an overall pass/fail judgement based on the trainee doctor's performance.
3. The candidate conducts a self-assessment of their performance by watching a recording of their PgWSE. This self-assessment informs the individualized feedback that is given to the trainee doctor when they meet with the assessment panel.

Establishing the realism of the PgWSE

Nine PgWSEs have been developed to reflect clinical practice in general surgery, general medicine and medicine for elderly people. The development of each PgWSE involves the shadowing of Foundation Year 1 and 2 doctors within a relevant clinical setting to identify the most frequent interruptions either from patients, their relatives, members of the healthcare team or from external sources such as the bleep system or telephone. Focus group sessions are held with members of the multidisciplinary team to

ensure realism is achieved. Each PgWSE is reviewed by clinical and education experts prior to be used in the assessment of junior doctors.

Identify the complexity of each PgWSE

Each PgWSE is mapped to the foundation curriculum [19] to ensure that the complexity of each PgWSE is measurable and should be attainable by a foundation year 1 and 2 junior doctor. Statistical analysis of the assessment tool and the PgWSE has been undertaken.

Results and outcome

The PgWSE has been shown to be a valuable addition to the diagnosis of junior doctors with performance issues. Since 2008, the national advisory group has received 38 trainee referrals from the four postgraduate deaneries in Scotland. Initial data analysis of the PgWSE has shown that this form of diagnostic assessment has proven reliability (Cronbach Alpha: 0.817) [20]. Multifaceted Rasch Modelling (MFRM) shows that the PgWSE was able to discriminate well between candidates on the basis of their performance.

Take-home messages

It is possible to develop a bank of standardized ward simulation exercises as a national resource which provides a reliable and cost-effective solution to the management and remediation of trainee doctors with performance issues.

What went well/worked well

The commitment of the management group to develop the PgWSE as a high-quality resource is one of the key achievements. Mapping each PgWSE scenario against the foundation curriculum and having the input of clinical experts into the design and testing of each ward simulation exercise has been critical to the creation of authentic immersive simulated environment.

Postgraduate Ward Simulation Exercise (PgWSE)

	Performance			
Task management Candidate has a good general overview and prioritises appropriately. Candidate conducts all essential tasks and clinical procedures. Delivers an appropriate handover	Very poor Outstanding 1 2 3 4 5 N/A			
Clinical skills Candidate demonstrates effective history taking skills. Candidate demonstrates appropriate examination technique and initiates appropriate investigations. Candidate interprets results and makes informed decisions	Very poor Outstanding 1 2 3 4 5 N/A			
Acutely ill patient Candidate recognises, and systematically assesses the patient using an ABCDE approach. Candidate manages the acutely ill patient appropriately and demonstrates good time management skills, recognizing when to get help from a senior colleague	Very poor Outstanding 1 2 3 4 5 N/A			
Prescribing technique Candidate demonstrates a safe and appropriate prescribing technique	Very poor Outstanding 1 2 3 4 5 N/A			
Written documentation Candidate completes written tasks appropriately	Very poor Outstanding 1 2 3 4 5 N/A			
Response to interruptions Candidate responds appropriately to interruptions and follows them up. Candidate responds appropriately/reacts to nursing observation	Very poor Outstanding 1 2 3 4 5 N/A			
Communication Candidate demonstrates good interpersonal skills and uses appropriate language. Candidate responds appropriately to each patients' care requirements, answering questions and keeping patients informed. Candidate communicates effectively with colleagues Relationship with patients/relatives Working with colleagues	Very poor Outstanding 1 2 3 4 5 N/A 1 2 3 4 5 N/A			
Health and safety Candidate demonstrates abilities in the following domains appropriate to their grade: Safe medical practice Preventing cross-infection	Very poor Outstanding 1 2 3 4 5 N/A 1 2 3 4 5 N/A			
Professionalism Candidate acts in a manner becoming of their actual grade of practice, is polite, considerate and honest. Candidate treats patients with dignity, respecting patients' privacy and right to confidentiality	Very poor Outstanding 1 2 3 4 5 N/A			

What behaviours does the candidate exhibit during the exercise?

What are the candidates strengths?

What areas does the candidate need to improve?

Overall global judgement of performance: Performance: Very poor   Outstanding
1   2   3   4   5   N/A

My overall judgement of this candidate is (please circle)   PASS   FAIL

Please sign and date your completed assessment form. Please complete the structured summary sheet with your colleagues prior to giving feedback to the candidate

Name (BLOCK CAPITALS) ....

Signature ....

Date (DD/MM/YY) ....

Figure 13.5 The PgWSE assessment tool.

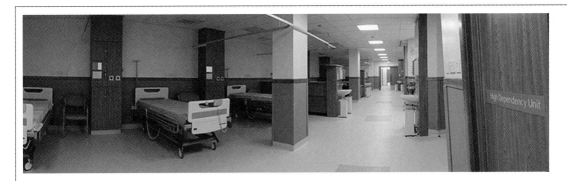

Figure 13.6   The Dow Clinical Simulation Suite.

What would you do differently

One of the challenges in any innovation is creating the resources both financial and time to develop the exercise and to have a system of dissemination in place from the outset. It is essential to spend time ensuring supervisors and educators and clinicians are on board.

ⓘ Hints and tips

Choose a management team with a range of both educational and clinical expertise. Seek out and engage with expert opinion at every stage of development to ensure that the simulation exercises created are based on quality clinical standards.

Simulation for remote and rural practice

Section contributors: Jerry Morse, Jean Ker[1,2] and Sarah Race[2] University of Aberdeen, [1]University of Dundee, [2]NHS Education for Scotland, UK

Background

Equity of access to healthcare training for all, irrespective of their geographical location is the tenet of the Scottish Clinical Skills Strategy. With the use of simulation in healthcare education continuing to increase, this must also extend to those one in five people who reside in the remote and rural areas of Scotland [24]. In conjunction with the Scottish Mobile Clinical Skills Unit, a wide range of simulation modalities can now be delivered on site, enabling multidisciplinary training with minimal disruption to working practice and at a fraction of the cost in sending staff to regional simulation centers.

What was done

This case describes a visit of the Mobile Skills Unit (Figure 13.7) and its onboard simulation facilities to one of the Scottish islands, where support and education was provided to locally based trainers.

Teams of multidisciplinary healthcare professionals including the cardiac arrest team from a remote and rural hospital, were given a series of simulated medical emergency scenarios to work through on the mobile skills unit. Each of the scenarios had a different set of learning outcomes which had been prearranged and tailored to the requirements of the local practitioners. All scenarios encompassed both technical and non-technical skills (structured communication tools) and prioritized clinical situations which did not occur as frequently as in larger hospitals, Participants were

informed that cameras would be recording the scenarios and consented to being observed and given feedback using video debrief techniques. In addition to the healthcare teams, the facilitators from the hospital were also trained in effectively running scenarios and, more importantly, debriefing skills. A semi-structured evaluation form was used to collect feedback on the sessions in the mobile skills unit from both the participants and facilitators. This was followed up six weeks after the event with a structured telephone interview with all participants.

Results and outcomes

The facilitators and local educators who delivered the sessions observed an enhanced use of structured handover by the remote and rural practitioners both during the exercise and in reviewing the videos. Participants commented on increased confidence in being able to cope with emergencies and an enhanced awareness of the different services and their roles when dealing with evolving situations.

The local educators identified an increased confidence in their roles following the customized training particularly in relation to debriefing scenarios. Both participants and facilitators reported that training did not always have to involve mid or high-fidelity simulators. The use of simulation for training especially in these remote and rural areas where access to such equipment can be problematic need not be a stumbling block. As long as clear aims and objectives are defined and agreed, simulated clinical scenarios can and have improved staff

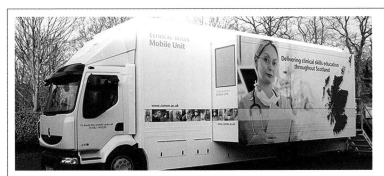

Figure 13.7 Picture of mobile unit.

training which ultimately can have a positive impact on patient safety.

Take-home messages

Practitioners in remote and rural settings are just as, if not more, enthusiastic about engaging in the use of simulation, particularly when there are trained facilitators and facilities available.

The ability to provide onsite simulation to the whole multidisciplinary team provides a unique opportunity for interprofessional education and awareness raising about the abilities and skills of others who work around them.

What went well/worked well

The scenarios worked well and were described by participants as 'realistic' due to being specifically tailored to their local situation. The local facilitators gained confidence not only in running scenarios but also in debriefing and feeding back to teams of healthcare professionals. This will and has had a knock-on effect that training in simulation continues in a structured manner in a remote area where previously only sporadic simulation training would have taken place.

What would you do differently

To improve future sessions it would be useful to build in more debriefing time for the local facilitators, so that they can also build on their experiences of running and providing debriefing to their colleagues. While in the sessions those who were the direct recipients of the 'training' benefited from practice in clinical emergencies, time also needs to be allocated for those who will provide similar training after the mobile skills unit has gone. As a result of providing simulation in remote and rural areas, the continued training of facilitators must be facilitated to ensure that the national strategies and regional standards are maintained.

ⓘ Hints and tips

As with all simulation, make it relevant to the participants. It is pointless running a pre-written scenario that they will never encounter. If the session is to be multidisciplinary, discuss with the relevant educators what aims and objectives and outcomes they want for their staff from the session.

The use of incognito standardized patients in general practice

Section contributor: Jan-Joost Rethans University of Maastricht, Maastricht, Netherlands

Background

A standardized patient (SP) is a simulated patient who has been trained to portray a patient in a standardized, consistent way. Standardized Patients' role-playing does not vary from physician to physician and does not vary from standardized patient to standardized patient. In this way standardized patient methodology represents an ideal method to assess the real practice (consultation) performance of physicians. An incognito (or unannounced) SP is a SP who enters a physician's surgery as if he/she is a real patient without the doctor knowing this is not a real patient.

What was done

In a number of studies in several European countries we sent incognito SPs (ISPs) to real surgery encounters of trainees in general practice, general practitioners, rheumatologists and primary care out-of-hours centres [21,22,23]. In each study we asked beforehand for the written consent of the healthcare professionals that were to be visited. Using refined techniques, we made sure that the ISPs were not detected, that they were able to report on the practitioner's practice performance in a valid and consistent way and that (in most studies) the physicians visited received feedback on their performance.

Results and outcomes

The ISP methodology was well accepted by all health care practitioners. Less than 1% of our ISPs were detected. Practice results show that real practice performance in most cases does not meet evidence-based standards of care, with a wide variation in physicians' clinical practice. Interestingly however ISPs were very content with the care received, especially when taking the 'human side' of consultations into consideration.

Take-home messages

ISP methodology is acceptable, valid, reliable and feasible after good ISP training, if the healthcare professionals to be visited are asked beforehand for consent, if their anonymity is guaranteed and feedback is given.

What went well/worked well

It is important to have a long time-lag between the consent of the physicians to be visited and the actual practice visits.

What would you do differently

Instead of training the ISPs to fill out a checklist, modern mobile technology devices should be used to record the consultations.

> ⓘ **Hints and tips**
>
> Be sure to take time for a careful and detailed preparation for the visits, both in terms of SP training and in obtaining information about the actual visit sites.

Integration of simulation-based training for the trauma team in a university hospital

Section contributors: Anne-Mette Helsø and Doris Østergaard Danish Institute of Medical Simulation, Copenhagen, Denmark

Background

The treatment of the multi-traumatized patient demands a coordinated effort from the trauma team. This requires aspects of medical expertise/practical skills as well as teamwork, leadership, communication, decision-making and situation awareness. Advanced trauma courses such as ATLS™ address the individuals' medical expertise and practical skills but, to function as a team, the multidisciplinary trauma team should be trained in their own environment and with the real team members. In this study we describe the development and implementation of a trauma team training course in a large university hospital.

What was done

A one-day course was developed comprising:
• introduction and house rules (create a safe learning environment)
• a mini-lecture of ATLS principles
• three or four trauma cases (discuss treatment)
• video-assisted group discussion of teamwork, leadership and communication
• skill stations (immobilization and log-roll)
• two full-scale simulations in the emergency room using a simulated patient and a simulator
• two debriefing sessions including video clips.
The course was developed by anaesthetists, surgeons, nurses and experts from the simulation centre. The hospital's trauma manual was used in the planning of the course. The participants filled in an evaluation form at the end of the course. A questionnaire was developed and the participants

self-assessed their competences after the first and second scenario.

Results and outcomes

Sixteen multidisciplinary trauma teams (165 participants) participated in the course. The training was evaluated as good or very good by all participants. Overall, the participants rated their communication, team work and leadership skills higher after the second scenario than the first scenario.

The course has now been implemented throughout our organization.

Take-home messages

• Train the full multi-professional team.
• Train in the real clinical environment (makes it possible to test manuals, action cards, etc.).
• Use a combination of methods to address the learning objectives.
• Continuously develop the course according to evaluations, changes in the organization and new medical knowledge/devices.

⚠ Hints and tips

• Commitment of leaders is required to free staff from clinical duties.
• Collaboration is required between departments in conducting the course and planning the course dates.

Conclusion

Simulation-based education as demonstrated by Scalese's example highlights how simulation-based education can enhance skills not only in the local context but also on a global scale and presents a pathway for collaboration and multicentre studies. Technological advances in recent years provide opportunities to take simulation to the workplace. This is exemplified by the cases from Morse and colleagues in the UK, who use a mobile unit to provide SBE to healthcare practitioners' to facilitate practitioners' technical and non-technical skills and Rethans in the Netherlands, who describes the use of incognito patients in different workplace settings to assess standards in the workplace. The case example from Helsø and Østergaard demonstrates the power of testing the use of hospital manuals and protocols as part of a simulation exercise with multiple teams who work together, so enhancing transfer of learning. Immersing the use of simulation as a norm in the workplace whether in primary or secondary care can improve standards in clinical practice as well enhancing transfer.

The last 15 years have seen enormous advances in our knowledge of why and how adverse events occur in clinical practice. For example the reports from the Institute of Medicine – *To err is Human* [25] – in the USA and from the UK Department of Health – *An organisation with a Memory* [26] highlighted the cost of adverse events in terms of both finances and harm to patients. Safety at all levels of the organization can be enhanced by the use of simulation. The case examples from O'Sullivan and colleagues in relation to the use of simulation for leadership skills development in the undergraduate curriculum and Marshall in relation to front-line team training share how errors in the system can be addressed and disseminated in a timely fashion using scenarios developed from critical incidents in the system. The use of live clinical incidents provides a reality both in terms of content and context particularly for experienced practitioners as they have the opportunity to reflect on their own individual and team performance. Simulation can uncover unintended consequences of a systems change in the health care organization and can provide evidence for leverage to address these.

Another common theme from the examples in this chapter is the concept of professional role modeling in simulation based education. The loss of the apprenticeship system as a result of both education and healthcare service delivery changes has highlighted the need for simulation-based education educators to remain in active clinical service to enhance learning from role modelling. The role of the facilitator both as a clinician and as a educator however highlights the staff development challenges currently faced in most countries by the lack of trained simulation-based educators.

Simulation can provide not only the opportunity to rehearse and relearn a wide variety of skills but it can also be used to regulate and diagnose difficulties in practice in relation to both the individual and the system. Lopreiato, through the use of simulation to assess specialists in child health and Stirling and Ker, through running a national programme for newly qualified doctors in difficulty share how simulation can be used both to diagnose and provide evidence for decisions on standards of practice.

The case studies in this chapter also demonstrate the need to pay attention to the theoretical and pedagogical underpinnning of simulation activities such as behaviourism for over-learning, social constructivism for resolving cognitive conflicts (as exemplified by Marshall) and transformative learning (as shared by Rethans). Simulation-based education enables all domains of learning (cognitive, psychomotor and affective) to be considered in the reconstruction. All the cases highlight the role of feedback which underpins all successful simulation-based education.

In a systematic review of high fidelity simulation, Issenberg [27] reported a number of key features which consistently facilitated learning in the use of high fidelity simulators including:

- providing feedback
- allowing repetitive practice
- integrating the use of simulation events within a curricular programme
- providing a range of difficulties and scenarios
- defining learning outcomes.

One criticism of simulation has been the added cost to education in both financial and human expertise. However, the example from Shilkofski demonstrates how simulation using low cost simulators can be used to enhance skills delivery in under-resourced settings in Africa. She highlights the need to consider sustainability and for identifying local champions in simulation based education.

All these examples can be viewed from perspectives of the different educational methods used to develop simulation interventions, the different contexts in which simulation takes place and the level of expertise of either the individuals or the organizations involved. A common thread through all the examples is that in every case the use of simulation has enhanced the deliberate learning of the individuals and/or the team where a clear purpose for the educational intervention is defined.

SUMMARY

This chapter has provided selected examples of where simulation has been used to great effect. The examples highlight how effective simulation can be a technique for teaching technical and non-technical skills and demonstrates how it enhances standards of practice through providing protected yet realistic scenarios for the learner which can be timed to maximize learning around identified learning outcomes. What is required to embed the use of simulation in health care education is, as Helsø and Østergaard so succinctly put it, 'the commitment of leaders to free staff from clinical duties'.

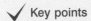

Key points

- Simulation-based education does not replace the reality of practice but has a clear role in preparation of the individual and team for healthcare delivery.
- Simulation can be an effective technique where resources are limited.
- Simulation-based education can be effective at all levels of the organization.
- Simulation-based education provides a safe opportunity to explore unintended consequences of systems design.

Acknowledgements

The following people contributed to this chapter: Jerry Morse, University of Aberdeen, UK; Nicole Shilkofski, John Hopkins University, USA; Jan Joost Rethans, University of Maastricht, Netherlands; Ross Scalese, University of Miami, USA; Joe Lopreiato, Uniformed Services University, USA; Helen O'Sullivan, University of Liverpool, UK; Kevin Stirling, University of Dundee, UK; Stuart Marshall, Monash University, Australia; Arpan Guha, University of Liverpool, UK; Jean Ker, University of Dundee and NHS Education for Scotland, UK; Sarah Race, NHS Education for Scotland, UK; Michael Moneypenny, University of Liverpool, UK; Anne-Mette Helsø, Danish Institute of Medical Simulation, Denmark; and Doris Østergaard Danish Institute of Medical Simulation, Denmark.

REFERENCES

1. Mangione S, Nieman LZ (1997) Cardiac auscultation skills of internal medicine and family practice trainees: a comparison of diagnostic proficiency (published erratum appears in *Journal of the American Medical Association* 1998; **279:** 1444). *Journal of the American Medical Association* **278:** 717–722.

2. Issenberg SB, Gordon DL, Stewart GM, Felner JM (2000) Bedside cardiology skills training for the physician assistant using simulation technology. *Perspectives on Physician Assistant Education* **11:** 99–103.

3. Issenberg SB, Petrusa ER, McGaghie WC, *et al.* (1999) Effectiveness of a computer-based system to teach bedside cardiology. *Academic Medicine* **74:** S93–95.

4. Issenberg SB, McGaghie WC, Gordon DL, *et al.* (2002) Effectiveness of a cardiology review course for Internal Medicine residents using simulation technology and deliberate practice. *Teaching and Learning in Medicine* **14:** 223–228.

5. Ewy GA, Felner JM, Juul D, *et al.* (1987) Test of a cardiology patient simulator with students in fourth-year electives. *Journal of Medical Education* **62:** 738–743.

6. Ericsson KA (2006) The influence of experience and deliberate practice on the development of superior expert performance. In: *The Cambridge Handbook of Expertise and Expert Performance* (KA Ericsson, N Charness, PJ Feltovich, RR Hoffman, eds). New York: Cambridge University Press, 683–703.

7. Issenberg SB, McGaghie WC, Petrusa ER, *et al.* (2005) Features and uses of high-fidelity medical simulations that lead to effective learning: a BEME Systematic Review. *Medical Teacher* **27:** 10–28.

8. Royal College of Physicians (2010) *Future Physicians: Changing Doctors in Changing Times.* Report of a working party. London: RCP.

9. General Medical (2009) *Council Tomorrow's Doctors: Outcomes and Standards for Undergraduate Medical Education.* London: GMC.

10. NHS Institute for Innovation and Improvement and Academy of Medical Royal Colleges (2010) *Medical Leadership Competency Framework*, 3rd edn. Coventry: NHS Institute for Innovation and Improvement.

11. Jones G, Steketee R, Black R, Bhtta Z, Morris S (2003) Bellagio child survival study group: How many child deaths can we prevent this year? *Lancet* **362:** 65–71.

12. Bindal T, Wall D, Goodyear HM (2011) Trainee doctors' views on workplace-based assessments: Are they just a tick box exercise? *Medical Teacher* **33:** 919–927.

13. Carraccio, C, Englander R (2000) The objective structured clinical examination: a step in the direction of competency-based evaluation. *Archives Pediatric and Adolescent Medicine* **154:** 736–741.

14. Hilliard RI, Tallett SE (1998) The use of an objective structured clinical examination with postgraduate residents in pediatrics. *Archives Pediatric and Adolescent Medicine* **152:** 74–78.

15. Frost GJ, Cater JI, Forsyth JS (1986) The use of the Objective Structured Clinical Examination (OSCE) in paediatrics. *Medical Teacher* **8:** 261–269.

16. Postgraduate Medical Education in Scotland: Management of Trainee Doctors in Difficulty. Operational Framework. NHS Education for Scotland. 2008. Available from http://www.nes.scot.nhs.uk/media/182663/mgmt_of_doctors_in_difficulty_framework_may_2009.pdf (accessed 6 March 2013).

17. Baker R (2005) Commentary: Can poorly performing doctors blame their assessment tools? **330:**1254. Available from http://bmj.

com/cgi/doi/10.1136/bmj.38469.406597. 0B (accessed 6 March 2013).

18. Ker JS, Hesketh EA, Anderson F, Johnston DA (2006) Can a ward simulation exercise achieve the realism that reflects the complexity of everyday practice junior doctors encounter? *Medical Teacher* **28:** 330–334.

19. The UK Foundation Programme Office. The foundation programme: about the programme. Available from http://www. foundationprogramme.nhs.uk/pages/home/ about-the-foundation-programme (accessed 6 March 2013)

20. McIlwaine L, Mcaleer J, Ker J (2007) Assessment of final year medical students in a simulated ward: developing content validity for an assessment instrument. *International Journal of Clinical Skills* **1:** 33–35.

21. Peremans L, Rethans JJ, Verhoeven V, *et al.* (2010) Empowering patients or general practitioners? A randomized clinical trial to improve quality in reproductive health care in Belgium. *European Journal of Contraception and Reproductive Health Care* **15:** 280–289.

22. Derkx H, Rethans JJ, Maiburg B, *et al.* (2009) New methodology for using incognito standardized patients for telephone consultation in primary care. *Medical Education* **43:** 82–88.

23. Rethans JJ, Gorter S, Bokken L, Morrison L (2007) Unannounced standardised patients in real practice: a systematic literature review. *Medical Education* **41:** 537–549.

24. Scottish Funding Council and NHS Education for Scotland (2007) *Scottish Clinical Skills Strategy, 2007*. London: HMSO.

25. Kohn L, Corrigan J, Donaldson M (eds) (1999) *To Err Is Human: Building a Safer Health System*. Washington, DC: Committee on Quality of Health Care in America, Institute of Medicine. National Academies Press.

26. DH 2000. Available from http://www. dh.gov.uk/prod_consum_dh/groups/dh_ digitalassets/@dh/@en/documents/ digitalasset/dh_4065086.pdf.

27. Issenberg SB, McGaghie WC, Petrusa ER, *et al.* (2005) Features and uses of high-fidelity medical simulations that lead to effective learning: a BEME systematic review. *Medical Teacher* **27:** 10–28.

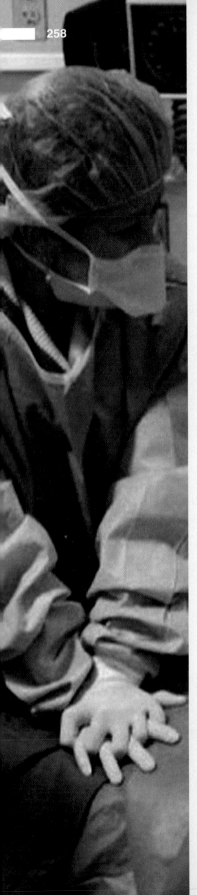

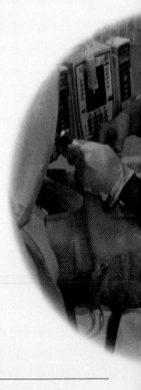

CHAPTER 14
The future for simulation

Overview

The final chapter comprises three sections. In each section the authors give their personal perspective on what they see as some of the key developments in simulation and how these will impact on future development and implementation.

Essential Simulation in Clinical Education, First Edition. Edited by Kirsty Forrest, Judy McKimm, and Simon Edgar.
© 2013 John Wiley & Sons, Ltd. Published 2013 by John Wiley & Sons, Ltd.

Horizon scanning: the impact of technological change

Section contributors: Iliana Harrysson, Rajesh Aggarwal and Ara Darzi Imperial College London, London, UK

Surgical simulation has come far since its beginning in the 1960s. A significant amount of research shows the benefit of simulation for technical skills, in the operating theatre, the procedure suite and on the wards [1,2,3,4,5,6]. Unfortunately, the incorporation of simulation into training and education has been slower than expected. Simulation technology, and the methodology with which it is used, will continue to develop, but for its full potential to be reached simulation needs to be easily accessible and Gaba [7] has suggested that curricular implementation of new simulation technologies is paramount to the success of simulation.

In the landmark report *To Err is Human* [8], it was noted that up to 98 000 people die unnecessarily because of medical errors in the USA alone. Simulation will be a growing part of the solution to combat these patients' deaths. For example, some medical errors could be eliminated and patient safety improved though repeated, simulated practice by medical staff, such as handovers and how to handle emergency situations. Traditionally, surgeons were taught how to operate by practising their skills on patients. This is no longer acceptable. Simulation is an ideal way for surgeons to practise before operating, thus removing the effects of the learning curve on patients.

This section examines the future of simulation, and, in particular, how technology can be developed to improve patient care. Future improvements and potential areas of simulation use are reviewed from the viewpoint of a patient's journey through the surgical environment as well as a surgeon's journey through his/her career.

A patient's journey

Figure 14.1 and the following text depicts and describes some of the potential uses of simulation as associated with the patient pathway through surgery.

In the clinic

In the first 20 years of its development, the focus of surgical simulation was on individual technical skills; then, with mounting clinical evidence, the medical community realized the importance of non-technical skills. Non-technical skills are usually the first that a patient encounters and affect much of how a patient feels about a doctor. Communication with the patient and family, within the care team, as well as with the hospital administration affects clinical care [9,10]. For the last 10 years, simulation has been used as a tool to practice communication, teamwork and collaboration. In the future, team-based simulation will become more important as the effectiveness of medical care is further scrutinized.

Simulation already plays an important role in undergraduate education through the use of standardized patient encounters. This educational methodology has not been used as extensively in surgical training, but with the incorporation of more simulation activities into the curriculum, this area is

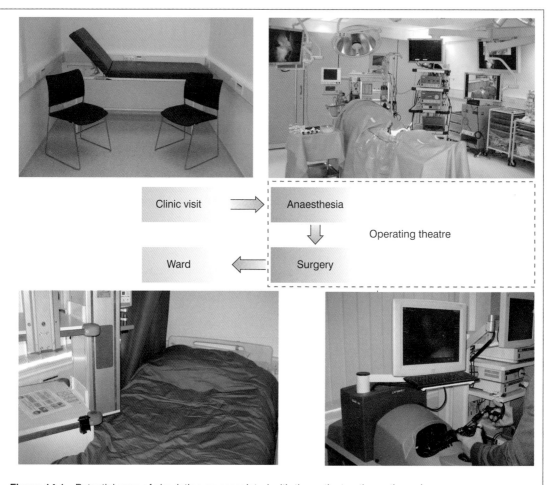

Figure 14.1   Potential uses of simulation as associated with the patient pathway through surgery.

growing. With improving technology, it is likely that standardized patients will be used less and the virtual patient will be used more. A virtual patient can be a manikin that talks, reacts and has physical findings or it can be a three-dimensional (3D) image of a patient with the specific physical findings recorded for the practising surgeon to examine. A trainee will be able to have a conversation with the virtual patient as if they were examining the patient in the clinic. In a virtual world, no two cases will have to be the same and the scenario can change each time the trainee sees the patient. Learning and the potential for any accompanying error will be removed from the patient encounter and the trainee

will first practise examinations and patient consultations on virtual reality simulators before encountering real patients.

From clinic to operating theatre

CT and MRI scans are commonplace before any major surgery to identify lesions and vessel morphology. Identifying vessels, dissection planes and densities will become more automated in the future. Two-dimensional (2D) images will be turned into 3D renderings that can be used not only for diagnosis but also for planning the surgery. Currently, this has been done with individual patients in laparoscopic liver surgery [11,12,13]. In addition to technical skills, the teamwork required in an operation can also be practised. For example, Willaert *et al.* simulated carotid artery stenting in an operating suite with the full team practicing the scenario before the actual case [14]. In the future, this will be able to be done quickly for all patients in an automated fashion. An example of how this may work is seen in Case study 14.1.

 Case study 14.1

Mr Jones has an enlarged liver that is being examined by Mr Scrub, a surgical consultant, during a clinic visit. The consultant orders blood tests and a CT scan of Mr Jones' abdomen for the next clinic visit. After the CT scan is done, a 3D rendering automatically appears in Mr Scrub's computer. Mr Scrub inspects the 3D image with his colleagues, a radiologist and pathologist. They conclude that this is most likely a complex liver cancer that will need surgery as soon as possible. After going back and reviewing the findings with Mr Jones, Mr Scrub schedules the surgery. Before the surgery, he imports the case into the virtual reality simulator and practices the technical skills of the operation. Because of the complexity of the case, he invites the whole operating team, including anaesthetist, scrub nurse, circulating nurse and surgical trainees to come to the simulated operating theatre to practise the case. Aberrant blood vessels and an additional cancer focus are identified in the practice session. When Mr Jones has his surgery, the surgery goes smoothly with minimal blood loss and clear margins around the tumour.

This automated process can be used for laparoscopic and robotic surgery, where the surgeon will practice on a virtual reality simulator, and in open surgery. With decreasing costs of 3D printing and improved materials, a replica of a patient's individual anatomy will be made, and the surgeon can practice on this 3D printed patient before going into the operating theatre. Work on holographic simulation is already under way, taking CT and MRI images and turning them into a holographic image. A holographic surgery with real-time changes during an operation is yet another way that surgery can be simulated.

By incorporating imaging, surgery and pathology, multidisciplinary review and decisions can be made with the improved ability to predict complications and thus improve safety and health outcomes.

In the operating theatre

Technical skills

Simulation has been shown to improve technical skills in the operating theatre. Seymour *et al.* [2]

showed that residents who practised on a virtual reality simulator were faster and performed better in the operating theatre when dissecting the gallbladder from the liver bed. This was done using the Minimally Invasive Surgical Trainer (MIST) virtual reality simulator, which consists of tasks that familiarize the trainee with laparoscopic instrument and working in a 3D environment but on a 2D screen. The first virtual reality simulator did not have haptic feedback and did not simulate an actual operation, yet it increased the skill of the surgeon substantially.

Like all technology, the hardware is constantly improving, and faster and cheaper hardware and software will make high-fidelity virtual reality simulation more accessible. Currently, some virtual reality simulators have haptic feedback which enables the user to feel what they are doing as if it were a real manoeuvre. Newer simulators, such as the LapMentor, have also been shown to improve technical skills of trainees [15]. Andreatta *et al.* [15] showed that interns that were trained using the virtual reality simulator outperformed those who did not have the training in live porcine practice sessions. They had better camera and instrument control and more efficient movements. The improvements to simulators will continue; the next step in making virtual reality simulators even more realistic includes improving textures and software. Improved and cheaper graphics cards will be able to accommodate the more complex virtual reality software and close collaboration between clinicians and simulation development companies will fully utilize the progress being made in computer technology.

In addition to improving current simulators, new simulators and simulation techniques will follow the progress of surgery in the operating theatre. Simulation will become available for the new arenas of robotic surgery, high-definition and 3D laparoscopic surgery as surgeons explore them and they become commonplace. Its incorporation will move technical skills training away from the patient and into the classroom and laboratory. Though simulated technical skills training is focused on trainees, practising surgeons can also use it in their day-to-day practice. This is especially true for difficult or rare surgeries, where patient-specific simulation as described will be very useful.

Teamwork skills

Immersive simulation for all team members is one way to foster a team-based approach to patient care. A simulated operating theatre will, for example, be available for all parts of the medical care team, nurses, technicians, doctors and surgeons, so that they can practice teamwork skills in standard cases or cases with known frequent complications and difficulties. Communication, leadership and teamwork skills are already being taught in a simulated environment, but the scenarios usually only focus on one part of the team. For example, Gettman et al. [16] showed that teamwork skills improved when surgeons practised in a simulated operating theatre; however, the whole clinical team can benefit from this kind of training, not only the surgeons. Exceptionally difficult cases or those with novel approaches will not only be able to be practised technically before they are performed, but the teamwork required can also be rehearsed. The handovers between surgical subspecialties and shift changes for nurses and technicians can also be perfected before

the actual case begins. For example, the transitions in a long case that requires both urological and general surgeons could be practised on a holographic image of the patient. The timing of when urology should take over or if it is possible for both teams to work simultaneously could be established before the surgery begins.

Full team simulations in a simulated operating theatre are costly and other alternatives have been proposed. The inflatable operating theatre designed by Kneebone et al. [17], for example, can be set up at a fraction of the cost of a full operating theatre. A virtual operating theatre can also be imagined, where only a few pieces of equipment are needed for tactile sensation and the periphery is simulated. The team scenarios can consist of a full operating theatre team or just a few members with the other members being virtual characters. For example, a scrub nurse and circulating nurse can practice communications skills with a virtual surgeon and anaesthetist. This kind of simulation is less difficult to organize and can be incorporated into the daily training of surgical teams more easily.

In transition and on the ward

Once a patient's operation is complete, they will be transferred to the recovery ward and then either discharged or admitted to a hospital ward. A simulated ward can be used to rehearse these transfers, this ward does not have to be a physical place where the medical team goes to practice, but it can be done simply with access to a computer. Second life™ (see Figure 14.2), a virtual world, does just this [18] Any part of the hospital (or world) can be simulated and each surgeon, nurse or other healthcare worker can have his or her own avatar in the simulated world. They can interact with other people's avatars or with simulated avatars. This concept can be expanded to include handovers, medication orders and patient movements, which can be simulated and perfected. By incorporating a similar simulation into each hospital system, trainees and new employees can explore replicas of their work place or new environments so that once they are assigned to a workplace, the orientation phase will

Figure 14.2 An operating room in second life. With permission from Henry Fuller. http://secondlife6750.wordpress.com.

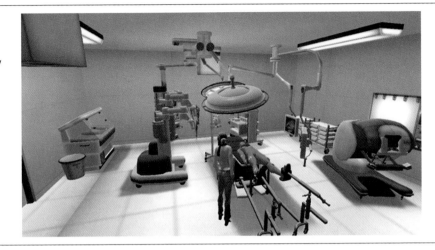

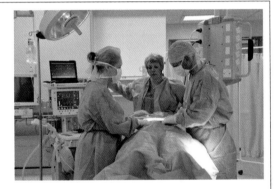

Figure 14.3 Team training can take place in the hospital setting. Courtesy of Jivendra Gosai, Hull Institute of Learning and Simulation.

A surgeon's journey

Simulation of the future will look and feel different from today and it will also be used in more ways. One of the many benefits of computer-based virtual reality simulation is that it provides an opportunity to record and assess what is being done objectively, which is important [20]. Multiple tools have been developed for raters to assess surgeons in the operating theatre such as a Global Rating Scale for technical skills [21] or Observational Teamwork Assessment for Surgery (OTAS) for non-technical skills [22]. With simulation, there is no need for a physical rater to be present at each training session and the assessment process can be more efficient. The data retrieved from a simulator can be used to evaluate the skills of an applicant to a surgical post, a trainee before performing a part of a real surgery in the operating theatre, or for revalidation of senior surgeons throughout their careers. While the data retrieved from a virtual reality simulator has been used in research, it is not yet being used regularly as a part of training or examination.

The possibilities of using simulation to assess individuals rely on the development of standardized scoring methods and test validation which requires collaboration between surgeons, academic centres and professional societies. Simulation will be used in all parts of the surgeon's career, from building his/her knowledge base, to improving technical and

be short and patients will have a more comfortable experience.

The simulated environment does not need to be constrained to a computer, skills laboratory or simulated operating theatre, but team training can be done in the hospital as well (Figure 14.3). *In situ* simulation has shown to not only improve skills of the trainees, but also identify larger systems issues [19]. In these simulations, administrators and hospital management can be involved to assess the risk and efficiency of certain practices.

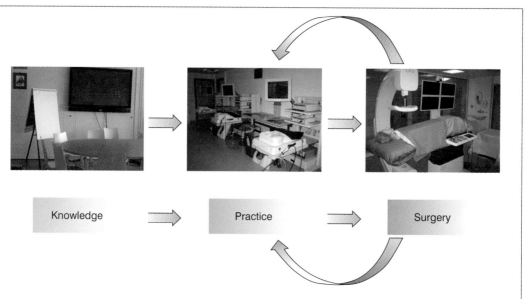

Knowledge ⟹ Practice ⟹ Surgery

Figure 14.4 The role of simulation in a surgeon's career path. © 2009 The Royal College of Physicians and Surgeons of Canada. http://rcpsc.medical.org/canmeds. Reproduced with permission.

non-technical skills, to actually performing surgery (Figure 14.4).

Before surgical training

Patient simulation is already used as a part of the assessment of medical students and, although a range of clinical skills are assessed before starting a residency programme, students' specific surgical technical skills are not assessed. Virtual reality simulation or box trainers can be used in an automated and (if required) anonymous application process to surgical posts. The actual technical skills of an applicant can be tested, but, also, each applicant's potential to learn and how much they improve after being taught about a procedure, can be measured.

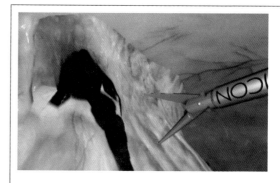

Figure 14.5 A haptic feedback virtual reality simulator. Courtesy of Jivendra Gosai, Hull Institute of Learning and Simulation.

During surgical training

Simulation will be used as both an educational and assessment tool throughout a surgeon's career. Different modules and methods will be used at different times in training. At the beginning of training, patient interactions and knot tying skills would be practised for example via a standardized patient, virtual reality patient or an avatar type environment

followed by knot tying skills via a suture board, laparoscopic box trainer or a haptic feedback virtual reality simulator (Figure 14.5). In this example, certain scores or benchmarks might have to be reached before being able to interview a patient or tie knots in the operating theatre. Surgery and team-based communication training will continue, using a variety of scenarios and types of simulation at different levels of training, with each level having defined passing criteria. As new technologies or techniques are introduced, simulation can also help equip surgeons, technicians and other staff with the necessary skills and competencies, not just handling instruments but also the finesse of surgery and being able to manoeuvre instruments in increasingly complex situations.

Feedback and learning will not be limited to the simulators, but a fully integrated educational programme can also record what happens in the operating theatre. The movements of the instruments can be recorded and this information can be used for later training purposes, like a football team watching and learning from the plays after the game is over. It can also be used as a black box, acting as an assessment tool if something goes wrong in the surgery in the way that an aircraft's or ship's black box recorder is used. This is a controversial aspect of real-time assessment which may or may not be utilized in the future.

As a consultant

With the development of more automated ways of creating patient specific simulation, surgeons can rehearse and practise difficult cases or the application of new technologies and techniques. Specific areas for improvement can also be identified which will be practised and perfected on a simulator.

Simulation can be used as an assessment tool for consultants as well. It might be a part of a job interview, a promotion pathway or revalidation. If surgeons have been on sabbatical or taken time off from work, simulation will be one way for them to get back to their baseline skills. As an objective measurement for the revalidation of surgeons, a combination of technical skills, non-technical skills and knowledge can be tested using the methods mentioned in this chapter.

Delivery and costs

The distribution and costs of simulation have been barriers to its incorporation into the surgical curriculum. In the future, while large simulators like a simulated operating theatre may only exist at large or academic institutions, other smaller scale simulators and virtual patient simulation will be available

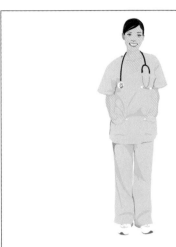

Figure 14.6 Avatar example. Courtesy of Henry Fuller. http://secondlife6750.wordpress.com.

in all centres. Simulation needs to be accessible to all parts of clinical teams in all locations so that, for example surgeons can practice laparoscopic knot tying in between clinical duties without having to leave the hospital. Nurses and surgeons can run through handovers at the end of the day using a virtual world or avatars (see Figure 14.6) from their office computers. The low-cost alternatives can be decentralized while the more expensive systems will be centralized. The full medical team can come to a larger centre on a regular basis to practice teamwork and communication in a simulated operating theatre.

The costs associated with a completely integrated simulation curriculum are large, but with a hub and spoke distribution system, the costs can be shared by many organizations. The costs saved by removing the effect of learning curve from the patient are also quite large. Bridges and Diamond [23] noted that training residents in the operating theatre costs US$47 970 per resident in extra operating time alone. McCashland et al. [24] noted that endoscopists who train fellows take 10–37% longer for procedures than those who do not. This loss in productivity costs between a half and one million dollars a year for 4000 cases. Training surgeons on simulators before they begin carrying out procedures can reduce, if not eliminate, these costs. Cohen et al. [5] noted that after incorporating central venous line placement simulation into the curriculum, the ICU ward reduced catheter infections by approximately 10 infections per year, saving $700000 [5]. The potential cost savings gained with simulation can help offset the costs of setting up centres throughout the country. With this in mind, the costs of simulation should no longer be an issue to its implementation, and it should have a wide distribution in the future.

Summary

If supported and integrated, simulation technology and methodology can grow into something much larger than it is today [25]. Technological advances will make it possible to make simulation more life-like and acceptable for its users. Training, teaching and patient care will improve with its incorporation into the healthcare system. If, on the other hand, simulation remains inaccessible to all parts of the surgical team or if it gets used haphazardly, without a clear vision, the potential progress described here will not be realized [7]. As seen throughout this section, simulation can be integrated into all parts of the patient and surgeon pathway. The future of simulation technology rests on its full implementation and acceptance by the medical community.

✓ Key points

- Simulation needs to be fully integrated into the healthcare system to reach its full potential.
- Improved graphics and software will create a more realistic simulated environment.
- The creation of 3D renderings and simulated operations from real patient cases will be automated.
- Full team simulation will be done in a simulated operating theatre but also in virtual worlds.
- Simulation will be used as an assessment tool in all parts of a surgeon's career from the application process to the revalidation of consultant surgeons.

Guiding the role of simulation through paradigm shifts in medical education

Section contributors: Viren N. Naik and Stanley J. Hamstra   University of Ottawa, Ottawa, Canada

The shift to competency-based education

Healthcare education today is facing several major paradigm shifts. Two of the most important changes for the future of simulation are the shift towards competency-based education (CBE) and a corresponding move towards a model of lifelong learning.

The accepted twentieth-century model of healthcare education conferring competence was 'time-based'. Time-based education focuses on curriculum and experience obtained over a certain time interval. The time-based model has been metaphorically compared to 'tea-steeping', where you put the trainee in the programme for a fixed period of time, and eventually you develop competence [26]. Unfortunately, in the twenty-first century, there are mounting barriers and challenges to this model. Institutional pressures for increased efficiency in the delivery of care limit the opportunities for trainees to interact with clinician-educators and their patients [27]. In addition, the growth of healthcare knowledge and skills is exponential; therefore, the most obvious logical solution to deliver this knowledge is curricular expansion. In conflict with curricular expansion are societal needs to graduate healthcare professionals, maintaining a fixed cost for training healthcare professionals, and an international call for work hour reform that limits the numbers of hours for both work and education for a trainee in a given week [28]. In fact, the current

model appears to be mostly determined on history and tradition rather than empirical evidence, and change appears inevitable.

CBE is proposed as an alternative to the time-based model [29]. In a recent publication from an international collaborative, CBE has been defined as 'an approach to preparing physicians for practice that is fundamentally oriented to graduate outcome abilities and organized around competencies derived from an analysis of societal and patient needs. It de-emphasizes time-based training and promises greater accountability, flexibility, and learner-centredness' [30, p. 636]. Until the 1980s, society required that physicians and other healthcare professionals displayed appropriate medical knowledge and technical expertise. The twenty-first century has seen the demand for a more holistic healthcare professional who embodies a broader set of competencies to address both patient and societal needs [31]. Multiple international approaches to competency have been defined (Table 14.1) [32,33,34]. In Canada, physicians are most familiar with the CanMEDs competency framework, which defines competence over seven domains of equal importance centred around 'medical expert' [35] (Figure 14.7). Simulation-based educators will quickly identify the medical expert domains to be very similar to the broad category of technical skills. Similarly, they would recognize that almost all the non-medical expert competencies map well to previously described non-technical skills [36]. The current struggle with all existing frameworks is that

Table 14.1 Contrasting competency frameworks: Canada, USA and UK

CanMEDS (Canada)	Good Medical Practice (UK)	ABMS/ACGME (USA)
Medical expert	Good clinical care	Patient care and procedural skills Medical knowledge
Communicator	Relationships with patients	Interpersonal and communication skills
Collaborator Manager Health advocate	Working with colleagues Maintain good medical practice	Systems-based practice
Scholar	Teaching and training, appraising and assessing	Practice-based learning and improvement
Professional	Probity Health	Professionalism

ACGME, Accreditation Council for Graduate Medical Education; ABMS, American Board of Medical Specialties.

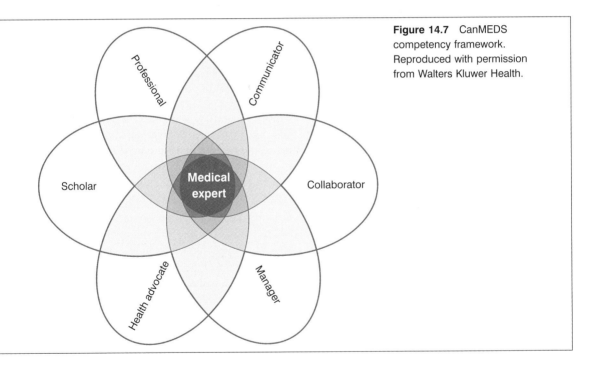

Figure 14.7 CanMEDS competency framework. Reproduced with permission from Walters Kluwer Health.

the description of the competencies are seen as too broad. This criticism affects the ability to define discrete outcomes for a competency that would help in enabling the development of valid assessment tools [37]. Having said that, the development of specific and tangible competency definitions are under way internationally, as are the development of assessment strategies for both technical and non-technical skills [38,39,40,41,42].

What are the implications of such a change in focus for healthcare education? Will the current trend towards CBE from a time-based model sweep across all specialties and jurisdictions without issue? Just as there are challenges to time-based models,

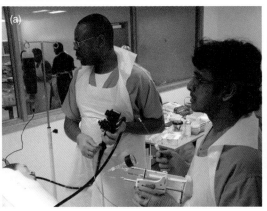 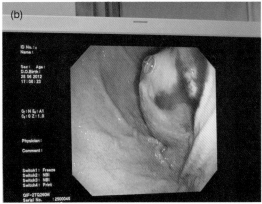

Figure 14.8 (a) Bronchoscopy simulation and (b) bleeding after a biopsy. Courtesy of Jivendra Gosai, Hull Institute of Learning and Simulation.

CBE faces formidable barriers in addition to defining the outcomes and assessment tools. Feedback and formative assessment needs to be virtually continuous in a CBE model. This in turn creates a shift towards goal-directed, deliberate practice.

Mastery learning

Deliberate practice is defined as practice undertaken over an extended period of time to attain excellence, and the ongoing efforts required to maintain it [43]. According to a widely accepted model of skill acquisition, the first stage in acquiring a skill is cognitive: learners develop an understanding of the task, describe the task and then demonstrate it [44]. In the next stage, learners integrate the task into their repertoire of skills through practice and feedback. In the final stage, learners are able to perform the task in an automated fashion with little cognitive input, and the focus then becomes fine-tuning the performance. Mastery can occur only at this level. Simulators have the potential to drive the learner toward integration and mastery, while reducing the need for the learner to practice on real patients while he or she is inexperienced. Through deliberate practice, the learner can focus on intensively practising specific tasks in a controlled setting, while receiving coaching and formative assessment through timely and thoughtful feedback from an expert supervisor (Figure 14.8). Therefore, learning and integration of skills may be accelerated in a way that may not be possible in the operating room or clinical setting given the barriers previously described. Using simulation to accelerate the learning of technical skills toward mastery and automation may also have the added benefit of allowing the development of the non-technical skills required for comprehensive patient care [45].

Continuing professional development

Most competency frameworks were created as a blueprint to create curricula for training programs and help address identified gaps in non-medical expert competencies. However, discussions of competence have found their way into debates of Maintenance of Certification (MOC), continuing professional development (CPD), revalidation, recertification or relicensing programmes for healthcare professionals. Competency-based experts promote the concept of 'progression of competence', meaning that learners advance along a series of defined milestones on their way to the explicit outcome goals of training. These definitions necessitate that competence must be conditional on and constrained by each healthcare professional's practice context, and that this required context needs to be dynamic and continually changing over time [46]. The shift towards lifelong learning emphasizes that healthcare professionals in practice must be comfortable not only with continuing education long after they pass their certification exams, but also with corresponding assessments of knowledge, skills and attitudes throughout their careers.

Most institutions, regulatory and statutory bodies (such as Medical Royal Colleges) and/or specialty boards require healthcare professionals to participate in a MOC or CPD program which are primarily designed to keep track of the number of hours a healthcare professional participates in continuing professional development. Prescribed minimums are required over a cycle of a set number of years. The inherent problem with the current system in maintaining competence and best practice is that it almost entirely depends on a healthcare professional's ability to self reflect on their current practice and critically decide how they will use new information to develop practice [47]. Unfortunately, we know that physicians' ability to self-assess is poor when compared with any existing valid measure of competence, and this is regardless of specialty or length in practice [48]. Unidirectional didactic lectures are the most common continuing professional activity and exemplify passive group learning. Systematic reviews have confirmed an almost negligible effect of these learning activities on altering clinical practice [49].

Both the government and public have called on the self-regulated healthcare professions for increased accountability to ensure their members maintain competence. In the UK, the call for increased accountability has led to the loss of self-regulation for physicians with increased oversight to regulators and employers with the inception of Revalidation in 2012. In the USA, cognitive written examinations for recertification are required by the American Board of Medical Specialties, which oversees all specialty certification boards [50]. In fact, recertification examinations are overwhelmingly supported by the public, who have mistakenly believed that they are already well established across North America [51]. Unfortunately, this solution to increase accountability for maintaining competence is somewhat flawed; it is widely acknowledged that high-stakes recertification written examinations, which focus on medical expert competencies, may not provide a comprehensive reflection of clinical ability, as they fail to value competencies or non-technical skills equally [52].

Assessment of competencies for lifelong learning

As mentioned, for the trainee, formative assessment and feedback is essential for a lifelong learning strategy. Assessment of broader competencies will likely necessitate operationalizing a breadth of assessment modalities to capture both medical expert and non-medical expert competencies [53]. Taxonomies of assessment such as Miller's pyramid are useful to enable us to identify different levels of performance that may be assessed with different tools [54]. Written tests such as MCQs and oral examinations can assess the 'knows' level of factual information. When designed to be rich in clinical context, the same tools probe the integration of that knowledge into clinical judgement and decision-making, the 'knows how' level of assessment [55]. It has been suggested that simulation has advantages over the oral examination in the domain of crisis management, because it can assess what trainees would actually do rather than what they say, the 'shows how' level of performance [56]. Simulation also has the potential to evaluate the competency of learners in a way that reflects actual clinical practice much more closely than other assessment methods. By better reflecting clinical practice, simulation allows for simultaneous assessment of multiple competencies, both technical and non-technical. In a realistic environment trainees must apply and integrate their knowledge, skills, teamwork and decision-making abilities in real time to manage a simulated patient, pathology or crisis situation. The 'does' level of assessment can only be performed in the workplace, and is challenged by logistical and patient safety issues in this complex and dynamic setting. Thus, simulation may offer the best alternative to workplace assessment by providing a relatively safe and standardized medium for work based assessment.

Scholarship in simulation-based education

The two future paradigm shifts described earlier are probably inevitable. As healthcare professionals, we must adopt a scholarly approach in order to successfully mediate the benefits and the challenges of these changes in an evidence-informed manner. Scholarship in education inevitably advances education by publically disseminating the innovation for adoption, review and critique by peers [57,58]. Research units with a mission of promoting innovation and scholarship in healthcare education can guide these shifts in paradigms with best evidence. These units are typically populated with full- or part-time educators with high-level qualifications and experience in education as a subject discipline and a core group of part-time clinician educators with a commitment to developing scholarship in healthcare education. Most of these units provide some type of support for the larger number of clinician educators at those institutions, for example education rounds, grant programmes, and support for fellowships and graduate degrees in education. Much of the activity of the educationalists involves direct collaboration and mentoring of healthcare educators who are starting out in the field, with individual consultation and education scholars' programmes to supplement the pursuit of postgraduate degrees in education. Many of these units also have an annual Education Research Day to highlight progress on projects and innovations and to further encourage scholarly work.

When used in combination with standard educational principles and practices, the Kirkpatrick hierarchy (adopted from the business literature) can be a powerful tool for assessing the impact of an educational innovation [59]. An example may help to illustrate the potential effectiveness of this approach. When a proposal is made to include simulation in an existing curriculum, we can determine whether the innovation warrants further support and adoption by asking the following four questions. (1) Is there a rationale or needs assessment for guiding how the proposed intervention addresses gaps in the current curriculum? (2) Are there well-defined learning objectives to help the teacher focus on essential constructs to be taught? (3) Is there a detailed lesson plan to ensure the identified needs are met? And, most importantly, in terms of scholarship: (4) is there a plan for evaluating the impact of the educational intervention?

This last question can be addressed directly by making use of the Kirkpatrick hierarchy described previously. For example, at the most basic level, 'reaction', we would want to know how many learners participated, both in terms of absolute numbers and relative to the population of learners available in that context. Moving to Level 2, 'learning', we would ask if the educators had evidence for a change in learners' attitudes or knowledge or skills as a direct result of the intervention. Note that such a question is strengthened if proper controls are present in the design of the intervention, such as a comparison group and/or random allocation to groups. At Level 3, 'behaviour', the educator should provide evidence for a change in behaviour, typically much harder information to obtain, as it suggests a follow up in data collection to determine if there has been a change in the learner's behaviour in the applied setting. At the highest level, 'results', participants are assessed as to what degree targeted outcomes occur as a result of the training event and subsequent reinforcement. This might consist of changes in practice or patient outcomes.

This hierarchy seems to have gained significant traction in healthcare education [60,61,62,63]. The advantage of the hierarchy is that it encourages scholars to consider raising the threshold for the type of evidence they accumulate in support of their innovations. The management and monitoring of innovations in this way, along with the collection of relevant data, fosters an accountability that not only ensures a thoughtful and rigorous approach to the implementation and accountability of educational interventions, but also prepares the way for reporting to stakeholders such as accreditation agencies. The message that simulation affects patient care is easily understandable to traditional scientists and appealing to government funding agencies. Translational science demands that we demonstrate further that simulation reduces morbidity and saves lives [64]. Simulation research must inform theory, policy and practice [65], to clarify how and when simulation can be best used cost-effectively to improve teaching and assessment, and ultimately measurably improve patient outcomes.

Summary

In conclusion, we have outlined an approach to addressing two major movements in medical education: CBE and lifelong learning through continuing professional development. Both forces demand a renewed individual accountability as both trainees and physicians in practice will be required to demonstrate competence according to external mandates. It appears there is an opportunity now to develop solid evidence to support specific recommendations for assessment of competence, for which the opportunities for simulation are evident. This response requires a scholarly approach, as we must be careful about how to define specific aspects of competence and how they are assessed. The support of educational scholars' programmes and fellowships in medical education can contribute meaningfully to addressing these challenges. By embracing educational scholarship, healthcare educators will be better able to navigate the exciting challenges and opportunities for simulation posed by these two major movements in medical education.

✓ Key points

- Medical education is on the verge of a paradigm shift from time-based to CBE, and a consequential need to embrace a culture of lifelong learning.
- Simulation-based education can accelerate learning to mastery and automation through deliberate practice.
- Simulation affords opportunities to assess a broader set of competencies at the 'shows how' level of Miller's pyramid.
- Medical education research units that are populated with qualified and experienced educators can support education scholarship by collaborating with and mentoring clinician educators.
- The Kirkpatrick hierarchy can help guide the rationale for education interventions, as well as the quality and impact of teaching innovations.

The future of training in simulation

Section contributor: Ronnie Glavin   Victoria Infirmary, Glasgow, UK

'It's tough to make predictions, especially about the future'. Yogi Berra

One hundred years from now robots will be capable of doing everything humans can do; humans will live lives of unbridled leisure and simulation will not be necessary because supercomputers will tell the robots what to do. Advances in stem cell therapy and genetic modification will eliminate all human disease and healthcare will consist of patching broken parts together. This sort of speculation belongs more to the world of science fiction than medical textbooks, and I would rather look at current trends and think about where we would like simulation to go and how we may go about reaching that destination.

Issenberg [66], in a review of the effectiveness of simulation training in healthcare, listed three necessary components:
1. Integration with curricula
2. Faculty to deliver the training
3. Resources – including equipment

Integration with curriculum

Education is about helping learners change the way they behave. This applies to both the capabilities they come to possess and the dispositions to act in certain ways under certain circumstances. Further discussion on the nature of education and training can be found elsewhere [67]. Stenhouse [68] has described the curriculum as sharing features with a recipe in that it describes content (the ingredients of a recipe or the competencies, abilities, capabilities, etc. – the changes in behaviour that the learner should be willing to adopt), processes (what teaching methods or experiences will help bring about the changes) and what to look for as evidence of satisfac-

tory progress (e.g. via assessment in which the learner should be able to recall the following information about safe dosages of local anaesthetic drugs).

Content

The medical curricula of Canada, USA and UK have changed over the last decade or so as frameworks have been introduced to give a broad idea of the main content areas. For example, the Canadian system – CanMEDS [69] – describes seven roles of a doctor (Figure 14.2 in Section 2) and curricula should identify where content, teaching methods and assessment tools relate to these roles.

As has been highlighted in previous chapters these roles take medical education beyond the biomedical model of the early twentieth century [70] to a much wider domain that encompasses the psychosocial realm. The biomedical model is necessary for doctor as medical expert but roles such as communicator and collaborator call on cognitive and social skills that fit more readily into the psychosocial realm.

One may imagine some sort of mission control where having defined the curriculum content the teaching methods and assessment tools are then developed; but I believe that instead of simulation being an afterthought to development of content, simulation has actually had a significant influence in the development of content. If we consider simulated patients or standardised patients featuring in teaching and Objective Structured Clinical Examinations (OSCE), the role of part task trainers in life support courses, the role of high-fidelity platform based simulation training in crew resource management training then we can see how the experience of working with such tools has allowed a body of expertise to develop. That body of expertise has in turn influenced how we populate the formal curricula. Would a curriculum development exercise carried out thirty years ago have been so confident in including roles such as communicator or collaborator? My hypothesis is that engagement with the different types of simulation listed earlier provoked, stimulated, challenged those pioneers in the field to explore beyond the confines of the traditional curriculum and began a process of engagement with psychologists, sociologists, anthropologists, ethnographers, etc., that has brought about a body of knowledge and expertise that can be applied to the curriculum.

Let me illustrate with one personal example. As an anaesthetist with an interest in education I have wanted to understand better the cognitive processes used by anaesthetists in their daily practice. When I was appointed to the Scottish Clinical Simulation Centre as one of the first co-directors, the Centre faculty recognized that if we were to teach and promote 'behavioural skills of anaesthetists' we would need a system that would allow us to study the impact of our educational interventions, not just in the simulation centre but also in the clinical workplace. The system that we developed – the Anaesthetists Non-Technical Skills (ANTS) [71] system now enjoys use beyond our centre; but I suspect that if we had not had the centre and the core faculty that constituted the initial critical mass then we would have been much less likely to have been successful in our grant applications and so less likely to have developed such close working relations with the Aberdeen University Industrial Psychology Research Centre. The collaborative process has been in two directions. The psychologists have come to have a better understanding of the different challenges of healthcare professionals from some of their other groups and so have been more able to collaborate more effectively with healthcare workers.

Non-technical skills systems such as ANTS are a way of populating curriculum content. The roles may still have been selected but without the awareness raising resulting from the body of work that had been accrued by people exploring what simulation could do we would not have so much psychosocial content.

Future curriculum development

The curricula referred to earlier have been aimed at doctors in training. While they also provide a template for maintenance of competence programmes they are applicable only to the medical specialty for which they have been developed. One future curriculum development could be those devised for use in healthcare institutions by the different healthcare professionals collaborating on different phases of clinical problems. These already exist to various degrees. For example, Draycott et al. [72] describe a monthly programme in an obstetric unit for the medical, nursing, midwifery and paediatric staff. The curriculum assumes that career grade staff members from whatever specialty, have acquired the relevant behaviours but need to apply them to a particular context. The concept of 'fire drills' is not new but whereas these have concentrated upon emergency events or complications (maternal haemorrhage, breech presentations) we are seeing the need for such training in more routine activities in the complex systems that characterize acute care in the developed world. The analogy I see is that of the pit crew of a formula one racing car team. Even someone not interested in F1 car racing cannot help but be impressed by the coordinated activities of the individuals in carrying out the various tasks such as tyre changes and loading fuel. Roger Kneebone has commented on the characteristics of rehearsal during presentations at various meetings (including the 2011 annual scientific meeting of the Society in Europe for Simulation Applied to Medicine, Granada, Spain). Rehearsal allows people to work together, iron out faults, spend more time on difficult sections and so on. He uses the analogy of a small music ensemble such as a string quartet. The individual musicians have a level of mastery over their own instruments but by working together in a safe space can develop their efforts towards a performance of high standard for public consumption.

One of my visions for the future of simulation training is that of groups of healthcare workers coming together to rehearse and practise and prepare for the introduction of new clinical challenges or new protocols or ways of implementing new practices. An example is a training programme that was devised by and for operating room staff in University College Hospital, London, to prepare for the introduction of the surgical brief and surgical pause as part of the World Health Organization (WHO) Safer Surgery Programme. Delivery of this programme entailed the closure of operating rooms to elective work during the rehearsal period but a combination of a far sighted Chief Executive Officer working with clinicians was prepared to take a short term hit for longer term benefits to both patients and budgets by implementing methods intended to reduce error and improve effectiveness.

Rehearsing such procedures is therefore not just about the continuing professional development of individual healthcare workers, it is an opportunity to review existing practices and look at ways in which efficiency can be enhanced without safety being compromised. As healthcare systems become more complex there will be a greater need to test the impact of new changes and so determine the content of the 'organization curriculum'.

Faculty

Faculty development has been described in a previous chapter. The abilities required to organize, run scenarios, debrief effectively and set up the next session apply beyond the simulation centre and classroom. As with content, I wonder how much of current educational practice was reinforced by simulation-based activity. I am sure that most medical staff of my generation first came across Pendleton's 'rules' (What went well? What could have gone better?) during educational activities with simulation-based activities, such as life support courses. The ability to help learners reflect on their performance, to help collections of healthcare workers reflect on their group performance is one that will be applied more and more often in an informal way. As an anaesthetist I would like to see more time spent at the end of a session in the operating room reviewing key issues and helping to form changes for the future sessions. These activities will only take place if they are seen as positive experiences by the participants – the operating room personnel. The skills, experience and ability to conduct this type of debrief in an efficient and effective manner require development and familiarity with

the frameworks that underpin human interaction with systems. Faculty development will not be confined to simulator-based education activities but will also extend to reviewing team performance in the workplace.

Experience and familiarity with change management will become of increasing importance for simulation faculty. I have already referred to the increased familiarity with psychosocial disciplines applied to clinical practice [70]. However, these are not the only areas that will form part of the faculty development curriculum. Kneebone [73] has referred to some of the other disciplines that will inform the practice of simulation faculty, including many from the performing arts.

Educational resources

In this section I shall concentrate upon the simulator equipment and technology but this is not to minimise the importance of essential resources such as time, space, administrative support, practical support, and so on. Future visions of technological developments certainly grab the imagination. Star Trek-like holodecks with anaesthetic trainees learning strategies for managing spinal anaesthesia in supermorbidly obese patients may be the stuff that such dreams are made off, but the reality is that the resources required to develop such devices cannot be committed without a clear idea of the educational role and the teaching and assessment requirements. Common criticisms of part task trainers relate to the lack of variation possible, whether in terms of underlying anatomy or other conditions that will tax the more experienced trainee or practitioner. If summative assessment of healthcare practitioners were to resemble the relicensing tests of civil aviation pilots then a whole industry of quality assurance provisions to ensure that consistent standards of production and testing would require to be put in place.

The existing partnership between simulation users, commissioners, manufacturers and even regulators will require more robust mechanisms to ensure that the resources required for investment are likely to bring about a significant return for that investment. I am not just talking about the financial investment but also the time and energy of the individuals from many roles who will be necessary to bring about the realization of such a vision. How will that occur? What roles will the various agencies currently on the scene take – the societies of practitioners, the regulators, the manufacturers? At this point in time I can only see discussion between these agencies leading to a bottom-up development.

There are plenty of examples of individual companies listening to the users, modifying their products and reaping the benefits of such collaboration but the ones I want to highlight reflect not so much the individual company as the importance of the purpose of the simulated device. My own background is that of a clinician working in a developed country at the sharp end of acute care. However, a large proportion of the world's population does not enjoy this level of healthcare. The 2006 WHO World Together for Health report highlighted the disparity of resources on the planet. Sub-Saharan Africa has 11% of the world's population and 24% of the global burden of disease but has only 3% of its health workers [74].

Initiatives such as those aimed at neonatal care and postpartum haemorrhage management targeted at care assistants in rural parts of the developing world have demonstrated how a high-tech approach to producing a low-tech product can incorporate simulation into educational programmes in the poorest parts of the world.

In the developed world we shall require resources targeted to help people in the voluntary sector develop their role in contributing to healthcare. Whether in acute healthcare or chronic healthcare, whether in the developing world or the developed world the three principles outlined by Issenberg [66] will set challenges for those of us involved in developing curricula, supporting faculty or designing resources.

How will we develop training?

I have shared my vision of where simulation-based education in healthcare may go. I have not yet addressed the question of how we may use simulation-based education to achieve those ends. The biggest challenge, at present, is building the educational framework that will underpin the uses of simulation mentioned earlier. Medical education itself has been under greater scrutiny [75] as we seek to better understand the theoretical basis that underpins our practice, whether simulation based or not. The development of that theoretical basis for simulation-based education is an iterative process; as we gain more experience and acquire more data we can undertake further analysis. However, we need some sense of framework or model against which we can test these data. Although we do not yet have answers we are beginning to formulate the questions. In June 2010 a meeting of 24 experienced simulation-based educators took place in Copenhagen [76]. This set up the basis for a larger research consensus in January 2011 [77]. The main research themes are listed in Box 14.1. This summit

---

Box 14.1 Topics explored at the society for simulation in healthcare research summit [77]

1. Using simulation for learning and practising skills and tasks
2. Using simulation learning in teams
3. Integration of systems design
4. Using simulation to understand and improve care environments and human team performance
5. Using simulation to study and validate tools, instruments and theories
6. Evaluating the impact of simulation on patient outcomes
7. Research regarding methods and integration of assessing learning
8. Research regarding debriefing and feedback as part of the learning process
9. Use of simulation for licensure, maintenance of credentialing and certification
10. Reporting inquiry

brought together many people at the cutting edge of simulation practice in healthcare and allowed them to work in groups to explore the literature and summarise where we are and where we might be going.

Gaba has written 'In the future it is likely that we will need to mobilise yet larger resources to provide more definitive answers to the big questions about simulation.' [78]. He, in turn, describes a model from those involved in astrophysics and space research – 'Science Traceability Structure' (Figures 14.9 and 14.10) [79]. This model links broad themes to relevant scientific goals. These are linked to specific objectives and thence to particular instruments on particular experiments. The whole is a matrix in which small or large studies can be mapped onto the relevant place in this hierarchical matrix. Such a model can be used when approaching funding bodies to show which part(s) of the matrix will be addressed by proposed work, or can be used more informally by individual groups of workers to show where their experimental research work can link in with the efforts of others. A science traceability structure matrix may not be a treasure map but it could help different units cooperate and coordinate their efforts more effectively as a contribution to larger questions.

If that quest can encourage collaboration, constructive effort and meaningful communication between simulation-based healthcare educators then we have a future worth pursuing.

Summary

Simulation-based education in healthcare has already exerted an influence on the content of the medical curriculum, the role and the attributes of teachers and the pattern of how that curriculum is delivered; which in turn has resource implications for medical education. These trends look likely to continue and future directions will be influenced by the developing theoretical basis underpinning current practice. A critical mass of people from many different domains, some within medicine,

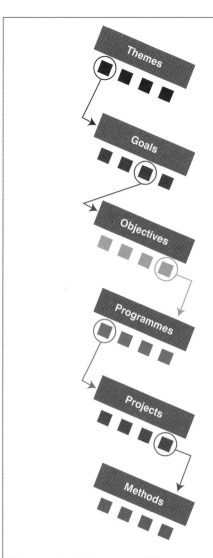

Figure 14.9 Science traceability structure model.

many from outside of medicine have brought not only new knowledge but also new perspectives; which, in turn, broaden the possibilities as simulation-based education continues to help prepare today's healthcare professionals for the global challenges of tomorrow's healthcare.

Level of traceability structure	Explanation of this level (using simulation classification)		Example of research thread in **planetary science**	Example of research thread in **simulation in healthcare**
Themes	Overarching questions	Wide agreement by scientific community	**Understand** Emergence of habitable worlds around gas giant planets	**Understand** simulation and its impact on quality and safety
Goals	Specific goals related to a question		**Explore** Europa (moon of Jupiter) to investigate habitability	Find out **how** does simulation training lead to learning
Objectives	Objectives to achieve the goal(s)		**Determine** surface composition and chemistry	Determine **what** debriefing adds to learning after simulations
Investigations Programmes	Interlocking set of projects to meet one or more objective		**Characterize** surface organic and inorganic chemistry	**Characterize** advantages and disadvantages to different systems of debriefing
Measurements Projects	Specific projects within the programme	Unique to project	**Measure** surface reflectance – through large spectral range	**Compare** debriefings by clinician vs non-clinician trained debriefers
Instruments Methods	Particular methods or techniques to be used in the project		**Use** infrared spectrometer	**Score** utterances of debriefer from recordings by blinded neutral expert

Figure 14.10   Science traceability structure matrix.

✓ Key points

- Simulation-based activities have encouraged the introduction of expert practice from other domains into healthcare.
- Such practices have helped broaden the curriculum by inclusion of the psychosocial realm into the biomedical world.
- The theoretical basis underpinning simulation-based activities in healthcare is already beginning to take form and structure.
- Close cooperation between those using the devices, those creating the devices and the healthcare community will be necessary to help simulation meet future challenges.

REFERENCES

1. Grantcharov T, Kristiansen V, Bendix J, *et al.* (2004) Randomized clinical trial of virtual reality simulation for laparoscopic skills training. *British Journal of Surgery* **91:** 146–150.

2. Seymour N, Gallagher A, Roman S, *et al.* (2002) Virtual reality training improves operating room performance: results of a randomized, double-blinded study. *Annals of Surgery* **236:** 458–463.

3. Aggarwal R, Ward J, Balasundaram I, *et al.* (2007) Proving the effectiveness of virtual reality simulation for training in laparoscopic surgery. *Annals of Surgery* **246:** 771–779.

4. Ahlberg G, Enochsson L, Gallagher A, *et al.* (2007) Proficiency-based virtual reality training significantly reduces the error rate for residents during their first 10 laparoscopic cholecystectomies. *American Journal of Surgery* **193:** 797–804.

5. Cohen E, Feinglass J, Barsuk J, *et al.* (2010) Cost savings from reduced catheter-related bloodstream infection after simulation-based education for residents in a medical intensive care unit. *Simulated Healthcare* **5:** 98–102.

6. McCulloch P, Mishra A, Handa A, *et al.* (2009) The effects of aviation-style non-technical skills training on technical performance and outcome in the operating theatre. *Quality & Safety in Health Care* **18:** 108–115.

7. Gaba D. (2004) The future vision of simulation in health care. *Quality & Safety in Health Care* **13:** i2–i10.

8. Kohn L, Corrigan J, Donaldson M. (eds) (1999) *To Err is Human: Building a Safer Health System*. Washington, DC: National Academy Press.

9. Pearson E, McLafferty I (2011) The use of simulation as a learning approach to non-technical skills awareness in final year student nurses. *Nurse Education in Practice* **11:** 399–405.

10. Belyansky I, Martin T, Prabhu A, *et al.* (2011) Poor resident-attending intraoperative communication may compromise patient safety. *Journal of Surgical Research* **171:** 386–394.

11. Mutter D, Dallemagne B, Bailey C, *et al.* (2009) 3D virtual reality and selective vascular control for laparoscopic left hepatic lobectomy. *Surgical Endoscopy* **23:** 432–435.

12. Marescaux J, Clement J, Tassetti V, *et al.* (1998) Virtual reality applied to hepatic surgery simulation: the next revolution. *Annals of Surgery* **228:** 627–634.

13. Soler L, Marescaux J (2008) Patient-specific surgical simulation. *World Journal of Surgery* **32:** 208–212.

14. Willaert W, Aggarwal R, Bicknell C, *et al.* (2010) Patient-specific simulation in carotid artery stenting. *Journal of Vascular Surgery* **52:** 1700–1705.

15. Andreatta P, Woodrum D, Birkmeyer J, *et al.* (2006) Laparoscopic skills are improved with LapMentor training: results of a randomized, double-blinded study. *Annals of Surgery* **243:** 854–860.

16. Gettman M, Pereira C, Lipsky K, *et al.* (2009) Use of high fidelity operating room simulation to assess and teach communication, teamwork and laparoscopic skills: initial experience. *Journal of Urology* **181:** 1289–1296.

17. Kneebone R, Arora S, King D, *et al.* (2010) Distributed simulation – accessible immersive training. *Medical Teacher* **32:** 65–70.

18. Conradi E, Kavia S, Burden D, *et al.* (2009) Virtual patients in a virtual world: Training paramedic students for practice *Medical Teacher* **31:** 713–720.

19. Guise J, Lowe N, Deering S, *et al.* (2010) Mobile in situ obstetric emergency simulation and teamwork training to improve maternal-fetal safety in hospitals. *Joint Commission Journal on Quality and Patient Safety* **36:** 443–453.

20. Darzi A, Smith S, Taffinder N (1999) Assessing operative skill. Needs to become more objective. *British Medical Journal* **318:** 887–888.

21. Martin J, Regehr G, Reznick R, *et al.* (1997) Objective structured assessment of technical skill (OSATS) for surgical residents. *British Journal of Surgery* **84:** 273–278.

22. Sevdalis N, Lyons M, Healey A, *et al.* (2009) Observational teamwork assessment for surgery: construct validation with expert versus novice raters. *Annals of Surgery* **249:** 1047–1051.

23. Bridges M, Diamond DL (1999) The financial impact of teaching surgical residents in the operating room. *American Journal of Surgery* **177:** 28–32.

24. McCashland T, Brand R, Lyden E, *et al.* (2000) The time and financial impact of training fellows in endoscopy. CORI Research Project. Clinical Outcomes Research Initiative. *American Journal of Gastroenterology* **95:** 3129–3132.

25. Aggarwal R, Mytton O, Derbrew M, *et al.* (2010) Training and simulation for patient safety. *Quality & Safety in Health Care* **19:** i34–i43.

26. Hodges B (2010) A tea-steeping or i-doc model for medical education? *Academic Medicine* **85:** s34–s44.

27. Ludmerer K (1999) *Time To Heal: American Medical Education from the Turn of the Century to the Era of Managed Care.* Oxford: Oxford University Press.

28. Philibert I, Chang B, Flynn T, *et al.* (2009) The 2003 common duty hour limits: process, outcome, and lessons learned. *Journal of Graduate Medical Education* **l1:** 334–337.

29. Whitehead C (2010) Recipes for medical education reform: will different ingredients create better doctors? *Social Science and Medicine* **70:** 1672–1676.

30. Frank JR, Mungroo R, Ahmad Y, *et al.* (2010) Toward a definition of competency-based education in medicine: a systematic review of published definitions. *Medical Teacher* **32:** 631–637.

31. Maudsley RF (1999) Content in context: medical education and society's needs. *Academic Medicine* **74:** 143–145.

32. The Medical School Objectives Writing Group (1999) Learning objectives for medical student education: Guidelines for medical schools: Report I of the Medical School Objectives Project. *Academic Medicine* **74:** 13–18.

33. Neufeld V, Maudsley R, Pickering R, *et al.* (1998) Educating future physicians for Ontario. *Academic Medicine* **73:** 1133–1148.

34. ACGME. The ACGME Competency Framework. Available from http://www.acgme.org/ (accessed July 28, 2011).

35. Frank JR, Danoff D (2007) The CanMEDS initiative: implementing an outcomes-based framework of physician competencies. *Medical Teacher* **29:** 642–647.

36. Gaba DM, Howard SK, Fish KJ, *et al.* (2001) Simulation-based training in anesthesia crisis resource management (ACRM): a decade of experience. *Simulation & Gaming* **32:** 175–193.

37. ten Cate O, Scheele F (2007) Competency-based postgraduate training: can we bridge the gap between theory and clinical practice? *Academic Medicine* **82:** 542–547.

38. Boulet JR, Murray DJ (2010) Simulation-based assessment in anesthesiology: requirements for practical implementation. *Anesthesiology* **112:** 1041–1052.

39. Murray DJ, Boulet JR, Avidan M, *et al.* (2007) Performance of residents and

anesthesiologists in a simulation-based skill assessment. *Anesthesiology* **107:** 705–713.

40. Fletcher G, Flin R, McGeorge P, *et al.* (2003) Anaesthetists' Non Technical Skills (ANTS): evaluation of a behavioural marker system. *Br J Anaesthesia* **90:** 580–588.

41. Malec JF, Torsher LC, Dunn WF, *et al.* (2007) The Mayo high performance teamwork scale: reliability and validity for evaluating key crew resource management skills. *Simulation in Healthcare* **2:** 4–10.

42. Morgan PJ, Pittini R, Regehr G, *et al.* (2007) Evaluating teamwork in a simulated obstetric environment. *Anesthesiology* **106:** 907–915.

43. Ericsson KA (2004) Deliberate practice and the acquisition and maintenance of expert performance in medicine and related domains. *Academic Medicine* **79:** S70–S81.

44. Reznick, RK, MacRae H (2006) Teaching surgical skills – changes in the wind. *New England Journal of Medicine* **355:** 2664–2669.

45. Ericsson K, Towne T (2010) Expertise. *Wiley Interdisciplinary Reviews: Cognitive Science* **1:** 404–416.

46. Campbell C, Silver I, Sherbino J, *et al.* (2010) Competency-based continuing professional development. *Medical Teacher* **32:** 657–662.

47. Eva KW, Regehr G (2008) "I'll never play professional football" and other fallacies of self-assessment. *Journal of Continuing Education in the Health Professions* **28:** 14–19.

48. Davis DA, Mazmanian PE, Fordis M (2006). Accuracy of physician self-assessment compared with observed measures of competence: a systematic review. *Journal of the American Medical Association* **296:** 1094–1102.

49. Mansouri M, Lockyer J (2007) A meta-analysis of continuing medical education

effectiveness. *Journal of Continuing Education in the Health Professions* **27:** 6–15.

50. Shaw K, Cassel CK, Black C, Levinson W (2009) Shared Medical regulation in a time of increasing calls for accountability and transparency comparison of recertification in the United States, Canada, and the United Kingdom. *Journal of the American Medical Association* **302:** 2008–2014.

51. Brennan TA, Horwitz RI, Duffy FD, *et al.* (2004) The role of physician specialty board certification status in the quality movement. *Journal of the American Medical Association* **292:** 1038–1043.

52. Savoldelli GL, Naik VN, Joo HS, *et al.* (2006) Evaluation of patient simulator performance as an adjunct to the oral examination for senior anesthesia residents. *Anesthesiology* **104:** 475–481.

53. Lockyer J, Blackmore D, Fidler H, *et al.* (2006) A study of a multi-source feedback system for international medical graduates holding defined licences. *Medical Education* **40:** 340–347.

54. Miller G (1990) The assessment of clinical skills/competence/performance. *Academic Medicine* **65:** S63.

55. Epstein R. Assessment in medical education (2007) *New England Journal of Medicine* **356:** 387.

56. Savoldelli GL, Naik VN, Joo HS, *et al.* (2006) Evaluation of patient simulator performance as an adjunct to the oral examination for senior anesthesia residents. *Anesthesiology* **104:** 475–481.

57. Glassick CE (2000) Boyer's expanded definitions of scholarship, the standards for assessing scholarship, and the elusiveness of the scholarship of teaching. *Academic Medicine* **75:** 877–880.

58. Fincher RM, Simpson DE, Mennin SP, *et al.* (2000) Scholarship in teaching: an imperative for the 21st century. *Academic Medicine* **75:** 887–894.

59. Kirkpatrick DL (1994) *Evaluating Training Programs: The Four Levels*. San Francisco: Berrett-Koehler.

60. Freeth D, Hammick M, Koppel I, *et al.* (2005) *Evaluating Interprofessional Education: A Self-Help Guide*. London: Higher Education Academy Learning and Teaching Support Network for Health Sciences and Practice. Available from http://www.health.ltsn.ac.uk/publications/occasionalpaper/occp5.pdf.

61. Curran VR, Fleet L (2005) A review of evaluation outcomes of web-based continuing medical education. *Medical Education* **39:** 561–557.

62. Steinert Y, Mann K, Centeno A, *et al.* (2006) A systematic review of faculty development initiatives designed to improve teaching effectiveness in medical education: BEME Guide No. 8. *Medical Teacher* **28:** 497–526.

63. Hammick M, Freeth D, Koppel I, *et al.* (2007) A best evidence systematic review of interprofessional education: BEME Guide no. 9. *Medical Teacher* **29:** 735–751.

64. McGaghie WC, Draycott TJ, Dunn WF, *et al.* (2011) Evaluating the impact of simulation on translational patient outcomes. *Simulation in Healthcare* **6:** S42.

65. Monrouxe LV, Rees CE (2009) Picking up the gauntlet: constructing medical education as a social science. *Medical Education* **43:** 196–198.

66. Issenberg SB (2006) The scope of simulation-based healthcare education. *Simulation in Healthcare* **1:** 203–206.

67. Glavin RJ (2011) Skills, training, and education. *Simulation in Healthcare* **6:** 4–7.

68. Stenhouse L (1975) *An Introduction to Curriculum Research and Development*. London: Heinemann.

69. Royal College of Physicians and Surgeons of Canada. CanMEDS 2005 framework. Available from http://rcpsc.medical.org/canmeds (accessed July 2011).

70. Kuper A, D'Eon M (2011) Rethinking the basis of medical knowledge. *Medical Education* **45:** 36–43.

71. Flin R, Patey R, Maran N, Glavin R (2010) Anaesthetists' non-technical skills. *British Journal of Anaesthesia* **105:** 38–44.

72. Draycott T, Sibanda T, Owen L, *et al.* (2006) Does training in obstetric emergencies improve neonatal outcome? *British Journal of Obstetrics and Gynaecology* **113:** 177–182.

73. Kneebone RL (2006) Crossing the line: Simulation and boundary areas. *Simulation in Healthcare* **1:** 160–163.

74. World Health Organization (2006) *The World Health Report*. Geneva, WHO. Available from http://www.who.int/whr/2006/en/ (accessed 6 March 2011).

75. Mann KV (2011) Theoretical perspectives in medical education: past experience and future possibilities. *Medical Education* **45:** 60–68.

76. Issenberg SB, Ringstead C, Østergaard D, Dieckmann P (2011) Setting a research agenda for simulation-based healthcare education: a synthesis of the outcome from an Utstein style meeting. *Simulation in Healthcare* **6:** 155–167.

77. Dieckmann P, Phero JC, Issenberg SB, *et al.* (2011) The first research consensus summit of the Society for Simulation in Healthcare: conduction and a synthesis of the results. *Simulation in Healthcare* **6:** S1–S9.

78. Gaba D (2011) Where do we come from? What are we? Where are we going? *Simulation in Healthcare* **6:** 195–196.

79. Gaba DM (2012) Adapting space science methods for describing and planning research in simulation in healthcare: traceability and decadal surveys. *Simulation in Healthcare* **7:** 27–31.

Index

Page numbers in *italics* denote figures, those in **bold** denote tables.

Essential Simulation in Clinical Education, First Edition. Edited by Kirsty Forrest, Judy McKimm, and Simon Edgar.
© 2013 John Wiley & Sons, Ltd. Published 2013 by John Wiley & Sons, Ltd.